Risk Management

Guest Editors
JOSEPH H. KAHN, MD, FACEP
BRENDAN G. MAGAURAN Jr, MD, MBA
JONATHAN S. OLSHAKER, MD, FACEP, FAAEM

EMERGENCY MEDICINE CLINICS OF NORTH AMERICA

www.emed.theclinics.com

Consulting Editor
AMAL MATTU, MD

November 2009 • Volume 27 • Number 4

SAUNDERS an imprint of ELSEVIER, Inc.

W.B. SAUNDERS COMPANY

A Division of Elsevier Inc.

1600 John F. Kennedy Boulevard • Suite 1800 • Philadelphia, Pennsylvania 19103-2899

http://www.theclinics.com

EMERGENCY MEDICINE CLINICS OF NORTH AMERICA Volume 27, Number 4
November 2009 ISSN 0733-8627, ISBN-13: 978-1-4377-1212-4, ISBN-10: 1-4377-1212-6

Editor: Patrick Manley
Developmental Editor: Theresa Collier

Emergency Medicine Clinics of North America (ISSN 0733-8627) is published quarterly by Elsevier Inc., 360 Park Avenue South, New York, NY, 10010-1710. Months of issue are February, May, August, and November. Business and Editorial Offices: 1600 John F. Kennedy Boulevard, Suite 1800, Philadelphia, PA 19103-2899. Customer Service Office: 6277 Sea Harbor Drive, Orlando, FL 32887-4800. Periodicals postage paid at New York, NY, and additional mailing offices. Subscription prices are $127.00 per year (US students), $247.00 per year (US individuals), $414.00 per year (US institutions), $180.00 per year (international students), $354.00 per year (international individuals), $499.00 per year (international institutions), $180.00 per year (Canadian students), $305.00 per year (Canadian individuals), and $499.00 per year (Canadian institutions). International air speed delivery is included in all *Clinics*' subscription prices. All prices are subject to change without notice. **POSTMASTER:** Send address changes to *Emergency Medicine Clinics of North America*, Elsevier Periodicals Customer Service, 11830 Westline Industrial Drive, St. Louis, MO 63146. Customer Service (orders, claims, online, change of address): Elsevier Periodicals Customer Service, 11830 Westline Industrial Drive, St. Louis, MO 63146. Tel: 1-800-654-2452 (U.S. and Canada); 314-453-7041 (outside U.S. and Canada). Fax: 314-453-5170. E-mail: journalscustomerservice-usa@elsevier.com (for print support); journalsonline support-usa@elsevier.com (for online support).

Reprints. For copies of 100 or more of articles in this publication, please contact the Commercial Reprints Department, Elsevier Inc., 360 Park Avenue South, New York, NY 10010-1710. Tel.: 212-633-3812; Fax: 212-462-1935; E-mail: reprints@elsevier.com.

Emergency Medicine Clinics of North America is covered in *MEDLINE/PubMed (Index Medicus), Current Contents/Clinical Medicine, EMBASE/Excerpta Medica, BIOSIS, SciSearch, CINAHL, ISI/BIOMED,* and *Research Alert*.

Printed in the United States of America.

Printed and bound by CPI Group (UK) Ltd, Croydon, CR0 4YY
Transferred to Digital Print 2011

Contributors

CONSULTING EDITOR

AMAL MATTU, MD, FAAEM, FACEP
Program Director, Emergency Medicine Residency; Associate Professor, Department of Emergency Medicine, University of Maryland School of Medicine, Baltimore, Maryland

GUEST EDITORS

JOSEPH H. KAHN, MD, FACEP
Associate Professor of Emergency Medicine; Director of Medical Student Education, Department of Emergency Medicine, Boston Medical Center, Boston University School of Medicine, Boston, Massachusetts

BRENDAN G. MAGAURAN Jr, MD, MBA
Assistant Clinical Professor, Department of Emergency Medicine; Vice Chair of Administration; Director of Clinical Operations, Emergency Department, Boston Medical Center, Boston University School of Medicine, Boston, Massachusetts

JONATHAN S. OLSHAKER, MD, FACEP, FAAEM
Chief, Boston Medical Center; Professor and Chair, Department of Emergency Medicine, Boston University School of Medicine, Boston, Massachusetts

AUTHORS

POOJA AGRAWAL, MD
Department of Emergency Medicine, Brigham and Women's Hospital and Harvard Medical School, Boston, Massachusetts

WILLIAM E. BAKER, MD
Department of Emergency Medicine, Boston University School of Medicine; Department of Emergency Medicine, Boston Medical Center, Boston, Massachusetts

VICTORIA A. COBURN, MD
Department of Emergency Medicine, Boston University School of Medicine, Boston Medical Center, Boston, Massachusetts

MAUREEN GANG, MD
Assistant Professor, Department of Emergency Medicine, New York University School of Medicine, Bellevue Hospital Center; Director, Emergency Department, Tisch Hospital, NYU Langone Medical Center, New York, New York

ROBERT A. GREEN, MD, MPH
Associate Director, Department of Emergency Medicine, Quality and Patient Safety Officer, New York Presbyterian Hospital/Columbia University Medical Center, New York, New York

JOSEPH H. KAHN, MD, FACEP
Associate Professor of Emergency Medicine; Director of Medical Student Education, Department of Emergency Medicine, Boston Medical Center, Boston University School of Medicine, Boston, Massachusetts

JOSHUA M. KOSOWSKY, MD
Department of Emergency Medicine, Brigham and Women's Hospital and Harvard Medical School, Boston, Massachusetts

BRENDAN G. MAGAURAN Jr, MD, MBA
Assistant Clinical Professor, Department of Emergency Medicine; Vice Chair of Administration; Director of Clinical Operations, Emergency Department, Boston Medical Center, Boston University School of Medicine, Boston, Massachusetts

CHRISTOPHER M. MCSTAY, MD
Assistant Professor, Department of Emergency Medicine, New York University/Bellevue Hospital Center, New York, New York

MARK B. MYCYK, MD
Associate Professor, Department of Emergency Medicine, Boston University School of Medicine, Boston Medical Center, Boston, Massachusetts

LAUREN NENTWICH, MD
Research Fellow, Department of Neurology, Stroke Research Center, Massachusetts General Hospital, Boston, Massachusetts

JONATHAN S. OLSHAKER, MD, FACEP, FAAEM
Chief, Boston Medical Center; Professor and Chair, Department of Emergency Medicine, Boston University School of Medicine, Boston, Massachusetts

TARA RAVIPRAKASH SOOD, MD
Department of Emergency Medicine, New York University/Bellevue Hospital Center, New York, New York

JEFFREY I. SCHNEIDER, MD
Assistant Professor of Emergency Medicine, Boston University School of Medicine; Residency Program Director, Department of Emergency Medicine, Boston Medical Center, Boston, Massachusetts

RISHI SIKKA, MD
Medical Director, Performance Improvement, Department of Emergency Medicine, Advocate Christ Medical Center, Oak Lawn, Illinois

MORSAL R. TAHOUNI, MD
Department of Emergency Medicine, Boston Medical Center, Boston University School of Medicine, Boston, Massachusetts

KARIS TEKWANI, MD
Department of Emergency Medicine, Advocate Christ Medical Center, Oak Lawn, Illinois

PAUL A. TESTA, MD, JD, MPH
Instructor, Department of Emergency Medicine, New York University School of Medicine, Bellevue Hospital Center, New York, New York

ANDREW S. ULRICH, MD
Vice-chair and Associate Professor, Department of Emergency Medicine, Boston Medical Center, Boston University School of Medicine, Boston, Massachusetts

KAR-MUN C. WOO, MD
Resident, Department of Emergency Medicine, Boston Medical Center, Boston, Massachusetts

KENNETH T. YU, MD, MBA
Instructor in Medicine, Department of Emergency Medicine, New York Presbyterian Hospital/Weill Cornell Medical Center, New York, New York

RICHARD D. ZANE, MD, FAAEM
Department of Emergency Medicine, Brigham and Women's Hospital; Associate Professor, Harvard Medical School, Boston, Massachusetts

Contents

Foreword xv

Amal Mattu

Preface xvii

Joseph H. Kahn, Brendan G. Magauran Jr, and Jonathan S. Olshaker

Clinical Practice Guidelines in the Emergency Department 555

Pooja Agrawal and Joshua M. Kosowsky

Many professional societies publish clinical practice guidelines that pertain to the management of patients with specific diagnoses. This article explores clinical practice guidelines affecting emergency physicians, such as those published by the American College of Emergency Physicians and other medical specialty organizations, such as the American Heart Association. Examples of such guidelines include algorithms, such as those published in Advanced Cardiac Life Support, clinical decision rules, such as the Ottawa ankle rules, and pathways that describe the treatment of critical diseases such as acute myocardial infarction. This article discusses the relevance of these guidelines, algorithms, and protocols to the practicing emergency medicine specialist.

Professional Liability Insurance 569

Morsal R. Tahouni and Joseph H. Kahn

This article introduces the emergency physician to professional liability insurance: the type of insurance, whether it is the only type available in the region, and, if claims-made insurance, whether the tail coverage rate is reasonable; the limits of liability and whether these are appropriate for emergency medicine in the region; the policy exclusions and restrictions; the insurance company's financial strength; whether an attorney is provided for a claim, whether fees are covered by the policy, whether they are subtracted from the policy limit, whether the physician can choose a defense attorney, and whether the physician's consent is required for the insurance company to settle a case.

The Legal Process 583

Richard D. Zane

Being named in a malpractice case may be one of the most stressful events in a physician's career and participating in a trial is likely to be remembered for a lifetime. Despite the climate of tort reform, it is a system that is unlikely to change anytime soon. By understanding and knowing the system and proactively participating in one's own defense, the traumatic experience of being named in a malpractice case may be mitigated.

Managing Emergency Department Overcrowding 593

Jonathan S. Olshaker

Emergency department (ED) crowding and ambulance diversion has been an increasingly significant national problem for more than a decade. More than 90% of hospital ED directors reported overcrowding as a problem resulting in patients in hallways, full occupancy of ED beds, and long waits, occurring several times a week. Overcrowding has many other potential detrimental effects including diversion of ambulances, frustration for patients and ED personnel, lesser patient satisfaction, and most importantly, greater risk for poor outcomes. This article gives a basic blueprint for successfully making hospital-wide changes using principles of operational management. It briefly covers the causes, significance, and dangers of overcrowding, and then focuses primarily on specific solutions.

Risk Management for the Emergency Physician: Competency and Decision-Making Capacity, Informed Consent, and Refusal of Care Against Medical Advice 605

Brendan G. Magauran Jr

This article focuses on those times that the emergency physician (EP) and patient do not agree on a treatment option. Attention is placed on the risk management issues relevant to the patient's unexpected choice. Emphasis is placed on determining a patient's competency or capability of making clinical decisions, with particular focus on the EP deciding that patient competency requires a formal evaluation. The EP should have a strategy for assessing clinical decision-making capability and an understanding of what circumstances should act as a trigger for considering such an assessment. Attention to documentation issues around informed consent, common barriers to consent, refusal of care, and ED discharge against medical advice are examined.

Evaluation of Physician Competency and Clinical Performance in Emergency Medicine 615

William E. Baker

This article (1) provides the background history of assessing health care quality; (2) presents an overview of current interest and importance of measuring physician competency and performance, including requirements related to certifying bodies and those integral to pay-for-performance programs; (3) describes some of the current methods of evaluating the practice performance of emergency physicians, including peer review and use of health care quality measures; and (4) discusses the state of the literature as it pertains to health care quality and individual emergency physician performance.

Triage, EMTALA, Consultations, and Prehospital Medical Control 627

Paul A. Testa and Maureen Gang

Medical control of prehospital emergency services, triage in the emergency department, and the dual duties within the Emergency Medical Treatment and Active Labor Act challenge emergency medicine physicians with both statutory obligations and liabilities. Each independently

may seem to present a definable boundary of liability for the practitioner. Under the Emergency Medical Treatment and Active Labor Act, the sequential duties of the medical screening examination and subsequent stabilization or transfer are confounded by the potential for tremendous sanction for a mechanistic violation. Nevertheless, the true obligation is to provide appropriate care to all who present to the emergency department and not simply weigh the totality of risk to the emergency medicine physician.

Critical Aspects of Emergency Department Documentation and Communication **641**

Kenneth T. Yu and Robert A. Green

This article focuses on the unique environment of the emergency department (ED) and the issues that place the provider at increased risk of liability actions. Patient care, quality, and safety should always be the primary focus of ED providers. However, the ED chart is the only lasting record of an ED visit, and attention must be paid to proper and accurate documentation. This article introduces the important aspects of ED documentation and communication, with specific focus on key areas of medico-legal risk, the advantages and disadvantages of the available types of ED medical records, the critical transition points of patient handoffs and changes of shift, and the ideal manner to craft effective discharge and follow-up instructions.

Physical and Chemical Restraints **655**

Victoria A. Coburn and Mark B. Mycyk

The combative or uncooperative patient is a growing problem in the emergency department. Restrained patients are at especially high risk of adverse outcomes. Particular attention has been given to de-escalation techniques to reduce the need for patient restraint. This article examines these techniques and the need for and risks of physical and chemical restraints in managing patients in the emergency department.

Evaluation of the Psychiatric Patient **669**

Tara Raviprakash Sood and Christopher M. Mcstay

Patients presenting to the emergency department (ED) with behavioral disturbances account for approximately 6% of all ED visits. Emergency physicians are often responsible for the initial assessment of these patients' psychiatric complaints, which might include homicidal and suicidal behavior and acute psychosis. The emergency physician might be asked to provide medical clearance before transfer to definitive psychiatric care. The purpose of the medical screening is to identify medical conditions that might be causing or contributing to the psychiatric emergency or that might be dangerous or inappropriate to treat in a psychiatric facility. Appropriate treatment in the ED is essential to avoid morbidity and mortality resulting from misdiagnosis of medical conditions as psychiatric illnesses and from mismanagement of psychiatric illnesses.

FORTHCOMING ISSUES

February 2010

High Risk Emergencies

Jeffrey Tabas, MD, and
Teri Reynolds, MD,
Guest Editors

May 2010

HIV in the Emergency Department

Mercedes Torres, MD, and
Rachel Chin, MD,
Guest Editors

August 2010

Altered States of Consciousness

Chad Kessler, MD, *Guest Editor*

RECENT ISSUES

August 2009

Cancer Emergencies, Part II

David M. Spiro, MD, and
Mohamud Daya, MD,
Guest Editors

May 2009

Cancer Emergencies, Part I

Mohamud Daya, MD, and
Charles R. Thomas Jr, MD,
Guest Editors

February 2009

Neurologic Emergencies

Robert Silbergleit, MD, and
Romergryko G. Geocadin, MD,
Guest Editors

RELATED INTEREST

Ultrasound Clinics, January 2008, Vol. 5, No. 1 (pages 1–178)
Emergency Ultrasound
V.S. Dogra and S. Bhatt, *Guest Editors*
www.ultrasound.theclinics.com

GOAL STATEMENT

The goal of *Emergency Medicine Clinics of North America* is to keep practicing physicians up to date with current clinical practice in emergency medicine by providing timely articles reviewing the state of the art in patient care.

ACCREDITATION

The *Emergency Medical Clinics of North America* is planned and implemented in accordance with the Essential Areas and Policies of the Accreditation Council for Continuing Medical Education (ACCME) through the joint sponsorship of the University of Virginia School of Medicine and Elsevier. The University of Virginia School of Medicine is accredited by the ACCME to provide continuing medical education for physicians.

The University of Virginia School of Medicine designates this educational activity for a maximum of 15 *AMA PRA Category 1 Credits*™ for each issue, 60 credits per year. Physicians should only claim credit commensurate with the extent of their participation in the activity.

The American Medical Association has determined that physicians not licensed in the US who participate in this CME activity are eligible for a maximum of 15 *AMA PRA Category 1 Credits*™ for each issue, 60 credits per year.

The Emergency Medicine Clinics of North America CME program is approved by the American College of Emergency Physicians for 60 hours of ACEP Category I Credit per year.

Credit can be earned by reading the text material, taking the CME examination online at http://www.theclinics.com/home/cme, and completing the evaluation. After taking the test, you will be required to review any and all incorrect answers. Following completion of the test and evaluation, your credit will be awarded and you may print your certificate.

FACULTY DISCLOSURE/CONFLICT OF INTEREST

The University of Virginia School of Medicine, as an ACCME accredited provider, endorses and strives to comply with the Accreditation Council for Continuing Medical Education (ACCME) Standards of Commercial Support, Commonwealth of Virginia statutes, University of Virginia policies and procedures, and associated federal and private regulations and guidelines on the need for disclosure and monitoring of proprietary and financial interests that may affect the scientific integrity and balance of content delivered in continuing medical education activities under our auspices.

The University of Virginia School of Medicine requires that all CME activities accredited through this institution be developed independently and be scientifically rigorous, balanced and objective in the presentation/discussion of its content, theories and practices.

All authors/editors participating in an accredited CME activity are expected to disclose to the readers relevant financial relationships with commercial entities occurring within the past 12 months (such as grants or research support, employee, consultant, stock holder, member of speakers bureau, etc.). The University of Virginia School of Medicine will employ appropriate mechanisms to resolve potential conflicts of interest to maintain the standards of fair and balanced education to the reader. Questions about specific strategies can be directed to the Office of Continuing Medical Education, University of Virginia School of Medicine, Charlottesville, Virginia.

The faculty and staff of the University of Virginia Office of Continuing Medical Education have no financial affiliations to disclose.

The authors/editors listed below have identified no professional or financial affiliations for themselves or their spouse/partner:

Pooja Agrawal, MD; William E. Baker, MD; Victoria A. Coburn, MD; Maureen Gang, MD; Robert A. Green, MD, MPH; Joseph H. Kahn, MD, FACEP (Guest Editor); Brendan G. Magauran Jr., MD, MBA (Guest Editor); Patrick Manley (Acquisitions Editor); Amal Mattu, MD, FAAEM, FACEP (Consulting Editor); Christopher M. McStay, MD; Mark B. Mycyk, MD; Lauren Nentwich, MD; Jonathan S. Olshaker, MD, FAAEM, FACEP (Guest Editor); Tara Raviprakash Sood, MD; Jeffrey I. Schneider, MD; Morsal R. Tahouni, MD; Karis Tekwani, MD; Paul A. Testa, MD, JD, MPH; Andrew S. Ulrich, MD; Kar-mun C. Woo, MD; Bill Woods, MD (Test Author); Kenneth T. Yu, MD, MBA; and, Richard D. Zane, MD, FAAEM.

The authors/editors listed below have identified the following professional or financial affiliations for themselves of their spouse/partner:

Joshua M. Kosowsky, MD is on the Speakers' Bureau and the Advisory Committee/Board for Sanofi Aventis/BMS, Daiichi Sankyo/Lilly, Schering Plough, and The Medicines Company.
Rishi Sikka, MD is a patent holder and has stock/ownership in Praxeon.

Disclosure of Discussion of Non-FDA Approved Uses for Pharmaceutical Products and/or Medical Devices

The University of Virginia School of Medicine, as an ACCME provider, requires that all faculty presenters identify and disclose any off-label uses for pharmaceutical and medical device products. The University of Virginia School of Medicine recommends that each physician fully review all the available data on new products or procedures prior to clinical use.

TO ENROLL

To enroll in the Emergency Medicine Clinics of North America Continuing Medical Education program, call customer service at 1-800-654-2452 or visit us online at www.theclinics.com/home/cme. The CME program is available to subscribers for an additional fee of $195.00.

Foreword

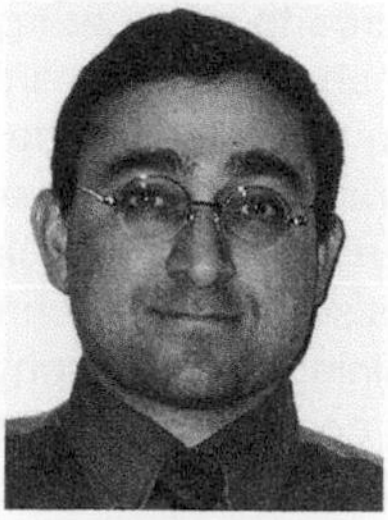

Amal Mattu, MD, FAAEM, FACEP
Consulting Editor

Emergency medicine is a high-risk specialty. "High-risk" implies danger to patients—typical conditions that are worked up and diagnosed in an emergency department (ED) include acute cardiac ischemia or infarction, stroke, intracranial bleeds, appendicitis, aortic catastrophes, meningitis, sepsis, multisystem trauma, life-threatening asthma, and so forth. Every patient that presents to an ED must be assumed at risk for serious morbidity or mortality. Patients are not the only people at risk in an ED, however; every physician-patient encounter represents not only health risk for the patient but also legal risk for the physician. The constant threat of malpractice in the US health care system, especially in high-risk specialties, such as emergency medicine, is an ever-present issue that affects physician work-ups, practice patterns, and dispositions on a daily basis.

There are many factors that produce medicolegal risk to emergency care providers. Foremost among them is that patients presenting to an ED often have life-threatening conditions. There is no guarantee of a good outcome for every patient visit. Societal expectations for modern health care practice, however, are unrealistically optimistic. These unrealistic expectations are largely fueled by the popular media—television, in particular, portrays physicians as capable of incredible "saves" in any situation. Studies have documented, for example, the influence of television on the lay public's expectations of survival from cardiac arrest.[1,2] When a bad outcome occurs, a patient or family may assume that malpractice was committed because the outcome did not meet expectations. Another major reason for medicolegal risk is the political power of the trial lawyers associations, which is likely a major reason for delays in or absence of tort reform in many states. This is also a likely reason why the judicial system in the United States favors the rights of potential plaintiffs to file a suit over the rights of defendants to file countersuit against plaintiffs for frivolous lawsuits. Other reasons for increasing medicolegal risk to emergency care providers are hospital overcrowding, which is decreasing even further the available time that emergency physicians have to communicate well and create rapport with patients; dwindling resources and

Emerg Med Clin N Am 27 (2009) xv–xvi
doi:10.1016/j.emc.2009.09.001

on-call consultant availability; and increasing patient acuity, which is largely attributable to the aging ED population.

In this issue of *Emergency Medicine Clinics of North America*, guest editors, Drs Kahn, Magauran, and Olshaker, provide a valuable resource to help emergency care providers learn about the medicolegal risk they face and about how to minimize that risk. Articles also address general topics in risk management, such as the legal process, documentation and communication, liability insurance, and triage and consultations. Authors also address many specific high-risk chief complaints, including chest pain, abdominal pain, and headache. They also address scenarios in which medicolegal risk is increased, including issues pertaining to use of physical and chemical restraints, clearance of the psychiatric patient, consent and refusal of care, and medical screening requirements. Finally, authors address problems of ED overcrowding and suggest some solutions.

This issue of *Emergency Medicine Clinics of North America* represents an important overview of the most important topics pertaining to emergency medicine risk management. This issue should be considered essential reading not only for practicing emergency physicians but also for emergency medicine trainees and for any other health care providers who care for patients in an ED. After completing this issue of *Emergency Medicine Clinics*, readers are certain to understand not only the risk they face but also simple and important methods of minimizing that risk. Kudos to the guest editors and authors for providing this valuable resource.

Amal Mattu, MD, FAAEM, FACEP
Department of Emergency Medicine
University of Maryland School of Medicine
110 S. Paca Street, 6th Floor, Suite 200
Baltimore, MD 21201, USA

E-mail address:
amattu@smail.umaryland.edu (A. Mattu)

REFERENCES

1. Diem SJ, Lantos JD, Tulsky JA. Cardiopulmonary resuscitation on television: miracles and misinformation. N Engl J Med 1996;334:1578–82.
2. Roberts D, Hirschman D, Scheltema K. Adults and pediatric CPR: attitudes and expectations of health professionals and laypersons. Am J Emerg Med 2000;18: 465–8.

Preface

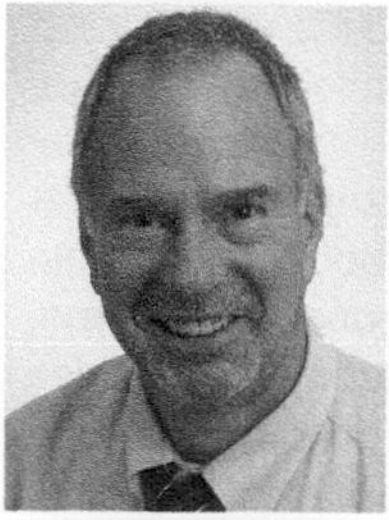
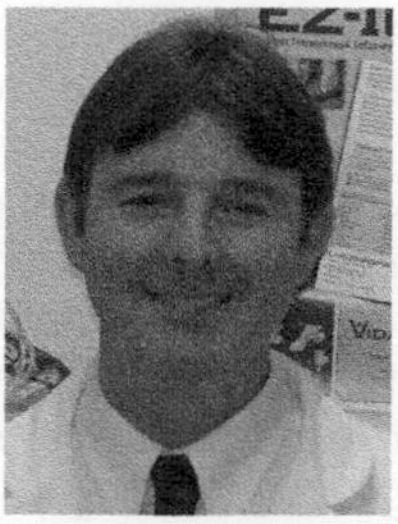
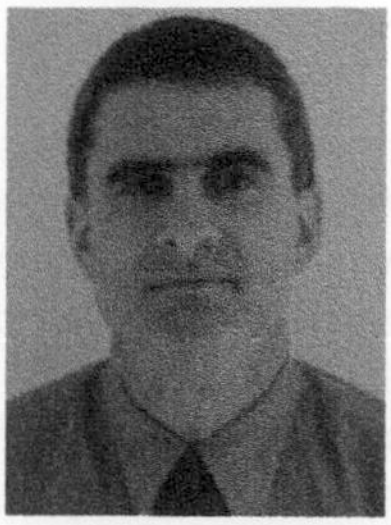

Joseph H. Kahn, MD, FACEP
Brendan G. Magauran Jr, MD, MBA
Jonathan S. Olshaker, MD, FACEP, FAAEM
Guest Editors

The vast majority of emergency physicians are well trained, highly skilled, competent, and compassionate. Nevertheless, litigation is a constant threat to the practicing emergency physician. The very nature of the practice of emergency medicine makes adverse outcomes unavoidable. We often have no knowledge of the preexisting medical conditions of the patients we treat. Many of our patients have no access to essential medical care, causing them to present late in the course of disease. Further complicating the picture is the high number of repeat emergency department patients who often lull us into a false sense of security because of absence of serious medical conditions on prior visits. Lack of an ongoing relationship with the patient and family makes litigation more likely when adverse outcomes occur.

In this issue, we have attempted to provide some principles of emergency medical practice that may help avoid litigation. The article on clinical practice guidelines provides a framework for when guidelines should be followed and when it is acceptable to deviate from them. The article on professional liability insurance discusses what types of malpractice insurance is available to emergency practitioners, and reviews the amount of settlements and judgments issued in recent years. The article on the legal process describes in detail the process of being a defendant or an expert witness in a malpractice action. The article on emergency department overcrowding describes perhaps the most pervasive problem in emergency medicine today, with strategies for lowering risk. The article on informed consent provides insights into dealing with patients who refuse treatment and for determining whether these patients have the capacity to refuse treatment. The article also touches on alternative care plans and implied consent.

Physician review will soon become a required component of board certification and hospital credentialing in emergency medicine, and the article on this important topic describes the latest state and federal agency requirements. The article on the Emergency Medical Treatment and Active Labor Act (EMTALA) gives a current description of what emergency physicians should do to remain in compliance of this federal "anti-dumping law." The article on documentation and communication covers the key issues of how to minimize risk and bad outcomes during change of shift, admission, and discharge of patients. It also focuses on the importance of thorough, concise, and clear charting, which is too often ignored in the practice of emergency medicine.

Emerg Med Clin N Am 27 (2009) xvii–xviii
doi:10.1016/j.emc.2009.08.003

The article on physical and chemical restraints covers the management of the very high risk group of patients who are combative and uncooperative. The article on the psychiatric patient discusses two very high risk areas in emergency medicine: the area related to psychiatric patients requiring a medical evaluation, and the area related to the question of involuntary hospitalization of patients with suicidal ideation, homicidal ideation, and acute psychosis.

The final three articles describe how to avoid medical legal pitfalls in the management of patients with high-risk chief complaints. The article about chest pain describes in detail management strategies to avoid missing acute coronary syndrome, thoracic aortic dissection, and pulmonary embolism, as well as other serious entities that present as chest pain. The article on high-risk complaints of the head and neck is a review of successful management strategies for dealing with headache, cervical spine injury, the difficult airway, and high-risk ophthalmologic complaints. The article on high-risk complaints of the abdomen and extremities provides strategies to avoid missing such entities as abdominal aortic aneurysm, mesenteric ischemia, appendicitis, and bowel obstruction, as well as compartment syndromes, foreign bodies, fractures, and nerve and tendon injuries.

Finally, the afterword summarizes the strategies outlined in the rest of this issue. It is hoped that these strategies will be effective in enabling the practicing emergency physician to reduce both adverse outcomes and malpractice risks.

In expressing our appreciation for the work associated with this issue, we first and foremost thank all of the authors who made this issue on risk management possible. Special thanks are due to Patrick Manley and the staff at Elsevier for their patience and support. We also thank our families for allowing us the time to edit and assemble this issue. Most of all, we thank those of you who read this issue of *Emergency Medicine Clinics of North America*.

Joseph H. Kahn, MD, FACEP
Department of Emergency Medicine
Boston Medical Center
Boston University School of Medicine
1 Boston Medical Center Place
Boston, MA 02118, USA

Brendan G. Magauran Jr, MD, MBA
Department of Emergency Medicine
Boston Medical Center
Boston University School of Medicine
1 Boston Medical Center Place
Boston, MA 02118, USA

Jonathan S. Olshaker, MD, FACEP, FAAEM
Department of Emergency Medicine
Boston Medical Center
Boston University School of Medicine
1 Boston Medical Center Place
Boston, MA 02118, USA

E-mail addresses:
joseph.kahn@bmc.org (J.H. Kahn)
brendan.magauran@bmc.org (B.G. Magauran Jr)
jonathan.olshaker@bmc.org (J.S. Olshaker)

Clinical Practice Guidelines in the Emergency Department

Pooja Agrawal, MD, Joshua M. Kosowsky, MD*

KEYWORDS

- Guidelines • Critical pathways • Protocols
- Clinical decision rules • Algorithms

In an era of proliferating scientific investigation and discovery, complicated disease pathologies, and increasing pressure on clinicians to deliver swift, efficient, and precise health care, physicians have had to find better ways to streamline the delivery of high-quality medical care to their patients. In the specialty of emergency medicine, these pressures are arguably more significant than anywhere else. These demands have prompted many emergency medicine physicians (EMPs) to turn to established protocols, algorithms, and guidelines to facilitate the complicated diagnostic and therapeutic decision-making process.

Clinical practice guidelines are consensus statements about specific clinical topics or diagnoses that have been "systematically developed to assist practitioners in making decisions about patient diagnoses and management."[1] Their successful and appropriate implementation is thought to improve the quality of patient care by reducing inappropriate variation between practice styles and by expediting the application of effective and validated treatments in everyday practice.[2,3]

In recent years, clinical guidelines have become an increasingly familiar part of medical practice. The driving force behind the groundswell of interest in clinical guidelines lies in several issues that reflect the changing needs and demands of the health care system. These issues include rising health care costs; increased burden of care with an aging population; more expensive technologies; variations in treatments among providers, hospitals, and geographic regions; misuse (over or under) of services; and the intrinsic desire of health care professionals to provide and patients' desire to receive the best health care possible.[4] Clinical guidelines are the industry's way of attempting to meet these demands while achieving a universally high standard of health care. Ideal topics for which clinical guidelines are created are generally chosen from complaints that present with high frequency, high risk, or high cost.

Department of Emergency Medicine, Brigham and Women's Hospital, Harvard Medical School, 75 Francis Street, Boston, MA 02115, USA
* Corresponding author.
E-mail address: jmkosowsky@partners.org (J.M. Kosowsky).

Emerg Med Clin N Am 27 (2009) 555–567
doi:10.1016/j.emc.2009.07.001
emed.theclinics.com

Although it may seem that abiding by clinical practice guidelines should be a voluntary decision, more and more regulatory pressure is being imposed to ensure physician and hospital compliance. Since the 1970s, various governmental organizations have been charged with the task of improving the quality and standardization of health care and responding to rising health care costs. In the 1980s, Peer Review Organizations, later called Quality Improvement Organizations, were created focusing on specific medical conditions that affected the Medicare population preferentially, such as acute myocardial infarctions, pneumonia, heart failure, and stroke. They were tasked with demonstrating measurable outcome improvements by standardizing treatments for these and several other conditions.[5]

The Joint Commission on Accreditation of Healthcare Organizations (JCAHO) was created to serve the role as the foremost quality monitoring organization and to establish minimum standards for hospitals to abide by. To this day, the Joint Commission continues to perform periodic audits of health care organizations to ensure that those minimum standards are being met and to encourage hospitals to strive for the highest level of quality. To qualify for Joint Commission accreditation, hospitals and other health care facilities must meet 20 specific minimum performance and hospital quality measures.[6] Departments of Public Health and other state and local governing bodies grade hospital performance using similar standards. As an added incentive, the governing bodies that regulate Social Security require that hospitals meet Joint Commission standards to be eligible for Medicare and Medicaid funding.

Almost every medical specialty society, including the American College of Emergency Physicians (ACEP), the American Heart Association (AHA), and the American College of Cardiology (ACC), creates and publishes specialty-specific practice guidelines, with recommendations relevant to their specialty. These practice guidelines range from specific algorithms, such as Advanced Cardiac Life Support (ACLS), Pediatric Advanced Life Support (PALS), and Advanced Trauma Life Support (ATLS) algorithms, to more general recommendations that provide assistance in answering a specific question or guiding a physician down a particular treatment pathway. These clinical recommendations are published in various forms and are called by a variety of names: policies, guidelines, protocols, pathways, and rules, to name a few. Each of these terms carries with it its own connotation, purpose, and format.

At one end of the spectrum, a "policy" suggests an absolute rule-based approach, presumably, although not always, on the basis of clear and convincing scientific evidence. Many organizations have moved away from the term "policy" out of concern for the medicolegal and other societal implications, should a clinician decide to deviate in some way from the recommended management. Over the years, ACEP has convened several working groups to create clinical policies for EMPs. Many of the early ACEP policies were too broad to be useful for the practicing clinician. Newer ACEP clinical policies have focused on specific clinical issues about which there is active interest or debate. For example, the current ACEP clinical policy on acetaminophen overdose addresses the use of *N*-acetylcysteine in detail but does not discuss the utility of activated charcoal.[7]

A "guideline" implies a somewhat more flexible standard aimed at eliminating discrepancy between what the scientific evidence supports and what clinicians actually do.[8] Guidelines are usually published by specialty-specific organizations.[9] For example, the American Medical Association has published a compendium of 1800 policies to assist clinicians in decision making. The ACC/AHA has meticulous and rigorously supported guidelines detailing many clinical presentations, for example, the management of patients with unstable angina and non–ST-elevation myocardial infarctions.[10] The National Guideline Clearinghouse database (www.guideline.gov) is a central repository for policies created by several organizations that allows clinicians to easily access recommendations from a variety of sources. More than 600 guidelines have been registered there to date.

A "pathway" is an algorithm that details, often visually, a sequence of actions designed to achieve a treatment outcome with optimum efficiency.[11] Pathways spell out the order of each specific task to be completed and identify the specific individual responsible for performing each of those tasks. Pathways are often designed to promote an appropriate and timely response to critical diagnoses, such as ST-elevation myocardial infarction or acute stroke. In a sense, all ACLS protocols are also examples of pathways (**Fig. 1**). Following established pathways for specific conditions has been shown to be effective in improving patient outcomes.[12]

A clinical decision rule (CDR) is a specific type of algorithm designed to answer a particular clinical question. CDRs ask the practitioner to use clinical factors, such as a patient's history, physical examination, and laboratory results, to determine the likelihood of a particular diagnosis or clinical outcome. Depending on the circumstances, a CDR may be used to establish the pretest probability of a diagnostic test, predict a patient's prognosis, or suggest a particular course of treatment.[13,14] CDRs are designed to simplify diagnoses and to improve clinical accuracy and efficiency. Examples include the Ottawa ankle rules (**Fig. 2**),[15] the Canadian cervical spine rule,[16] the National Emergency X-radiography Utilization Study (NEXUS) cervical spine rules,[17] the Canadian head computed tomography rule,[18] and the thrombolysis in myocardial infarction (TIMI) risk score (**Box 1**).[19]

There are several factors involved in the development of a scientifically rigorous guideline. Careful assessment of the evidence supporting each recommendation, of the applicability of the evidence to the population of interest, and of the cost-benefit implications is essential. If the methodology of a study is flawed, if the study design does not have sufficient power, or if there are hidden biases, then the guidelines based on their findings have the potential to do more harm than good. It is difficult to achieve uniformly high standards, and many guidelines do not, although they may be widely used.[20] The ideal practice guideline should be evidence-based, derived from peer-reviewed literature, consistent with other relevant policies, and supportive of practices shown to improve patient outcome.[21]

Understanding the criteria used for grading evidence and assessing the strength of each recommendation is important. Different groups may use slightly different nomenclature, and although each scheme has its merits, there are fundamental differences in philosophy that should be understood. These differences have the potential to create opposing recommendations, and unless a clinician is aware of those differences they may be perplexed by potentially conflicting guidelines. For example, the ACEP classification scheme (A, B, or C) looks only to the quality of evidence on which recommendations are made. Class I evidence (the best evidence) is defined as the evidence that comes from randomized controlled blinded trials and subsequent meta-analyses of those trials. Class II evidence comes from retrospective cohort studies, case control studies, or cross-sectional studies. Class III evidence is derived from observational reports and consensus statements (**Table 1**).[22]

The applicability of the evidence base to the emergency department (ED) setting is also an important factor in determining the strength of the evidence of studies evaluated to create an ACEP recommendation.[23] For example, in the ACEP grading scheme, a study that would otherwise be considered class I would be downgraded to a lower level if it is not directly applicable to practice in the ED.

The ACC/AHA, on the other hand, uses a two-pronged approach to classification, grading not only the evidence to support a recommendation but also the potential

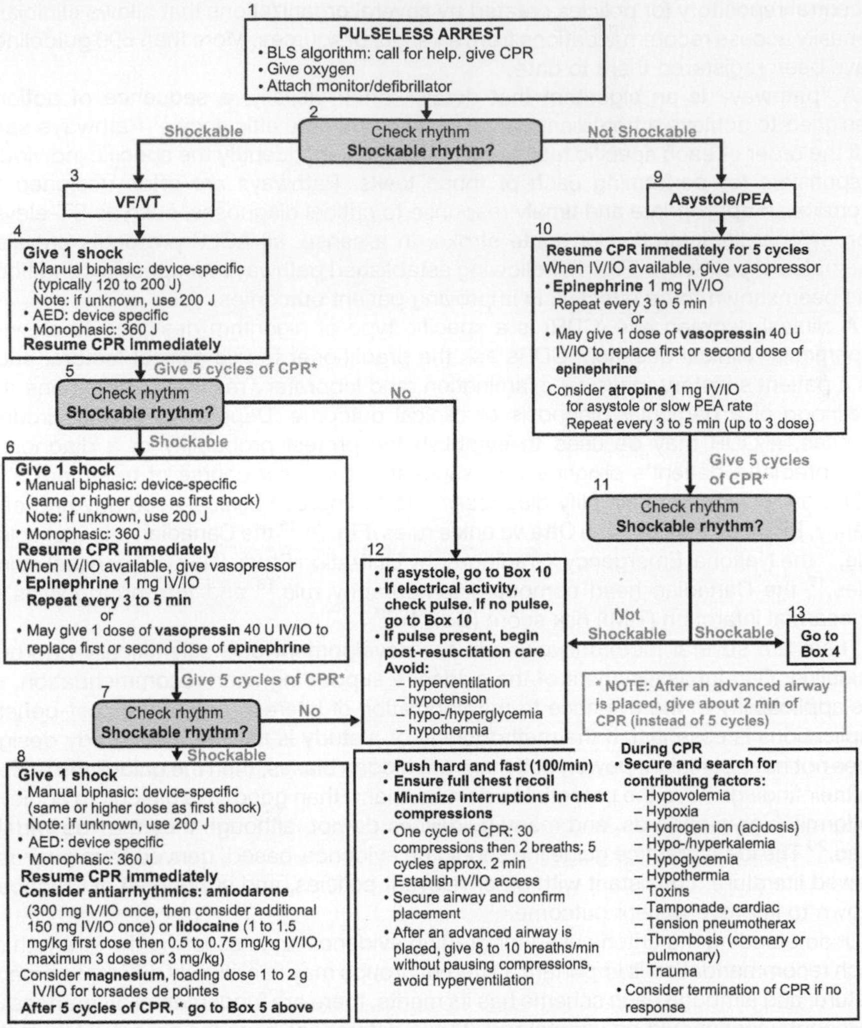

Fig. 1. ACLS protocol. AED, automated external defibrillator; BLS, basic life support; CPR, cardiopulmonary resuscitation; IO, intraosseous; IV, intravenous; PEA, pulseless electrical activity; VF, ventricular fibrillation; VT, ventricular tachycardia. (*From* Zipes DP, Camm AJ, Borggrefe M, et al. ACC/AHA/ESC 2006 guidelines for management of patients with ventricular arrhythmias and the prevention of sudden cardiac death. Circulation 2006;114:e385–484; with permission.)

effect of a recommendation on outcomes. The evidence that supports each study classified by ACC/AHA standards is graded from A to C. Level A evidence is derived from large studies with several levels of risk stratification, whereas level C evidence comes from a limited number of subjects. ACC/AHA recommendations include a further classification scheme that comments on the risk-to-benefit ratio of following the treatment suggested by a particular study. A class I recommendation implies that the benefit of following a study's recommendation greatly outweighs the risk of not doing so, whereas a class III recommendation suggests the opposite (**Fig. 3**).[10]

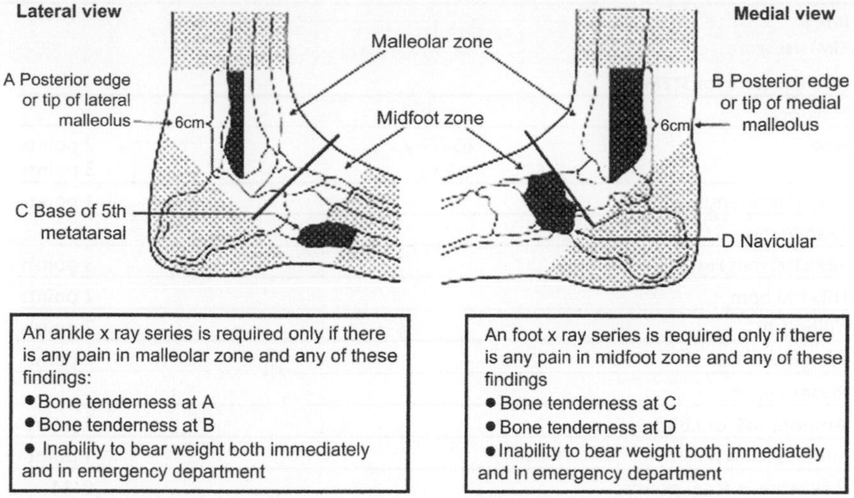
Lateral view
Medial view
Malleolar zone
Midfoot zone
A Posterior edge or tip of lateral malleolus
6cm
B Posterior edge or tip of medial malleolus
6cm
C Base of 5th metatarsal
D Navicular
An ankle x ray series is required only if there is any pain in malleolar zone and any of these findings:
• Bone tenderness at A
• Bone tenderness at B
• Inability to bear weight both immediately and in emergency department
An foot x ray series is required only if there is any pain in midfoot zone and any of these findings
• Bone tenderness at C
• Bone tenderness at D
• Inability to bear weight both immediately and in emergency department

Fig. 2. Ottawa ankle rules. (*From* Stiell IG, Greenberg GH, McKnight RD, et al. A study to develop clinical decision rules for the use of radiography in acute ankle injuries. Ann Emerg Med 1992;21(4):384–90; with permission.)

When using the ACC/AHA classification scheme to evaluate a study, it is necessary to be cognizant of both of these systems.

Published guidelines need to be assessed for internal and external validity.[24,25] Internal validity is the degree to which a causal relationship exists between the variables being assessed. The treatment being evaluated should be directly responsible for the outcome, and the study should be assessed for any confounding factors. External validity refers to the generalizability of the results of a study to other populations. A clinician needs to ensure that the reference population from which the guidelines were derived mirrors their patients, and that the rules can be applied to different populations with the same outcomes.[26]

Validation studies can be informative and can add to the clinical significance of a guideline. With new information about disease states, diagnoses, and treatments emerging on a regular basis, it is essential that clinical guidelines be reassessed with some frequency.[27] Some organizations use the concept of a "living guideline committee," a panel of experts charged with the responsibility of monitoring ongoing publications, to incorporate and update relevant discoveries or advances into previously published practice guidelines.[28]

Expert opinion and clinical experiences influence recommendations, and therefore guidelines have the potential to be susceptible to pressure from political interests.[29,30] In addition, each member of a writing committee tasked with creating guidelines must provide full disclosure of their potential conflicts of interest; this is paramount to the integrity and credibility of the guideline writing process.[31]

The ultimate goal for using clinical guidelines is to improve patient outcomes. A successful and appropriately applied clinical guideline has the potential to confer benefit to patients, health care providers, quality-assurance teams, and medical researchers (**Box 2**).[32]

From the patient's perspective, guidelines have been shown to improve quality of care and to benefit health outcomes, arguably the most important indication for their use.[33] Studies from around the world have shown that when guidelines are not used,

Box 1
TIMI risk score

TIMI risk score for STEMI		
Historical		
Age	65–74 y	2 points
	≥75 y	3 points
DM/HTN or angina		1 point
Examination		
SBP<100 mm Hg		3 points
HR>100 bpm		2 points
Killip II–IV		2 points
Weight<67 kg		1 point
Presentation		
Anterior STE or LBBB		1 point
Time to Rx>4 h		1 point
Risk score = total points		0–14

Risk score	**Odds of death by 30 days**[a]	
0	0.1	(0.1–0.2)
1	0.3	(0.2–0.3)
2	0.4	(0.3–0.5)
3	0.7	(0.6–0.9)
4	1.2	(1.0–1.5)
5	2.2	(1.9–2.6)
6	3.0	(2.5–3.6)
7	4.8	(3.8–6.1)
8	5.8	(4.2–7.8)
>8	8.8	(6.3–12)

Abbreviations: DM, diabetes mellitus; HR, heart rate; HTN, hypertension; LBBB, left bundle branch block; SBP, systolic blood pressure; STE, ST-segment elevation; STEMI, ST-segment elevation myocardial infarction.

[a] Referenced to average mortality (95% confidence intervals).

Data from Morrow DA, Antman EM, Charlesworth A, et al. TIMI risk score for ST-elevation myocardial infarction: a convenient, bedside, clinical score for risk assessment at presentation: an intravenous nPA for treatment of infarcting myocardium early II trial substudy. Circulation 2000;102:2031–7.

there is significant variation among doctors, specialists, and geographic regions in the frequency with which lifesaving procedures are performed.[34] Clinical guidelines have the potential to assist in the delivery of uniform care regardless of the type of facility, available resources, or clinician providing treatment. Whether they actually assist in the delivery of uniform care is unclear, however, because patients, doctors, payers, and managers define the concept of quality differently.[35]

Health care providers also benefit from guidelines because they can streamline the process of clinical decision making. Guidelines offer explicit recommendations for clinicians who may not be sure about how to best diagnose or treat a specific condition. Because EMPs are in some sense generalists, clinical guidelines developed by other specialty organizations can assist in the management of conditions that may

Table 1
ACEP literature classification scheme

Design/Class[a]	Therapy[b]	Diagnosis[c]	Prognosis[d]
1	Randomized controlled trial or meta-analyses of randomized trials	Prospective cohort using a criterion standard	Population prospective cohort
2	Nonrandomized trial	Retrospective observational	Retrospective cohort case control
3	Case series Case report Other (eg, consensus, review)	Case series Case report Other (eg, consensus, review)	Case series Case report Other (eg, consensus review)

[a] Some designs (eg, surveys) will not fit this scheme and should be assessed individually.
[b] Objective is to measure therapeutic efficacy comparing two or more interventions.
[c] Objective is to determine the sensitivity and specificity of diagnostic tests.
[d] Objective is to predict outcome, including mortality and morbidity.
Data from Jagoda AS, Bazarian JJ, Bruns JJ, et al. Clinical policy: neuroimaging and decision making in adult mild traumatic brain injury in the acute setting. Ann Emerg Med 2008;52(6):714–48.

not be familiar or common. Particularly in situations that require a practitioner to act in a decisive and almost reflexive action (such as myocardial infarction, stroke, or multi-trauma), pathways can help keep the clinician's attention focused on the most vital steps of care in a critical patient.

EMPs are specialists in the delivery of emergency care of patients who present with acute clinical presentations. However, they are also confronted with essentially every disease process from every other specialty field in medicine on an almost daily basis. It would be unrealistic to expect an EMP to know all the management details and research updates of every disease process.

The use of guidelines can improve communications among physicians, their patients, and their peers. Guidelines provide a common language for establishing protocols and standards of care. Because medicine is a team effort, having every member of the team understand and be familiar with established protocols leads to fewer deviations from proven algorithms and ultimately provides better care for patients.

From a standpoint of quality management, adherence to a guideline is often taken as a proxy for the standard of care, and can simplify the process of auditing and reporting on various process and outcome measures.

Guidelines may also have an influence on public policy, particularly by highlighting gaps in knowledge or by practice within a particular field, or as related to a specific patient population. In some instances, adoption of a clinical guideline may result in payment from health insurance providers or funding from governmental bodies.

Health care systems benefit from guidelines on the theory that efficiency of care is improved by standardization.[36] Implementation of guidelines may cut down on costs for hospitalization, diagnostic testing, therapeutic modalities, and procedures. Publicizing an institution's adherence to guidelines also improves public image, demonstrating commitment to quality and excellence through promoting good will, political support, and, ultimately, revenue.

Guidelines do have limitations, however, and emergency physicians have not universally embraced the use of guideline-based management.[37,38] As with any tool, to use an algorithm effectively requires a basic level of training and an

SIZE OF TREATMENT EFFECT →

ESTIMATE OF CERTAINTY (PRECISION) OF TREATMENT EFFECT

	CLASS I *Benefit > > > Risk* Procedure/Treatment SHOULD be performed/ administered	CLASS IIa *Benefit > > Risk* *Additional studies with focused objectives needed* IT IS REASONABLE to perform procedure/administer treatment	CLASS IIb *Benefit ≥ Risk* *Additional studies with broad objectives needed; additional registry data would be helpful* Procedure/Treatment MAY BE CONSIDERED	CLASS III *Risk ≥ Benefit* *No additional studies needed* Procedure/Treatment should NOT be performed/administered SINCE IT IS NOT HELPFUL AND MAY BE HARMFUL
LEVEL A Multiple (3-5) population risk strata evaluted* General consistency of direction and magnitude of effect	■ Recommendation that procedure or treatment is useful/effective ■ Sufficient evidence from multiple randomized trials or meta-analyses	■ Recommendation in favor of treatment or procedure being useful/effective ■ Some conflicting evidence from multiple randomized trials or meta-analyses	■ Recommendation's usefulness/efficacy less well established ■ Greater conflicting evidence from multiple randomized trials or meta-analyses	■ Recommendation that procedure or treatment is not useful/effective and may be harmful ■ Sufficient evidence from multiple randomized trials or meta-analyses
LEVEL B Limited (2-3) population risk strata evaluted*	■ Recommendation that procedure or treatment is useful/effective ■ Limited evidence from single randomized trials or nonrandomized studies	■ Recommendation in favor of treatment or procedure being useful/effective ■ Some conflicting evidence from single randomized trials or nonrandomized studies	■ Recommendation's usefulness/efficacy less well established ■ Greater conflicting evidence from single randomized trials or nonrandomized studies	■ Recommendation that procedure or treatment is not useful/effective and may be harmful ■ Limited evidence from single randomized trials or nonrandomized studies
LEVEL C Very limited (1-2) population risk strata evaluated*	■ Recommendation that procedure or treatment is useful/effective ■ Only expert opinion, case studies, or standard-of-care	■ Recommendation in favor of treatment or procedure being useful/effective ■ Only diverging expert opinion, case studies, or standard-of-care	■ Recommendation's usefulness/efficacy less well established ■ Only diverging expert opinion, case studies, or standard-of-care	■ Recommendation that procedure or treatment is not useful/effective and may be harmful ■ Only expert opinion, case studies, or standard-of-care
Suggested phrases for writing recommendations†	should is recommended is indicated is useful/effective/beneficial	is reasonable can be useful/effective /beneficial is probably recommended or indicated	may/might be considered may/might be reasonable usefulness/effectiveness is unknown/unclear/uncertain or not well established	is not recommended is not indicated should not is useful/effective/beneficial may be harmful

Fig. 3. ACC/AHA literature classification scheme. (*From* ACC/AHA task force on practice guidelines. ACC/AHA 2007 guidelines for the management of patients with unstable angina/non-ST-elevation myocardial infarction: executive summary. Circulation 2007;116:803–77; with permission.)

Box 2
Goals of clinical guidelines

- Selecting the "best practice" when practice varies unnecessarily
- Defining standards for the expected length of hospital stay and for the use of tests and therapies
- Examining interactions between steps in a care algorithm to coordinate steps and decrease delay at the rate-limiting step
- Providing a common pathway for all staff to view and understand their individual roles in the care process
- Providing a framework for data collection to troubleshoot and improve efficiency in the pathway
- Decreasing documentation burdens
- Improving patient satisfaction through education about plan for care

Data from Pearson SD, Goulart-Fisher D, Lee TH. Critical pathways as a strategy for improving care: problems and potential. Ann Intern Med 1995;123(12):941–8.

understanding as to when to follow the guideline, when to deviate from it, and when it may not be applicable at all.

The existence of a guideline has the potential to simplify decision making for a clinician. However, reflexive compliance with a guideline or pathway risks premature closure. The presence of a guideline or pathway may prevent a physician from considering an alternative diagnosis or concurrent condition. Thus, clinicians must continue to be vigilant about assessing a patient's complete presentation and not fall into an easy, predetermined algorithm without first performing a complete critical assessment of that patient.

Individual patient preferences and values are difficult to capture in a guideline, and assumptions about patients' best interests may be built into a guideline. Algorithms and pathways are not meant to keep patients from participating in the decision-making process regarding their own health care. Clinical pathways are often devised based on pooled data from trials that sample a large population. They suggest the best course of action for the average patient or institution and are not necessarily tailored to an individual's needs. When data are derived from a population, they tend to be more relevant to a typical and uncomplicated patient. However, certain individuals may lie outside the norm or have certain predisposing or complicating factors that make a particular guideline irrelevant to them specifically. They may not take specific comorbidities into account that could be relevant to a particular patient. The indiscriminate application of a clinical pathway may lead to inappropriate treatment and potential harm. In particular, recommendations that are based on cost-effectiveness analysis generally do not take into account economic factors that may be regional, institutional, or patient specific.

Some authors have expressed concern that algorithms and pathways may tend to stifle independent thinking and critical analysis. This could be particularly relevant for training medical students and house staff who are still developing their personal clinical judgment. In truth, however, an integral part of guideline-based education is teaching when and how to apply algorithms and pathways, as described earlier.

Practice guidelines have played a "relevant or pivotal role in the proof of negligence" in fewer than 7% of malpractice claims nationwide.[39] A study that surveyed attorneys reported that the existence of established clinical guidelines prompted them not to bring forth a malpractice suit in the first place; other surveys found that critical pathways actually decrease a physician's overall malpractice risk and may reduce the cost of settling cases that actually do get legal attention.[40,41] In general, when malpractice suits reach trial, it is because of disagreement over the definition of "standard of care."

Debate still exists regarding the effect that the use of clinical guidelines has on litigation. An Australian paper concluded that the use of guidelines does not directly prevent or encourage litigation, and that clinical guidelines are regarded as a form of expert opinion or a representation of the standard of care to the courts.[42] However, a study in the obstetrics literature concluded that following established clinical guidelines potentially protects physicians against malpractice litigation and that not doing so increases that risk.[43]

Although the legal system has accepted many clinical guidelines as representations of the standard of care, they do not regard these guidelines as indisputable. On the contrary, when they are disputed in court, even established and widely used clinical guidelines are often subjected to careful examination to establish their validity and relevance to the specific case in question. When there is controversy regarding the question of reasonable practice, courts continue to place more weight on the testimony of expert witnesses than on the recommendations of validated clinical guidelines.[44]

From a medicolegal perspective, it is sometimes assumed that the existence of a practice guideline establishes the standard of care, and that any deviation is presumptive malpractice. However, in most jurisdictions and in most cases, guidelines are not dispositive. Nevertheless, there is legitimate concern on the part of practicing clinicians that they will be held to standards that may encourage the inappropriate use of resources.

At the same time, one must recognize that simply following a guideline does not guarantee protection from a medicolegal standpoint. No reasonable person would advocate blind adherence to a guideline solely for medicolegal reasons. Nevertheless, to the extent that one's management deviates from an accepted pathway, it is certainly prudent to document one's rationale explicitly in the medical record in the event that a less-than-optimal outcome should result in legal action.

Increasingly, guidelines dictate reimbursement policies for governmental or private payers. Guidelines are seen as a way to standardize treatments to achieve cost savings, and deviation from a clinical practice guideline can be used as the basis for denying payment.

Clinicians may be concerned that the clinical practice guidelines threaten their clinical autonomy and do not allow them the freedom to practice in their own developed style.[45] However, lack of familiarity with guidelines and how they are meant to be applied may be the underlying issue in many cases.

SUMMARY

The use and sheer number of clinical practice guidelines are proliferating at a rapid rate and have become an important part of clinical practice in the ED setting. The effective use of guidelines requires the appropriate application of relevant decision trees, a critical understanding of the clinical pathology and research methodology involved, and acknowledgment of the reasons to use the guidelines in the first place. Although these guidelines have the potential for improving the standard of health care, there are limitations in their use, and any clinician should be cognizant of their potential medical, legal, and financial implications. Overall, the need for quick decision making and expeditious interventions make algorithms and pathways invaluable in the ED setting.

REFERENCES

1. Field MJ, Lohr KN. Clinical practice guidelines: direction of a new program. Washington, DC: National Academy Press; 1999.
2. Audet AM, Greenfield S, Field M. Medical practice guidelines: current activities and future directions. Ann Intern Med 1990;113(9):709–14.
3. Chassin MR. Practice guidelines: best hope for quality improvement in the 1990s. J Occup Med 1990;32:1199–206.
4. Every NR, Hochman J, Becker R, et al. Critical pathways: a review. Circulation 2000;101:461–5.
5. Jencks SF, Cuerdon T, Burwen DR, et al. Quality of medical care delivered to medicare beneficiaries: a profile at state and national levels. JAMA 2000;284:1670–6.
6. Griffey RT, Kosowsky JM. CMS/Joint Commission hospital quality measures: is it the federal grade for quality? Emerg Med Rep 2007;28(19):225–36.
7. Wolf SJ, Heard K, Sloan EP, et al. Clinical policy: critical issues in the management of patients presenting to the emergency department with acetaminophen overdose. Ann Emerg Med 2007;50:292–313.
8. Woolf SH, Grol R, Hutchinson A, et al. Clinical guidelines: potential benefit, limitations and harms of clinical guidelines. BMJ 1999;318:527–30.
9. Dunham CM, Barraco RD, Clark DE, et al. Guidelines for emergency tracheal intubation immediately after traumatic injury. J Trauma 2003;55:162–79.
10. ACC/AHA Task Force on Practice Guidelines. ACC/AHA 2007 guidelines for the management of patients with unstable angina/non-ST-elevation myocardial infarction: executive summary. Circulation 2007;116:803–77.
11. Campbell H, Hotchkiss R, Bradshaw N, et al. Integrated care pathways. Br Med J 1998;316:133–7.
12. Giugliano RP, Lloyd-Jones DM, Camargo CA, et al. Association of unstable angina guideline care with improved survival. Arch Intern Med 2000;160:1775–80.
13. Laupacis A, Sekar N, Stiell I. Clinical prediction rules: a review and suggested modifications of methodological standards. JAMA 1997;277(6):488–94.
14. McGinn TG, Guyatt GH, Wyer PC, et al. Users' guides to the medical literature XXII: how to use articles about clinical decision rules. JAMA 2000;284(1):79–84.
15. Stiell IG, Greenberg GH, McKnight RD, et al. A study to develop clinical decision rules for the use of radiography in acute ankle injuries. Ann Emerg Med 1992;21(4):384–90.
16. Stiell IF, Wells GA, Vandemheen K, et al. The Canadian C-spine rule for radiography in alert and stable trauma patients. JAMA 2001;286:1841–8.
17. Hoffman JR, Mower WR, Wolfson AB, et al. Validity of a set of clinical criteria to rule out injury to the cervical spine in patients with blunt trauma. N Engl J Med 2000;343:94–9.
18. Stiell IG, Wells GA, Vandemheen K, et al. The Canadian CT head rule for patients with minor head injury. Lancet 2001;357:1391–6.
19. Morrow DA, Antman EM, Charlesworth A, et al. TIMI risk score for ST-elevation myocardial infarction: a convenient, bedside, clinical score for risk assessment at presentation: an intravenous nPA for treatment of infarcting myocardium early II trial substudy. Circulation 2000;102:2031–7.
20. Shaneyfelt TM, Mayo-Smith MF, Rothwangl J. Are guidelines following guidelines? The methodological quality of clinical practice guidelines in the peer-reviewed medical literature. JAMA 1999;281(20):1900–5.

21. Gibbons RJ, Smith SC, Antman E. American College of Cardiology/American Heart Association clinical practice guidelines: part I: where do they come from? Circulation 2003;107(23):2979–86.
22. Jagoda AS, Bazarian JJ, Bruns JJ, et al. Clinical policy: neuroimaging and decision making in adult mild traumatic brain injury in the acute setting. Ann Emerg Med 2008;52(6):714–48.
23. Fesmire FM, Jagoda A. Are we putting the cart ahead of the horse: who determines the standard of care for the management of patients in the emergency department? Ann Emerg Med 2005;46(2):198–200.
24. Gallagher EJ. Shooting an elephant. Ann Emerg Med 2004;43(2):233–7.
25. Steyerberg EW, Harrell FE Jr, Borsboom GJ, et al. Internal validation of predictive models: efficiency of some procedures for logistic regression analysis. J Clin Epidemiol 2001;54:774–81.
26. Aldrich R, Kemp L, Williams JS, et al. Using socioeconomic evidence in clinical practice guidelines. Br Med J 2003;327:1283–5.
27. Shekelle PG, Ortiz E, Rhodes S, et al. Validity of the agency for healthcare research and quality clinical practice guidelines: how quickly do guidelines become outdated? JAMA 2001;286:1461–7.
28. Gibbons RJ, Smith SC, Antman E. American College of Cardiology/American Heart Association clinical practice guidelines: part II: evolutionary changes in a continuous quality improvement project. Circulation 2003;107(24):3101–7.
29. Lim W, Arnold DM, Bachanova V, et al. Evidence-based guidelines: an introduction. Hematology 2008;1:26–30.
30. Kane RL. Creating practice guidelines: the dangers of over-reliance on expert judgment. J Law Med Ethics 1995;23:62–4.
31. Choudhry NK, Stelfox HT, Detsky AS. Relationships between authors of clinical practice guidelines and the pharmaceutical industry. JAMA 2002;287(5):612–7.
32. Pearson SD, Goulart-Fisher D, Lee TH. Critical pathways as a strategy for improving care: problems and potential. Ann Intern Med 1995;123(12):941–8.
33. Bohan JS. Guidelines in emergency medicine. In: Marx JA, Hockberger RS, Walls RM, editors. Rosen's emergency medicine: concepts and clinical practice. 6th edition. Philadelphia: Mosby Elsevier; 2006. p. 3034–45.
34. Chassin MR, Brook RH, Park RE, et al. Variations in the use of medical and surgical services by the Medicare population. N Engl J Med 1986;314:285–90.
35. Grimshaw JM, Russell IT. Effect of clinical guidelines on medical practice: a systematic review of rigorous evaluations. Lancet 1993;342:1317–22.
36. Shapiro DW, Lasker RD, Bindman AB, et al. Containing costs while improving quality of care: the role of profiling and practice guidelines. Annu Rev Public Health 1993;14:219–41.
37. Holroyd BR, Wilson D, Rowe BH, et al. Uptake of validated clinical practice guidelines: experience with implementing the Ottawa ankle rules. Am J Emerg Med 2004;22(3):149–55.
38. Cameron C, Naylor CD. No impact from active dissemination of the Ottawa ankle rules: further evidence of the need for local implementation of practice guidelines. CMAJ 1999;160:1165–8.
39. Hyams AL, Brandenburg JA, Lipsitz SR, et al. Practice guidelines and malpractice litigation: a two way street. Ann Intern Med 1995;122(6):450–5.
40. Garnick DW, Hendricks AM, Brennan TA. Can practice guidelines reduce the number and costs of malpractice claims? JAMA 1991;266(20):2856–60.
41. Nolin CE. Malpractice claims, patient communication, and critical paths: a lawyer's perspective. Qual Manag Health Care 1995;3:65–70.

42. Tito F, Newby L. Medico-legal implications of clinical practice guidelines. Sydney: NHMRC National Breast Cancer Centre; 1998.
43. Ransom SB, Studdert DM, Dombrowski MP, et al. Reduced medicolegal risk by compliance with obstetric clinical pathways: a case-control study. Obstet Gynecol 2003;101(4):751–5.
44. Hurwitz B. Clinical guidelines: proliferation and medicolegal significance. Qual Saf Health Care 1994;3:37–44.
45. Tunis SR, Hayward RSA, Wilson MC, et al. Internists' attitudes about clinical practice guidelines. Ann Intern Med 1994;120(11):956–63.

Professional Liability Insurance

Morsal R. Tahouni, MD, Joseph H. Kahn, MD, FACEP*

KEYWORDS

- Liability • Insurance • Risk • Risk management
- Tail coverage • Nose coverage

Essentially all emergency medical practitioners carry some form of professional liability insurance. Most hospitals, clinics, and health centers will not allow a physician to practice in the absence of professional liability insurance.[1]

In the United States, medical liability insurance has been in a state of crisis repeatedly over the past 40 years. The first crisis occurred in the early 1970s, when malpractice insurance became unavailable to some physicians because the increase in malpractice claims drove many insurance carriers from the market.[2,3] In the 1980s, the second crisis occurred, as another increase in the size and frequency of claims sent the premiums for malpractice insurance to a level that was unaffordable for many practitioners.[2,3] A third crisis started in 2003, again due to decreased availability and affordability of malpractice insurance policies. The increasing number and size of claims with the resultant increase in malpractice policy premiums, particularly in high-risk specialties, has led to an exodus of physicians from high-risk specialties and a crisis of specialty care access for patients.[2–8]

The process of choosing a stable malpractice insurance carrier, the type of coverage, and the limits of liability can be daunting for the emergency practitioner. Even if malpractice insurance is provided by the hospital, clinic, urgent care center, or physician group, it behooves the practitioner to have a working knowledge of professional liability insurance. The practitioner not only needs insurance coverage but also needs to know if there are exclusions to this coverage, what the reporting requirements are, and whether the insurance will continue to cover claims of alleged malpractice that occur after the practitioner has left that facility. Furthermore, it is essential for the practitioner to know whether the liability insurance carrier will assign a defense attorney and if the practitioner can choose an independent defense attorney. The physician also needs to know whether the insurance carrier can settle a claim against the physician without the physician's consent.[9]

Department of Emergency Medicine, Boston Medical Center, Boston University School of Medicine, 1 Boston Medical Center Place, Boston, MA 02118, USA
* Corresponding author.
E-mail address: jkahn@bu.edu (J.H. Kahn).

Emerg Med Clin N Am 27 (2009) 569–581
doi:10.1016/j.emc.2009.07.002
emed.theclinics.com

With approximately 25,000 board-certified emergency physicians practicing in the United States (as of 2005),[10] and at least 80 medical professional liability insurance companies underwriting policies in the United States (many being state-specific), the choices are confusing.[11] Keeping abreast of malpractice awards and settlements in a practitioner's area may be helpful in choosing limits of liability. Knowledge of strengths and weaknesses of different policy types is also helpful in making an intelligent choice.

ANATOMY OF A POLICY

Indemnity

Indemnity protects the medical practitioner from claims filed by a patient, patient's family, or patient's estate.[12] The medical malpractice liability policy should clearly state what is covered by the policy.[13] Generally, the policy will provide coverage for damage sustained by a patient while receiving professional medical services from a health care provider or facility.[13]

The policy may also cover the cost of defense counsel for the practitioner who is the target of the lawsuit, but this must be stated in the policy. It is important to clarify whether the cost of providing a defense is subtracted from the policy limits.[13]

Finally, the practitioner should ascertain whether interest on an award for a plaintiff is covered, because interest can be substantial in a case that is decided years after the alleged malpractice occurred.[13]

Declarations

The declarations page of a professional liability insurance policy includes the name of the insured, the date that the policy is effective, the policy period, the limits of liability, the amount of the insurance premium, and the coverage restrictions, if any.[14] The declarations page summarizes the policy and is often required by hospitals and licensing boards when applying for privileges.

The limits of liability stated in the policy's declarations usually include 2 figures. The first figure is the limit of liability for the practitioner for a patient, and the second is the limit of liability for the practitioner for the policy period, which is usually 1 year. Limits of liability should be adequate to protect the physician's assets in the event of an award. What the limits of liability should be is a topic of some debate. Some practitioners mistakenly think that keeping the limits of liability low will reduce the size of the award to fit the policy. Finding out what limits other emergency physicians carry in the same area may serve as a guide to selecting limits of liability. In group practices, the practitioner should clarify that the limits apply to the individual and not to the group.[13]

Conditions

Carefully understanding the conditions of coverage of a medical liability insurance policy may be the most important aspect of a medical practitioner's review of the policy. The practitioner must meet the conditions to be covered by the insurance policy.

Many policies require the condition of notice, which means that the physician must notify the insurance company as soon as possible when an adverse event occurs that the physician believes may result in a claim.[15] Failure to notify the insurance carrier in a reasonable time after the event can constitute grounds for the carrier to deny coverage.[13] It may be confusing for a physician to determine which events should prompt notification of the insurance carrier. Not every poor patient outcome warrants notifying the carrier, but cases in which the physician or administrator thinks that a malpractice claim is likely should prompt notification.

Another condition of a professional liability insurance policy may be that the physician cooperates with the insurance company in defending the claim. Not cooperating and assisting in discovery and trial, and in preparations for discovery and trial, may be grounds for an insurance company to deny coverage.[13]

Insured

The professional liability insurance policy may be in the name of an individual or a group. Policies issued in an individual's name definitely cover that individual.[16] If, however, the policy is issued in the name of an emergency medicine group or health care facility, then the physician should be listed as an "additional insured."[13] If the practitioner is not listed as such, then the policy should state that all physicians are covered while they are practicing medicine for the physician group.[13]

Endorsements

An endorsement can add to or limit the scope of coverage of a professional liability insurance policy. It may be called an amendment or a rider.[14] An endorsement can add coverage for a person, a procedure, or a geographic location. It can also exclude coverage for an individual, a procedure, or a location. The policy holder should carefully review endorsements to see that they meet the needs of the insured.

Exclusions

The exclusions of a professional liability insurance policy can significantly reduce the coverage provided by it. Exclusions may state that a physician will not be covered for procedures outside of the physician's scope of practice, or they may exclude coverage for punitive damages[13] or for nonclinical activities, such as administration or emergency medical service activities, that the physician performs within the hospital or physician group.[17] Furthermore, physicians who choose to participate as expert witnesses in legal proceedings may be liable for any testimony given, depending on the jurisdiction, and they should consult with their insurance carrier regarding whether such practices are covered under their policy.[18] Physicians need to be aware of coverage exclusions, to ascertain whether the hospital's insurance covers the activity or if an endorsement can be added to the policy to cover it.[13]

Occurrence

An occurrence is an unexpected event that happens in the course of medical practice, which may or may not result in harm to the patient.[13] Depending on the nature of the occurrence, the hospital administration may need to be notified with an incident report.[19] If the hospital or the practitioner thinks that a lawsuit may result from the event, then the professional liability insurance company should be notified.

Incident

An incident is an event that the patient, or someone acting on behalf of the patient, claims caused harm to the patient.[14]

Claim

A claim occurs when a patient or a patient's guardian, proxy, or estate makes a written demand for money. This demand may be through a lawsuit or through another avenue, such as a state malpractice screening board.[14] Once the practitioner is notified of a claim, immediate notification of the liability insurance carrier is required, so that the insurance company and the defense attorney can begin their investigation with the cooperation of the practitioner.

Limits of liability

Limits of liability generally consist of a per-case limit and annual limit. Determining the acceptable limits of liability that a given physician requires is a difficult task; limits probably should be based on the recent average payment from the top 10% of malpractice payments made in the physician's specialty and the region in which that physician practices.[20] It is not practical to base the limits on the top 1% of awards, as these are outliers that generally exceed available insurance limits.

The average malpractice payment (including awards and settlements) for US physicians across all specialties has increased from $173,018 in 1991 to $263,101 in 2003 (**Table 1**).[20] These figures are misleading when choosing limits, because the average highest 10% of malpractice payments (including awards and settlements), for US physicians across all specialties, has increased from $867,792 in 1991 to $1,115,031 in 2003 (see **Table 1**).[20,21] In 2001, the average payment for the highest 10% of awards (not including settlements) was $2,827,785, but this figure had retreated to $1,850,294 by 2003 (**Table 2**).[20]

When choosing limits of liability, physicians should consider the malpractice environment of the state in which they practice (**Fig. 1**).[22] Some states have taken steps to improve the medical liability environment, such as limiting the size of punitive damages, creating medical malpractice screening panels, and creating state-funded patient compensation funds.[2]

Table 1
Change in medical malpractice payments made on behalf of physicians, 1991–2003

		Judgments and Settlements	
Year	**Number of Payments in NPDB**	**Average Payment ($)**	**Average Payment for Highest 10% of All Payments ($)**
1991	13,365	173,018	867,792
1992	14,119	194,893	972,65
1993	14,151	197,152	955,292
1994	14,568	200,908	995,174
1995	13,511	207,863	999,689
1996	14,240	220,062	913,449
1997	13,845	219,881	973,642
1998	13,305	225,187	985,769
1999	14,175	232,711	1,050,898
2000	14,626	247,651	1,054,807
2001	15,694	258,965	1,130,976
2002	14,539	262,629	1,127,478
2003	14,368	263,101	1,155,031
Test for trend		*P*<.000	*P*<.000
1991–2003 growth		52.1% (4.0%)	33.1% (2.5%)
2000–2003 growth		6.2% (1.6%)	9.5% (2.4%)

Abbreviation: NPDB, National Practitioner Data Bank.

Data from Chandra A, Nundy S, Seabury SA. The growth of physician medical malpractice payments: evidence from the National Practitioner Data Bank. Health Aff (Millwood) 2005:Suppl Web Exclusives:W5-240–9.

Table 2
Change in medical malpractice payments made on behalf of physicians, 1991–2003

Year	Number of Payments in NPDB	Average Payment ($)	Average Payment for Highest 10% of All Payments ($)
	Judgements		
1991	459	320,917	1,472,779
1992	413	398,890	2,111,009
1993	444	422,652	2,034,162
1994	419	353,326	1,542,976
1995	398	369,793	1,798,806
1996	578	387,264	1,634,023
1997	453	384,905	1,594,561
1998	401	425,663	1,764,773
1999	404	387,782	1,447,200
2000	537	474,821	1,840,507
2001	533	601,155	2,827,785
2002	411	488,020	1,903,668
2003	430	460,736	1,850,294
Test for trend		*P*<.006	*P*<.295
1991–2003 growth		43.6% (3.4%)	25.6% (2.0%)
2000–2003 growth		-3.0% (0.7%)	0.5% (0.1%)
Settlements			
1991	12,906	167,758	853,373
1992	13,706	188,746	918,424
1993	13,707	189,847	894,590
1994	14,149	196,395	908,393
1995	13,113	202,948	997,338
1996	13,662	212,988	898,364
1997	13,392	214,298	945,389
1998	12,904	218,958	949,778
1999	13,771	228,162	1,015,759
2000	14,089	238,992	1,023,973
2001	15,161	246,935	1,064,999
2002	14,128	256,072	1,095,691
2003	13,938	257,004	1,080,121
Test for trend		*P*<.006	*P*<.000
1991–2003 growth		53.2% (4.1%)	26.6% (2.0%)
2000–2003 growth		7.5% (1.9%)	5.5% (1.4%)

Data are for all payments (judgments or settlements) involving a physician defendant in the 50 states between January 1, 1991 and December 31, 2003. All dollar values are converted to year 2000 dollars using the implicit gross domestic product price deflator and are rounded to the nearest dollar. Numbers in parentheses are average annual growth rates.

Based on data from Chandra A, Nundy S, Seabury SA. The growth of physician medical malpractice payments: evidence from the National Practitioner Data Bank. Health Aff (Millwood) 2005:Suppl Web Exclusives:W5-240–9.

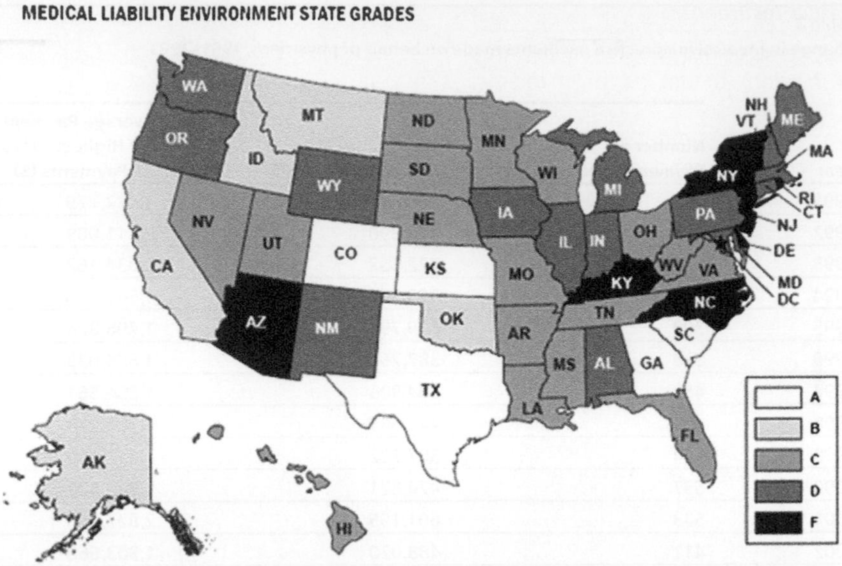

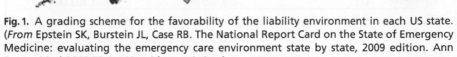

Fig. 1. A grading scheme for the favorability of the liability environment in each US state. (*From* Epstein SK, Burstein JL, Case RB. The National Report Card on the State of Emergency Medicine: evaluating the emergency care environment state by state, 2009 edition. Ann Emerg Med 2009;53:4–148; with permission.)

TYPES OF INSURANCE

The current professional liability environment provides a broad array of insurance options for the emergency medicine provider, depending on the provider's specific needs. Although not meant to be all-inclusive, this section introduces many of the basic concepts in the different forms of insurance coverage available.

Primary Insurance

Primary insurance is the insured's first line of protection from liability claims, covering losses up to the monetary limits defined in the insurance policy.

Excess Insurance

Excess insurance is a secondary policy purchased by the insured to cover losses greater than the limits listed in the primary policy. This type of policy may be used to increase current monetary coverage or to temporarily provide extended coverage in times of increased financial risk.

Commercial Insurance

The most common type of professional liability protection, commercial insurance, is purchased from one of many insurance providers that operate inside the United States. Commercial carriers provide a wide range of insurance options that are easily accessible and reliable. Increasing litigation in recent years has created some disadvantages for the provider purchasing from commercial carriers, because most insurers have limited the areas in which they provide insurance (either by specialty or geography) or have drastically increased premiums to help cover the increase in litigation.[3]

Captive Insurance

When a provider creates a separate legal entity (such as a sister or subsidiary corporation) to act as a limited-purpose insurance company, this is known as captive insurance.[23] Such programs require either internal or external personnel to manage the different functions of the company, and they are often created off-shore. The company usually enters into a reinsurance agreement with a commercial insurer, to reduce the risk of the company and provide additional financial coverage in exchange for a portion of the premiums paid.[23] Captive insurance offers providers decreased premiums and easier reinsurance; however, it is associated with a much higher start-up and management cost than self-insurance trusts. Captive insurance companies include those that insure only their parent company and affiliates or insure external groups and providers operating under the same professional risks.

Risk Retention Groups

A risk retention group (RRG) is a distinct type of captive insurance company that allies groups or persons engaged in similar business practices to provide liability coverage for its members.[13,23] Because of the Federal Risk Retention Act of 1986, once an RRG is licensed in one state, it may cover members in any other state regardless of differing liability and licensing laws. RRGs also allow group members to control the amount and rate of liability coverage and to participate actively in risk management for the group.

Channeled Insurance Programs

Channeled insurance programs (CIPs) are another form of captive insurance company and are created to provide liability coverage solely to a hospital or group of hospitals, including affiliates and employees.[13] CIPs do not generally assume risk from any outside individuals or institutions. Liability risk is channeled to a third party, the CIP, thereby obviating the need for the numerous employees of a hospital or a hospital system to obtain individual liability insurance.

Self-insurance Trusts

A self-insurance trust is insurance created when a provider contributes money into a trust fund that is created for the purpose of covering professional liability losses.[23] The fund is managed exclusively by the provider with the aid of a fiduciary, usually a financial institution (lawyer, bank, or investment firm). This provides certain advantages for the provider, including reduced costs of coverage and increased control in management of claims and settlements.[23] However, the provider must also determine the amount of money required to maintain the trust, evaluate the potential risk of those involved, and assume overall management of the trust. Providers can create self-insurance trusts as a form of primary insurance, thereby decreasing the cost of liability insurance and freeing up funds to purchase excess insurance from a commercial provider.[23]

Off-shore Insurance

This term pertains to any insurer whose location of business is outside the United States.[13] Captive insurance companies and self-insurance trusts are sometimes created in these jurisdictions, with beneficial tax laws and financial incentives, to decrease the monetary burden of operating such an institution.[23]

TYPE OF COVERAGE

The 2 most common forms of professional liability insurance are claims-made and occurrence coverage. Each form carries its own complexities, advantages, and disadvantages. Therefore, it is important for the emergency medicine provider to understand the differences and subtleties of each form, to ensure complete protection from litigation. The main difference revolves around what the insurer defines as the coverage trigger, the event that activates insurance coverage.

Claims-made

The most common form of professional liability insurance, claims-made insurance, defines the coverage trigger as the moment the insured becomes aware of a potential or real claim. It is the insured's responsibility to notify the insurer of such claims immediately. Therefore, the policy only covers those claims that the insured became aware of during the policy period. One advantage to this form is that it covers claims regardless of the time during which the event occurred, providing that the inciting event occurred before a date named in the policy.[24] The insured must be cautious in following the reporting procedures outlined in the insurance policy. Failure to follow the procedures could result in the insurer withdrawing coverage for that claim. Furthermore, this form of policy will not cover any claims that the insured becomes aware of after the policy period has ended, leaving the insured potentially unprotected if no further coverage is acquired.[24]

Occurrence

Occurrence policies define the coverage trigger as the date the event leading to a claim occurred. Therefore, the insured is protected regardless of when a claim is made and has fewer responsibilities in reporting the claim to the insurer. Protection is for the event, regardless of when a claim is made and even if the policy is long expired, as long as it occurred during the coverage period, thus obviating extended coverage.[24] Occurrence policies tend to be more expensive, however, and are less readily available from commercial insurers.

Modified Claims-made

Some insurance providers have begun to offer a form of claims-made insurance entitled modified claims-made coverage. This type of coverage is geared toward groups with a low-risk profile and minimal claims history.[25] These policies usually include built-in prior acts coverage and tail coverage, at a substantially reduced price from usual occurrence policies.[25] However, modified claims-made polices are not offered in all areas and can be difficult to obtain for providers with a history of prior claims.

Nose Coverage

Nose coverage is also known as prior-acts coverage. Physicians using claims-made coverage may, at times, find themselves in need of a limited-term policy to cover gaps in coverage between new and old insurance policies. This type of coverage is termed a "nose" when it is purchased from a physician's new insurer. It will cover any claims made against the insured for a specified amount of time, starting when the prior policy expires and extending until the new policy takes effect. Nose coverage costs less than tail coverage, because the insured will have to pay rates similar to the premium of their new coverage. Unfortunately, nose coverage is not always offered from the new insurer. Physicians leaving group practices, for instance, are often not eligible for nose coverage if they are covered under a group policy.[26] This is because it can be difficult for the new insurer to separate out the individual physician's risk from the rest of the group.[26] Availability will also vary depending on the individual physician's risk profile and the location of practice.[26]

Tail Coverage

Also referred to as an "extending reporting endorsement," tail coverage is similar in function and scope to nose coverage. It is purchased from the previous insurer as opposed to a new insurer. Most primary insurers will offer tail coverage when a physician is near the end of a policy's term or chooses to leave a group policy. Physicians must purchase this coverage, usually within 30 days, or the offer will be rescinded.[26,27] However, tail insurance comes at a much higher cost than nose coverage.

Given the high cost of tail coverage, responsibility for the coverage can vary depending on a physician's contract. Some contracts force physicians to pay the cost of the tail and enforce a time limit for arranging it.[27] This serves the employer's interests by protecting its assets once a physician has left and by devolving the costs of such protection to the leaving employee. Other employer contracts may provide for payment of some or all of the cost or provide for negotiating payment depending on the circumstances surrounding the physician's end of employment.[27]

There are circumstances in which physicians are eligible for "free" tail coverage. For example, when a physician's risk profile decreases dramatically, it is prudent for the insurer to provide this free coverage. When a physician dies, the insurer may assign free tail coverage to protect the deceased's estate.[27] Furthermore, if a physician becomes disabled and is no longer able to practice, the insurer may also offer a free tail to the physician.[27] Finally, some physicians are eligible when they retire from clinical practice. However, the definition of retirement may differ depending on the insurer and may not cover all circumstances.[27]

INSURANCE OPTIONS

To cater to the expanding business of medical practice, insurance carriers now offer a greater variety of malpractice coverage options for the emergency medicine practitioner. Although not appropriate for every physician, these options provide extended coverage for special situations depending on the physician's practicing environment.

Billing Errors and Omissions

This optional coverage provides protection for physicians accused of Medicare or Medicaid fraud.[28] Depth of coverage varies per insurance provider. Some policies may cover only legal expenses associated with the instance, whereas others may pay a portion or all of the associated penalties or settlements.

Legal Expense

Most malpractice policies provide coverage for legal expenses occurring in situations wherein the physician is directly named in legal action. However, this special coverage option provides legal expense reimbursement when a physician is required to participate in legal processes, resulting from action taken against a colleague or coworker. In certain instances, it may also cover expenses associated with disciplinary or licensing processes.[28]

Loss of Income

Medical liability policies typically provide reimbursement for loss of income incurred during legal processes. This type of coverage includes participation in hearings, depositions, and trial proceedings, and is usually assessed on a per day basis.

Sexual Misconduct

Expenses stemming from claims of sexual misconduct made toward a physician are not always covered by malpractice policies. This special coverage provides physicians with protection and reimbursement for claims made against them while they are providing health care services.[28] These policies are specifically intended to reimburse the physician for the cost of defense in a civil proceeding.[28]

Equipment Maintenance

The multiple contracts required for the preventative maintenance and repair of medical equipment can be difficult to manage for many hospitals and physician groups. This coverage option allows the policy holder to consolidate the various contracts for the care of medical equipment under 1 policy, usually decreasing overall cost and improving efficiency.

SELECTION OF COUNSEL

Insurance Counsel

Generally, the professional liability insurance carrier will assign an attorney to represent the physician in the event of a lawsuit and will pay the attorney's fees. It is advisable for the physician to have knowledge of medical malpractice defense attorneys in the community and to make a recommendation to the insurance carrier.[29] If the insurance carrier will not take input from the practitioner in selecting an attorney, then the physician should investigate the attorney's malpractice defense experience and record, looking particularly at experience with emergency medicine lawsuits.

Hospital Counsel

The hospital or other health care facility where the alleged incident occurred may also be named in the lawsuit. If the physician is an employee of the hospital, then the hospital attorney may be assigned to defend the physician. It is important for the physician to clarify whether the hospital attorney is representing the health care facility, the physician, or both, at the beginning of the case and before having in-depth discussions with the hospital attorney.[30]

Independent Counsel

Physicians must realize that the legal counsel assigned by the insurance company is representing the insurance company and themselves and that at times, the goal of the insurance company may differ from that of the physician. The physician may not want to admit any culpability in a case, whereas the malpractice insurance carrier may be willing to admit the physician's culpability and settle the suit for an amount which it thinks will be far less than a jury may award.[31] In this situation, the settlement will be reported to the National Practitioner Data Bank, the state medical licensing agency, and the hospital, even though the physician denies culpability and there has been no jury trial. In such situations, it may be preferable for the physician to hire independent counsel, even though the insurance carrier will not cover the legal fees. Another consideration for hiring independent legal counsel is a lawsuit with a probability of a high jury award exceeding the insurance policy limit of liability. In such cases, the physician defendant would be liable for the amount of the award above the limit of liability. Exploring all options including an offer to settle at the limit of liability should be considered, particularly if there are multiple named defending parties to the lawsuit, all being represented by one entity and carrier. The best interests of the individual physician may differ from those of the insurer or other named defending parties.

Independent counsel can address these situations solely from the individual physician's perspective.

Joint Counsel

Not infrequently, there may be more than one defendant in a case, and all defendants may be assigned the same counsel. A joint defense refers to 1 attorney representing both practitioners (joint counsel), or 2 different lawyers representing 2 different clients, but with the same defense strategy.[13]

Joint counsel may work to the advantage of a defendant through sharing of information and avoiding the situation wherein one defendant tries to convince the jury or the plaintiff that the other defendant is more culpable.[13] The disadvantage of joint counsel is that when one defendant is found liable, it makes both defendants more likely to be liable, because a single defense strategy is used. Furthermore, one party being underinsured may even result in a larger payout for the less culpable defendant.[13]

CONSENT TO SETTLE

When a patient or agent of the patient files a medical malpractice claim against a physician, it may sometimes benefit the physician to settle the claim without a jury trial. An example of such a situation is when a jury verdict in favor of the plaintiff is likely, and the jury award is likely to exceed the limits of the malpractice policy. There are times, however, when the insurance company may want to settle but the physician may not. The insurance company may think that a plaintiff verdict is likely in a jury trial and so may want to settle the case at a lower amount than a jury is likely to award. However, the physician accused of malpractice may believe that she or he is not culpable and may not want to settle the case.

The professional liability policy usually states whether the insurer needs the consent of the physician to settle the case.[29] This should be clarified by the practitioner when obtaining the coverage. Although it is preferable for the insurance carrier to need a physician's consent to settle, a refusal to settle in these circumstances does expose the physician to greater liability,[13] especially if the subsequent award exceeds the limits of liability of the policy.

Hammer Clause

There is another risk to the physician who chooses not to settle when the insurance company wants to do so. Some medical liability insurance policies have a "hammer clause," which states that if a physician refuses to settle at the amount that the insurance company has negotiated with a plaintiff who later wins at trial, then the physician is responsible for any award in excess of the negotiated settlement.[28]

FINANCIAL STRENGTH RATINGS

Multiple methods can be used by a practitioner to assess the quality and stability of an insurance carrier. One of the more commonly used is a financial strength rating. These ratings are issued by an independent third party known as a nationally recognized statistical rating organization (NRSRO). NRSROs are regulated by the Securities and Exchange Commission (SEC), and are allowed by the SEC to issue financial strength ratings for various financial institutions, including insurance carriers.[32] These ratings are in essence an assessment of a financial institution's creditworthiness, and they are used to guide investors, financial regulators, and other interested parties.[32]

Currently there are 10 NRSROs registered with the SEC; however, one deserves special mention in discussing professional liability insurance. A.M. Best Company, founded in 1899, with offices in New Jersey, Washington, DC, and other international locations, specializes in financial strength ratings for insurance companies.[33] A.M. Best issues reports regularly, assessing the financial health of insurance providers. The company evaluates the insurance carrier's balance sheet, operating performance, and business profile.[34] Using these factors, the company then assigns each carrier a letter grade (A++ to F, with special designations). These letter grades correlate with a further assessment of each carrier as secure or vulnerable.[34]

A.M. Best ratings, and those of other NRSROs, provide an objective, timely estimation of an insurer's relative financial stability and ability to cover the potential risks of the insured. Physicians who are considering the purchase of a policy from an insurance carrier should consider that company's financial strength rating among the many other factors involved in such a decision. Failure to do so can leave a physician without proper liability coverage, despite fully paid premiums, and scrambling to find a new insurer. Further information about the methodology used in creating these ratings and the proper use of these ratings can be found on the SEC's Web site and each NRSRO's Web site.

SUMMARY

The emergency physician needs to be aware of several issues regarding professional liability insurance. Firstly, the physician should know the type of insurance (occurrence or claims-made); whether this is the only type available in the physician's region; whether tail coverage is available at a reasonable rate, and who pays for it, if it is claims-made insurance. Secondly, the physician should know the limits of liability of the policy, and whether these are appropriate for emergency medicine in the practitioner's geographic region. Also, it is helpful to know whether the malpractice insurance company provides an attorney in the event of a claim, whether the attorney fees are covered by the policy, whether the attorney fees are subtracted from the limit of the policy, and whether the physician can choose a defense attorney. Other essential information includes policy exclusions and restrictions and whether the physician's consent is required for the insurance company to settle a case. The physician should be aware of the financial strength of the insurance company.[35] This article has attempted to introduce the emergency physician to these and other important issues regarding medical liability insurance.

REFERENCES

1. Shore EE. Going bare? Bad idea. Med Econ 2007;84:26.
2. American Medical Association. Medical Liability Reform – NOW! a compendium of facts supporting medical liability reform and debunking arguments against reform" 2008. Available at: http://www.ama-assn.org/go/m/rnow. Accessed February 22, 2009.
3. Mello MM, Studdert DM, Brennan TA. The new medical malpractice crisis. N Engl J Med 2003;348(23):2281–4.
4. Kessler DP, Sage WM, Becker DJ. Impact of malpractice reforms on the supply of physician services. JAMA 2005;293(21):2618–25.
5. Studdert DM, Mello MM, Brennan TA. Medical malpractice. N Engl J Med 2004; 350(3):283–92.
6. Coile RC Jr. 10 factors affecting the physician shortage of the future. Physician Exec 2003;29:62–5.
7. Special Report Insurance loss leaves doctors scrambling for coverage. Lancet 2003;362:376.
8. Darr K. The 'New' medical malpractice crisis – part 1. Hosp Top 2004;82:33–5.

9. Archambault WH. Will my malpractice case be settled? The physician-defendant's voice in the decision. Semin Diagn Pathol 2007;24:119–30.
10. Camargo CA, Ginde AA, Singer AH, et al. Assessment of emergency physician workforce needs in the United States, 2005. Acad Emerg Med 2008;15:1317–20.
11. Medical malpractice insurance information. Available at: http://www.zoominfo.com/Industries/insurance/insurance/medical-malpractice-insurance-2.htm. Accessed February 18, 2009.
12. What is indemnity? Available at: http://www.wisegeek.com/what-is-indemnity.htm. Accessed February 18, 2009.
13. Harris SM, Silverstein E. Insurance coverage. Emergency medicine risk management: a comprehensive review. 2nd edition. Dallas: ACEP; 1997. p. 131–8.
14. Medical malpractice insurance for medical professionals. Available at: http://www.camedicalmalpractice.net/glossary.htm. Accessed February 22, 2009.
15. Berry DB. The physician's guide to medical malpractice. Baylor University Medical Center Procedings. Available at: http://www.pubmedcentral.nih.gov/articlerender.fcgi?artid=1291321. Accessed April 21, 2009.
16. Insurance – Risky Business. American Academy of Physician Assistants. Available at: http://www.aapa.org/gandp/risky.html. Accessed April 21, 2009.
17. Dunn J. Professional liability insurance part II. ACEP foresight. 1987;5: p. 2–3.
18. Bender RL. Liability for the psychiatrist expert witness. Am J Psychiatry 2002;159: 1819–25.
19. Dunn J. Professional liability insurance part I. ACEP foresight.1987;4:4.
20. Chandra A, Nundy S, Seabury SA. The growth of physician medical malpractice payments: evidence from the National Practitioner Data Bank. Health Aff (Millwood) 2005;(Suppl Web Exclusives):W5-240–9.
21. Vukmir RB. Medical malpractice: managing the risk. Med Law 2004;23:495–513.
22. Epstein SK, Burstein JL, Case RB. The National Report Card on the State of Emergency Medicine: evaluating the emergency care environment state by state, 2009 edition. Ann Emerg Med 2009;53:4–148.
23. Hendrix GP, Mauriello K. Self-insurance trusts and captive insurance for institutional healthcare providers. Health Law News March 2004. Available at: http://www.agg.com/Contents/PublicationDetail.aspx?ID=921. Accessed February 22, 2009.
24. Smith B. Claims made v. occurrence malpractice coverage. Physician's News Digest, April 2005. Available at: http://www.physiciansnews.com/business/405.html. Accessed February 22, 2009.
25. Lawrence B. PIAM Malpractice Bulletin Spring 2009:10(1):2.
26. Murray D. Malpractice: the scary truth about tail coverage. Med Econ July 2004; 8:49–50.
27. Guglielmo WJ. Tail insurance: watch out for the gotcha! Med Econ February 2008; 85:35–6.
28. Marshall J. Liability insurance offers more than it used to. Med Econ 2001;78(9):112
29. Cantrill SV. "Evaluating medical malpractice insurance policies." ACEP foresight 1988;9:2
30. Liguori R, Jones DC. Report of the NAPNAP malpractice insurance survey: do you know if you are covered? J Pediatr Health Care 2006;20:143–7
31. Berlin L. Professional liability insurance. AJR Am J Roentgenol 1998;170:565–9
32. Available at: http://www.sec.gov/answers/nrsro.htm. Accessed February 22, 2009.
33. Available at: http://www.ambest.com/about. Accessed February 22, 2009.
34. Available at: http://www.ambest.com/ratings/guide.asp. Accessed February 22, 2009.
35. Rice B. When a malpractice insurer sinks, how do its doctors survive? Med Econ 1998;75:188–98

The Legal Process

Richard D. Zane, MD, FAAEM[a,b,*]

KEYWORDS

- Law suit • Malpractice • Expert witness
- Tort reform • Negligence

Medical malpractice litigation is pervasive in the United States and all physicians, regardless of specialty, are likely to be named in a malpractice claim at some point in their career.[1] Emergency physicians are at particular risk because the patient typically presents to an emergency department with high-acuity illness[2] and the delivery of emergency care is complex.[3] Also, emergency physicians rarely have an ongoing relationship with their patients, and care is frequently passed off from one provider to another.[4] Include emergency department (ED) and hospital overcrowding and it becomes clear that the ED is a legally risky environment.[5]

Although tort reform has had some effect on the current malpractice crisis, the effect has been variable and dependent on jurisdiction.[6] Litigation continues to exact an emotional toll on the health care providers involved and a financial one on the health care system as a whole, by raising malpractice insurance premiums and contributing to the practice and culture of defensive medicine.[7] By understanding the legal system and the medical litigation process, physicians may avoid litigation and, when named in a lawsuit, may better participate in their defense.

Before examining the specifics of the system and process, one must understand the intended societal goals of malpractice litigation: to deter unsafe practices, to compensate persons injured through negligence, and to exact corrective justice.[8] These laudable goals form the basis of our current system, although they may be difficult to recognize when monetary reward for attorneys and patients seems paramount. Equally important to recognize are the similarities and differences in the relationship between the physician and patient and between the attorney and client. Both relationships require professionalism, ethical conduct, extensive skill and training, and confidentiality, yet they are practiced in diametrically dissimilar fashions.[9] Although this description is overly simplistic and entire texts have been devoted to both types of relationship, in the physician-patient relationship, the physician's job is to prevent, diagnose, discover, and, if possible, remedy an illness and alleviate suffering. The legal system is based on an adversarial process; the attorney has an ethical duty to

[a] Department of Emergency Medicine, Brigham and Women's Hospital, 75 Francis Street, Boston, MA, 02117, USA
[b] Harvard Medical School, Boston, MA, USA
* Department of Emergency Medicine, Brigham and Women's Hospital, 75 Francis Street, Boston, MA, 02117.
E-mail address: rzane@partners.org

Emerg Med Clin N Am 27 (2009) 583–592
doi:10.1016/j.emc.2009.07.009 emed.theclinics.com
0733-8627/09/$ – see front matter

fervently represent a client and attempt to win the case or argument,[10] which is often decided by a third unaffected party: jury, judge, or mediator. Winning may not be synonymous with truth or justice. An adversarial process requires that a patient or client enters into a situation in which a former physician is now an adversary. Also a matter of some controversy and debate is that in most medical malpractice cases, attorneys representing patients are paid on contingency, collecting an agreed portion of the settlement or award after expenses only if they are successful. If the lawsuit is unsuccessful, the attorney not only is uncompensated for time and advocacy but also is likely to have incurred much expense in bringing the case to litigation. The expense of bringing a case to litigation is often in the hundreds of thousands of dollars.[11] Contrast this with the way in which physicians are compensated. Even though an argument could be made that neither relationship or system of compensation is ideal or even just, it is telling that they are so different.

BASICS

The legal system is based on the premise of trial advocacy, which relies on the adversarial arrangement of opposing parties, a judge, and a jury. The jury serves as the decider of fact, whereas the judge decides all questions of law. Some of the questions of law on which a judge may be asked to rule are which statutes or specific laws apply in a certain situation, what evidence is germane and allowable, who may or may not be permitted to testify in front of the jury, and to what they may testify. Although all of these issues can affect the outcome of a trial, the jury decides the facts, including whether a physician was or was not negligent and did or did not commit malpractice, whether there was any injury related to the said malpractice, and if that injury warrants monetary award. The jury will also decide the amount of that award, and the judge is only involved if the decision of the jury is unreasonable.[12]

Medical malpractice is generally categorized as the "failure of a physician or health care provider to deliver proper services, either intentionally or through negligence, or without obtaining informed consent."[13] Most medical malpractice litigation in the United States revolves around the concept of negligence[14] and liability, making this type of litigation part of tort law. The word *tort* comes from the Latin term *torquēre*, which means "twisted or wrong."[14] Tort law, as defined by West's *Encyclopedia of American Law*, is

> *"...a body of rights, obligations, and remedies that is applied by courts in civil proceedings to provide relief for persons who have suffered harm from the wrongful acts of others. The person who sustains injury or suffers pecuniary damage as the result of tortious conduct is known as the plaintiff, and the person who is responsible for inflicting the injury and incurs liability for the damage is known as the defendant or tortfeasor."*

Tort law is a combination of legislative enactments and common-law principles. These laws may vary substantially from state to state because they are often based on the precedents from previous rulings. In contrast to legal actions for breach of contract, tort actions do not depend on a previous contract or agreement between the disputing parties, and unlike criminal cases in which the government serves as the plaintiff, tort actions are brought by private individuals. The tortfeasor or defendant is not subject to incarceration or fines in civil court.

In a malpractice suit, the plaintiff is usually the patient or someone acting on behalf of the patient and the defendant is any medical provider, which may or may not include a hospital or health center. A plaintiff can bring a successful medical malpractice claim if 4 essential elements of an action are demonstrated. First, was there a duty owed to the plaintiff by the defendant? If a physician or health care provider treated the plaintiff as a patient, this element is usually clear. It is less clear when an emergency physician speaks to a specialist regarding the care and treatment of a specific patient, yet the specialist has not agreed to care for or has not yet cared for that patient. This may especially be true when a specialist is "curb-sided" and does not have a relationship with the patient or an obligation to care for the patient because of being on call. Second, was that duty breached; did the health care provider deviate from the prevailing standard of care in treating the patient? Although different from one state to another, the definition of standard of care is usually described as what a reasonably prudent health care provider would do under like or similar circumstances.[15] Most states describe the standard of care as a national standard although some specify that the standard is local with specific geographic boundaries. Most deviations in standard of care are proven using expert testimony or the doctrine of *res ipsa loquitur,* which means "the thing speaks for itself" in Latin. The doctrine of *res ipsa loquitur* signifies that further details are unnecessary and that the facts of the case are self-evident. This applies to cases in which there has been clear medical error that does not require an expert. An example would be wrong-side surgery, an egregious medication error, or a surgical instrument left in a patient. Third, did the breach in the standard of care cause the injury? Fourth, did the injury result in damage?[16] With no damage, there is no cause for action, regardless of the presence of negligence.

Unlike criminal law, which requires that the defendant be proven guilty beyond reasonable doubt, in a tort claim involving monetary damages, the defendant needs to be proven liable based on "a preponderance of the evidence."[17] This definition may vary slightly from one state to another and may include: "to a reasonable degree of medical certainty," "more likely than not," or "greater than 50% probability."

THE PROCESS

Claims and Suits

If a patient or a patients' estate believes or suspects that the patient was a victim of medical negligence, the patient or patient's estate typically consults with an attorney. The attorney interviews the patient and decides whether to proceed with investigating the case. Either the patient has the pertinent medical records or the attorney writes a letter to the physician or hospital requesting medical records. Most letters from attorneys requesting medical records are for insurance purposes. Occasionally, if an attorney requests medical records from a hospital and either the law firm is known to specialize in medical malpractice or the patient has been previously identified as a potential litigant by the risk management department, then this department may initiate an internal investigation if it has not already done so.[16]

Having received the medical records, the attorney usually has the records reviewed by a medical provider. Some large law firms have in-house employees who are general practice nurses or physicians and screen cases for medical negligence. For those who do not, there is an entire industry dedicated to performing these types of record reviews. When the screeners believe that there may be medical negligence, the attorney will usually send the records to an expert in the specific field related to the alleged malpractice to determine if there was indeed negligence on the part of the health care provider and if said negligence resulted in harm. Based on the opinions of the medical reviewers and experts, the attorney may decline participation in the case or engage in representing the plaintiff in a formal action. On initial review, the attorney may decline participation for multiple reasons other than lack of evidence of negligence or causation. As most malpractice attorneys are compensated based on contingency, they may decline a case if the potential damages do not warrant the likely time and expense involved. In contrast, an attorney may pursue a case, despite scant evidence of malpractice or causation, if the potential damages or awards are large. There is much discussion regarding the prevalence of frivolous lawsuits—those that lack evidence of damage, of deviation in standard of care, or both. A recent closed-case analysis showed that 3% of claims had no demonstrable injury associated with the alleged negligence and 37% were not associated with error. Although not as uncommon as one might hope, most of these cases were denied compensation.[11]

If the attorney representing the patient or estate believes that the case is meritorious, an allegation of malpractice is formally issued. The different types of allegations vary by jurisdiction but are generally in the form of either a claim or a suit. Formal claims are demands for payment or compensation by claimants who convey their intent to pursue a demand. This formal claim is made directly to the physician, group, hospital, or health care institution and may be communicated in writing, in person, or by phone. The claim usually includes details of the case and rationale for the claim. After a claim is received by a physician or hospital, it is investigated in conjunction with the health care providers' insurance carrier. Based on this investigation a decision is made to defend the claim or to negotiate a settlement on the claim. A negotiated settlement takes into account the allegations in the claim, the costs associated with litigating the claim, the likelihood of a verdict in favor of the plaintiff, and the potential award for the plaintiff. Physicians may or may not have the right to decline settlement, depending on the specific type of their malpractice insurance policy. If the demand is denied, then the claimant may drop the claim or proceed to a suit.[17,18]

In most states, a claim becomes a suit when a plaintiff files a formal complaint with the court, specifically seeking compensatory damages. Every state is slightly different in the way in which a claim becomes a suit, but most require that some proof is offered of a minimal degree of evidence that a suit is meritorious and should proceed. The formal complaint filed with the court usually includes a structured description of the case, naming the providers and institutions, explaining how or why each had a duty to the patient and failed to meet the standard of care, and showing that this deviation contributed to or caused an injury that is due compensatory damages. Many states will also require an expert physician who has reviewed the records to swear, in the form of an affidavit, that each of these providers or institutions failed to meet the standard of care. Depending on the state, this may be all that is required to move forward to a formal suit.

In efforts to screen for frivolous lawsuits, some states have added steps that involve a preliminary review by a physician, or expert member panel that may include a physician, to determine if there is sufficient proof to move the suit forward. In Massachusetts, for example, the state legislature established a Medical Malpractice Tribunal made up of a licensed physician, a justice of the Superior Court, and an attorney[19] The tribunal is charged with determining

> *"...if the evidence presented if properly substantiated is sufficient to raise a legitimate question of liability appropriate for judicial inquiry or whether the plaintiff's case is merely an unfortunate medical result."*[20]

To date the tribunal has rejected 16% of cases; however, even if the tribunal denies the suit, the plaintiff may override the rejection by posting a $6000 bond, which is returned if the plaintiff wins.[21]

The time between the alleged malpractice occurring and a claim or suit being filed may be several years, and it depends on the specific statute of limitations for that state. Most states define the statute of limitations as taking effect when a plaintiff has become aware or should have become aware of the alleged act of malpractice.[17] For example, if the allegation is a failure to interpret a chest radiograph and recognize an abnormal nodule that is eventually diagnosed as cancer, then the statute of limitations takes effect from the day that the cancer was diagnosed and the previous chest radiograph was determined to have been improperly interpreted. Most states have different statutes of limitations for pediatric and birth injury cases, which may remain in effect until the child is an adult. Consequently, the time between a physician's committing an alleged negligent act and being able to defend himself in a court of law may be quite long. Because of statutes of limitations, plaintiff attorneys may initially name any medical provider who may have had any role in the alleged malpractice. The rationale behind this practice is that if they have failed to name a specific individual, who may later be implicated in the alleged negligence, before the statute of limitations has passed, then it provides an opportunity for other defendants to assign blame to the unnamed clinician. Ironically, failing to name providers has led to attorneys being named in legal malpractice suits. Although potential claims are not reported to any regulatory agencies, if a physician is named in a formal suit, that physician is usually required to report this on hospital credentialing forms, and, depending on the state, medical license applications. Any payment made to a claimant on behalf of a health care provider must be reported to the National Practitioner Data Bank.[17]

After a complaint has been officially filed with the court, the named parties are formally notified of the complaint: that they have been named and, specifically, what their alleged role was. In most states, the notification is accomplished in the form of a subpoena, which is served upon the health care provider. Some hospitals have arrangements with the court that will allow them to accept the notice or subpoena on behalf of a provider and guarantee delivery, in the absence of which, an officer of the court will personally hand-deliver the subpoena to the health care provider. This can be a harrowing experience because it may be unexpected and the person hand-delivering the subpoena is unknown, may be in uniform, identifies the health care provider by name, hands them the document, and then says, "Dr Smith, you have been served." This event may occur anywhere, including the provider's place of employment, home, or other location. Once physicians have been served or notified of a pending complaint, they should immediately notify their risk management department and their insurance carrier. The risk management department and carrier will do an internal investigation if they have not already done so. The carrier will generally assign an attorney or instruct the provider on how to arrange for attorney representation.

At this point, the suit is officially in the discovery period. During this time, which may last months to years depending on the state, the plaintiff and defense will begin to obtain facts relevant to the case.[22] In addition to more medical records, hospital policies and procedures may be collected and a list of witnesses developed, including factual witnesses, such as coworkers and family members, and expert witnesses. During this phase of the suit, factual witnesses and the plaintiff are likely to be deposed. In many states, the defendants are requested to answer interrogatories, which are specific written questions used to establish the facts of the case.[17] Before being deposed, defendants may also have their unsworn statements taken. An unsworn statement is much like a deposition except that the statement is not evidence and may not be used in a court of law.

Expert witnesses review the case and communicate their opinions to the attorneys as to whether or not standard of care was breached and if that breach in the standard of care caused or contributed to the alleged damage. Initially, the experts review the medical records but may or may not have had an opportunity to review the depositions of the defendant and factual witnesses. After they have reviewed the evidence available, they are asked for their final opinion. The defendants and the plaintiff are required to disclose their respective experts to each other and are given the opportunity to investigate the specific opinions held by the experts. The manner in which this is done varies by state. In many states, experts must disclose their opinions in a written document that is submitted to the court; then the opposing side is given an opportunity to depose the experts to determine the details and basis of their opinions. Attorneys are not required to disclose expert witnesses whose opinions were sought and found not to have been favorable to their case. This occasionally results in an attorney "shopping" a case to multiple experts until a favorable opinion is found.

After the discovery phase is complete, the opposing parties may meet to discuss the possibility of resolving the case before it goes to trial. These settlement meetings may happen based on the desires of either of the parties or the carrier, or they may be required by some states before proceeding to trial. These meetings may involve an arbitrator who serves as an impartial third party, attempting to negotiate a settlement. Most arbitration meetings are nonbinding, neither party being required to accept the position or opinion of the arbitrator or to settle the action. In some states, the opposing parties may choose binding arbitration in lieu of a trial. In binding arbitration cases, there is usually more than one arbitrator who hears the case and decides the issues of law and fact. There is a decision, which includes any deviation in the standard of care and if that deviation caused harm. Damages are assigned and binding arbitration decisions are final. Physicians' insurance policies may or may not allow them to refuse to settle a case before going to trial.

If the case goes to trial, depending on the state and the agreement of the parties, the defendant physician may opt for a bench trial instead of a jury trial. In a bench trial, the judge serves as judge and jury. Should the case proceed to trial, it is the responsibility of the plaintiff to prove negligence and causation, although unlike in a criminal trial, negligence needs to be proven to a reasonable degree of certainty or a preponderance of the evidence, not beyond reasonable doubt. An attorney represents each physician and one represents the hospital if it is party to the suit. The plaintiff and defendant have the opportunity to make opening statements to the jury and then the plaintiff will present evidence to the jury, usually in the form of factual witnesses and expert witnesses. After the plaintiff rests his or her case, the defense has an opportunity to present evidence and witnesses to counter the plaintiff's evidence. Expert witnesses are offered by the plaintiff and defense. When experts are first called, they are asked a series of questions by the attorney who has retained their services. This is called direct testimony. The attorney representing the opposing party is then able to question, that is, cross-examine, that expert.

At any point during the trial, the parties may agree to settle the case; they may also consent to certain stipulations or agreements before the trial to mitigate potential losses. For instance, the parties may agree to a high-low agreement, meaning that no matter what the outcome, the plaintiff is guaranteed a minimum amount and the defense a maximum.[23] After closing statements by both parties, the jury deliberates and assigns a verdict and compensatory damages if there are any.

In certain circumstances, defendant physicians may consider retaining or hiring their own counsel, separate and distinct from counsel approved by their carrier. For instance, a physician may be provided counsel who is also assigned to represent co-defendants, including physicians from other specialties, or even the hospital. Although it may seem as if all of these parties should be aligned in their defense, attorneys representing multiple parties may be conflicted and not be able to vigorously represent one client when also representing another. For example, adequate representation of 2 emergency physicians by one attorney may be difficult if both cared for a patient during the same visit, the first transferring the case to the second after initial evaluation and testing, but not contributing to the medical decision making, and the second discharging the patient. Another instance in which a physician may consider hiring separate counsel is when a plaintiff has made an offer to settle a matter for less than the physician's coverage limits, yet the carrier wishes to proceed to trial. This counsel may make representation to the carrier, making an arrangement or statement so that (1) the physician is not held liable should a verdict be returned with an award that is greater than the policy limits, and (2) the physician is not personally responsible for the amount of the verdict in excess of policy limits.

Expert Witnesses

The role of the expert witness is a matter of much discussion nationally, and the debate is continually evolving. A medical expert is required to establish the standard of care and if there was a breach of that standard. Most physicians bring a tremendous amount of professionalism to the process and play an important role in explaining a complicated concept to a lay jury.[9] Regardless of whether they are testifying on behalf of the physician or the patient, experts have a duty to independently examine the facts and formulate an opinion, and at the time of trial, they must be able to interpret complex medical issues and present them in a cogent way, such that a layperson may understand.

In general, most states have minimum requirements for experts, including that they are licensed to practice medicine and possess sufficient experience, education, and training to opine on the standard of care. In addition, some states have specific requirements: having a minimum percentage of time spent in clinical practice in the specific field, having board certification in that specialty, and practicing in the same or similar geography or setting as the defendant. The required qualifications to be an expert are not universal; there remain states where a physician need only be licensed to qualify as an expert and testify for or against any physician, regardless of the expert's training, experience, board certification status, or practice setting. In some states, it is still possible for a physician who does not practice emergency medicine, and is not specialty trained or board certified, to opine on the standard of care for an emergency physician. This occurs in other specialties also.

The attorney, while presenting evidence, also presents witnesses whose opinions favor their argument in the case. The system is, by definition, adversarial, and therefore both sides collect and organize evidence as it is best presented to further their arguments,[9,16] including diametrically divergent opinions from experts. As neither side is obligated to show evidence that is not supportive of their argument, the jury, who is impartial, may not be exposed to the entirety of the evidence. After an attorney has presented an expert whose opinions have been outlined, the opposing counsel has the opportunity to cross-examine the expert. The cross-examination may serve to question or discredit the experts' medical opinions and their motivation for testifying. It is routine for experts to be questioned about how much of their income is derived from expert testimony, how often they are employed by the same firm, and how often they testify on behalf of patients or physicians.[12]

Expert witnesses are often the focus of much scrutiny regarding their motivation and the lack of impartiality of their testimony. It is not entirely uncommon for a witness to have testified in one manner for a defense attorney and in a contradictory manner for a plaintiff's attorney in a similar case. There have also been occasions on which a physician reviews the same case for both sides. A simple Internet search for expert witness services yields thousands of expert witnesses who advertise their services and companies who specialize in locating or providing medical experts. This has led many specialty societies to issue guidelines and position statements to their members regarding the role and obligations of the expert witness in malpractice cases; some societies and colleges have sanctioned members and even revoked membership because of questionable testimony.[24]

Although there is no governing body that oversees expert testimony, specialty societies have attempted to begin the process of oversight. The American Academy of Emergency Medicine (AAEM) published a *Position Statement on Ethical Expert Conduct and Testimony*[25] and the American College of Emergency Physicians (ACEP) issued *Expert Witness Guidelines*[26] in an attempt to address the issue of unethical expert testimony. Both include guidelines for testimony and descriptions of the minimum requirements to qualify as an expert. The requirements are similar, although ACEP does not recommend specialty board certification by a board recognized by the American Board of Medical Specialties, which is a requirement of virtually every other specialty society. Some authors and specialty societies have endorsed the obligations of experts and admonished them to be available to both plaintiff and defendant, to preserve their independence from undue influence, and to uphold their responsibility to the truth.

AAEM has a link on its Web site for "remarkable" testimony. The Web site allows physicians to submit testimony that "seems farfetched, unbelievable, or just plain wrong." The case and the testimony are then reviewed by the AAEM malpractice task force, to determine if the testimony is remarkable before posting it on the Web site. The expert will be contacted and given an opportunity to respond to the accusation that the testimony was remarkable. The testimony, the letter to the expert, and the expert's response to AAEM are then posted.

Tort Reform

The case for tort reform has waxed and waned for years, depending on the political will or interests at the time, most recently becoming a cause célèbre due to the efforts of the last Republican presidential administration's response to rapidly rising malpractice insurance premiums. To physicians who have been dealing with escalating insurance premiums in the face of decreasing reimbursement and the perception of a more litigious work environment, tort reform has come to symbolize a way to possibly relieve these pressures.[27] When speaking of tort reform, physicians are most commonly speaking of efforts to change the current medical malpractice system, which may include limits on damages, altering the ways plaintiff attorneys may be compensated, creating special malpractice courts in which a panel of experts would substitute for a lay jury, and many other ideas. Tort reform, however, is broader than an isolated, distinct theory, and depending on the interest, it could be applied to many subjects and systems[28] in addition to medical malpractice, including tobacco liability, construction, the automobile industry, and others.

The United States is not alone in attempting to use tort reform to stem a malpractice crisis; Canada, Australia, New Zealand, and Sweden, to name a few, have recently changed laws to limit medical liability. The California Medical Injury Compensation Reform Act of 1975 was one of the earliest models of tort reform aimed squarely at medical malpractice.[27] It addressed attorney fees and time limits on suits, capped noneconomic damages, and introduced binding arbitration as a way to resolve malpractice claims. Although malpractice premiums did decrease or stabilize, there remains much debate over the value of tort reform versus insurance regulation in reducing premiums.[29] Given the highly political nature of tort reform, national health care quality experts have advocated that efforts should be focused on injury prevention and insurance regulation restructuring, rather than on tort reform.[30]

SUMMARY

Being named in a malpractice case may be one of the most stressful events in a physician's career, and participating in a trial is likely to be remembered for a lifetime. Despite the climate of tort reform and the reported lack of real justice in the current system, it is a system that is unlikely to change anytime soon. By understanding and knowing the system and proactively participating in one's own defense, the traumatic experience of being named in a malpractice case may be mitigated.

REFERENCES

1. Nepps ME. The basics of medicine malpractice: a primer on navigating the system. Chest 2008;134(5):1051–5.
2. Fordyce J, Blank FSJ, Pekow P, et al. Errors in a busy emergency department. Ann Emerg Med 2003;42:324–33.
3. Kachalia A, Gandhi TK, Puopolo AL, et al. Missed and delayed diagnoses in the emergency department: a study of closed malpractice claims from 4 liability insurers. Ann Emerg Med 2007;49:196–205.
4. Kuhn G. Circadian rhythm, shift work, and emergency medicine. Ann Emerg Med 2001;37:88–98.
5. Trzeciak S, Rivers EP. Emergency department overcrowding in the United States: an emerging threat to patient safety and public health. Emerg Med J 2003;20: 402–5.
6. American Medical News. State of liability. Available at: http://www.ama-assn.org/amednews/2007/03/05/prca0305.htm.
7. Studdert DM, Mello MM, Sage WM, et al. Defensive medicine among high-risk specialist physicians in a volatile malpractice environment. JAMA 2005;293(21): 2609–17.
8. Keeton WP, Dobbs DB, Keeton RE, et al. Prosser and Keeton on the law of torts. 5th edition. St. Paul (MN): West Publishing; 1984.
9. Amon E. Expert witness testimony. Clin Perinatol 2007;34:473–88.
10. Wecht CH, Koehler SA. Book review. J Leg Med 2005;26:529–34.
11. Studdert DM, Mello MM, Gawande AA, et al. Claims, errors and compensation payments in medical malpractice litigation. N Engl J Med 2006;354:2024–33.
12. Jerrold L. The role of the expert witness. Surg Clin North Am 2007;87:889–901.
13. Luce JM. Medical malpractice and the chest physician. Chest 2008;134(5): 1044–50.
14. Sage WM, Kersh R. Medical malpractice and the U.S. Health Care System. 11–12. New York: Cambridge University Press; 2006.
15. Black HC. editor. Black's law dictionary. 5th edition. St. Paul (MN): West Publishing Co; 1981.
16. Danzon PM. Medical malpractice- theory, evidence and public policy. Cambridge (MA): Harvard University Press; 1985.
17. Claims Management and the Legal Process. Risk management foundation of the Harvard medical institutions. Cambridge (MA): Risk Management Foundation; 1994.
18. Sanbar SS. Legal medicine. 6th edition. Philadelphia: Mosby; 2004.
19. Norris DM. A medical malpractice tribunal experience. J Am Acad Psychiatry Law 2007;35(3):286–9.

20. Massachusetts General Law Annotated, Chapter 231: Section 60B. Malpractice actions against providers of health care; tribunal, 2007. Available at: http://www.mass.gov/legis/laws/mgl/231-60b.htm
21. Erskine B. Medical tribunals keep spurious malpractice cases out of court, law and ethics, vital signs. Waltham (MA): Massachusetts Medical Society; 2009.
22. Szalados JE. Legal issues in the practice of critical care medicine: a practical approach. Crit Care Med 2007;35(2 Suppl):S44–58.
23. Teichman PG. How high-low agreements work in a malpractice case. Fam Pract Manag 2007;43–5.
24. Blackett WB. AANS testimony rules rewritten: New rules for neurosurgical medical/legal expert opinion service. AANS Bulletin 2005;13(1):33.
25. Available at: http://www.aaem.org/positionstatements/ethicalexpert.php.
26. Available at: http://www.acep.org/practres.aspx?id=29446.
27. Millard WB. Elephants, blind sharpshooters, golddiggers, and beyond: the prospects for constructive tort reform (Part 1 of A 2-Part series). Ann Emerg Med 2007;50(1):59–63.
28. Studdert DM, Mello MM, Brennan TA. Medical malpractice. N Engl J Med 2004; 350:283–92.
29. How insurance reform lowered doctors' medical malpractice rates in California: and how malpractice caps failed. Presented by the Foundation for Taxpayer and Consumer Rights a nonprofit, nonpartisan organization. Santa Monica (CA); March 7, 2003.
30. Sage WM. Putting the patient in patient safety: linking patient complaints and malpractice risk. JAMA 2002;287:3003–5.

Managing Emergency Department Overcrowding

Jonathan S. Olshaker, MD, FACEP, FAAEM

KEYWORDS

- Emergency department • Overcrowding
- Ambulance diversion • Boarding • Adverse outcomes

OVERCROWDING

The issue of emergency department (ED) crowding and ambulance diversion first received national attention with sporadic reports in the late 1980s. It has been an increasingly significant national problem for more than a decade. Surveys of hospital directors have reported overcrowding in almost every state in the United States. Daily overcrowding has been reported by 10% to 30% of the hospitals surveyed. More than 90% of hospital ED directors reported overcrowding as a problem resulting in patients in hallways, full occupancy of ED beds, and long waits occurring several times a week.[1] Overcrowding has many other potential detrimental effects including diversion of ambulances, frustration for patients and ED personnel, lower patient satisfaction, and most importantly, greater risk for poor outcomes. Poor patient outcomes then create potentially significant risk management implications for providers. The combination of unhappy patients and adverse outcomes breeds an environment ripe for litigation. There is no evidence at present that "the ED was just too crowded" is a valid defense for medical malpractice claims.

Initial position statements from major organizations, including the Joint Commission on Accreditation of Healthcare Organizations (JCAHO) and the General Accounting Office (GAO), suggested that the problem of overcrowding was a result of inappropriate use of emergency services by those with nonurgent conditions, probably cyclical, and needed no specific policy response.

More recently, these and other organizations have more forcefully highlighted the problem of overcrowding and focused on the inability to transfer emergency patients to inpatient beds as the single most important factor contributing to ED overcrowding.

Department of Emergency Medicine, Boston Medical Center, Boston University School of Medicine, Dowling 1 South, Boston, MA 02118, USA
E-mail address: olshaker@bu.edu

Emerg Med Clin N Am 27 (2009) 593–603
doi:10.1016/j.emc.2009.07.004
emed.theclinics.com

Standard-of-care treatment for specific disease entities certainly lowers the risk to patients and providers. But to successfully combat overcrowding, it must be looked at as an overall hospital issue, not as a problem of the ED. To quote a leader in overcrowding research, Brent Asplin,[2] "if you want to fix crowding, start by fixing your hospital." ED leadership must work in concert with hospital senior management to make substantive changes. This article gives a basic blueprint for successfully making hospital-wide changes using principles of operational management. The causes, significance, and dangers of overcrowding are discussed briefly and then specific solutions are provided.

HOW DID IT HAPPEN?

The 1980s and 1990s saw a steady downsizing in hospital capacity. American Hospital Association data showed 1.36 million hospital beds in 6933 hospitals in 1981, 927,000 staffed beds in 5370 hospitals in 1991, and 829,000 beds in 4950 hospitals in 1999. There were 4547 hospital EDs in the United States in 1991, and only 4177 remained by 1999.[3]

The most reliable data on ED visits come from the National Hospital Ambulatory Medical Care Survey (NHAMCS), which has been conducted annually since 1992 by the Centers for Disease Control's (CDC) National Center for Health Statistics (NCHS). During the period from 1992 to 1999, the number of ED visits rose by 14%; from 89.9 million annual visits in 1992 to 102.2 million in 1999.[4] More than half of this increase came between 1997 and 1999. The 2006 CDC NCHS survey documented a continuing increase in the number of hospital ED visits even as other data showed a further decline in the actual number of hospital EDs. In 2006, Americans made 119.2 million visits to hospital EDs, a 32% increase over the 90 million visits made in 1992. During the same period, the number of hospital EDs decreased by more than 10%.[5]

During this time period, a number of laws, programs, and other factors contributed to increased volume with a simultaneous decrease in reimbursement:

1. The 1986 Emergency Medical Treatment and Active Labor Act (EMTALA),[6] the law upheld by the United States Supreme Court, guarantees emergency medical care as a civil right extended to all US residents. The Act requires screening and stabilization to be provided for all who seek emergency care, regardless of the ability to pay, and threatens physicians and hospitals with explicit legal and financial penalties for noncompliance. There are no accompanying requirements for payors, public or private, to support such a mandate. There is no guarantee of payment for hospitals, emergency physicians, or on-call specialists who provide these services.
2. The Balanced Budget Act of 1999 cut net Medicare reimbursement.
3. The number of uninsured and underinsured persons in the United States has increased steadily during the same time period; in 1990 there were 35.6 million nonelderly uninsured patients, whereas in 1998, about 43.9 million nonelderly were uninsured.[7]
4. There is limited availability of off-hour services by primary care physicians.
5. Increased use of technology has led to referrals to the ED for computed tomography (CT) scan, magnetic resonance imaging, ultrasound, and other new technologies. Even well-insured patients are increasingly using EDs when primary care physicians are unavailable and the urgency and complexity of the problems do not allow for a scheduled, elective evaluation.

In addition, the problem has become worse by a national work force nursing shortage. In some hospitals, the shortage of ED and critical care nurses has reached crisis proportions. Recognition of overcrowding as a significant national problem outside the emergency medicine community has occurred in the last few years only. In 1992, a nationwide study of hospital EDs by the US Senate Committee on Finance, based on the GAO Survey of 689 US hospitals, was published with the following conclusions:

1. ED visits had increased significantly during the preceding decade.
2. The problem was most prevalent in large urban hospitals and was exacerbated by inappropriate use of emergency services by those with nonurgent conditions as defined by discharge diagnosis (estimated at up to 43% of all visits).
3. Overall, 89% of patients appeared to be receiving timely care, and only 7% of patients with urgent conditions experienced significant delays.
4. No national policy interventions were recommended.[8]

In November 2000, a Boston Globe article published comments by the US Surgeon General and the president of JCAHO indicating that ambulance diversion may be only a "cyclical phenomenon" that would not require a dedicated policy response.[9]

The GAO put out a new report in March 2003 with some of its conclusions markedly different from 11 years earlier. The 2003 Government Accounting Office Report to the US Senate, titled "Hospital Emergency Departments: Crowded Conditions vary among Hospitals and Communities. Survey of 2000 hospitals with EDs" found that crowding was most severe in metropolitan areas with large populations, areas with high population growth, and areas with a high percentage of people without health insurance.

The report stated, "While no single factor stands out as the reason why crowding occurs, GAO found the factor most commonly associated with crowding was the inability to transfer emergency patients to inpatient beds once a decision has been made to admit them as hospital patients rather than to treat and release them. Hospitals attempt to match staffed bed with revenue rather than licensed capacity and tend to give priority to scheduled admissions. Of Medicare patients being admitted from the ED, 19/20 of the most common diagnosis-related groups are for medical conditions that are regarded as less profitable than surgical admissions."[10]

The GAO report further goes on to state, "While there are no comprehensive studies on the consequences of crowded conditions, health care researchers and clinicians report that crowding has multiple effects including prolonged pain and suffering for some patients, long patient waits, increased transport times for ambulance patients, inconvenience and dissatisfaction for the patients and their families, and an increased frustration among medical staff. In addition to delays in treatment, some EDs have reported that patient care has been compromised and patients experienced poor outcomes as a result of crowded conditions in EDs."

The report found three major crowding indicators: diversion, boarding, and leaving before a medical evaluation.

Two-thirds of the hospitals in the GAO survey went on diversion at least once during fiscal year 2001. Diversion status was in effect in 2 of every 10 institutions for more than 10% of the time, and 1 in 10 were on diversion for more than 20% of the time.

GAO also concluded that senior hospital leadership committees dedicated to solving the problem of ED throughput and output can result in significant improvements.

INSTITUTE OF MEDICINE REPORT

The Institute of Medicine published a major report in 2006, titled "The Future of Emergency Care in the United States. Hospital-Based Emergency Care: At the Breaking Point." Its main summary points were:

- Serious overcrowding exists
- Boarding more than 48 hours is not uncommon
- 500,000 ambulance diversions occur a year
- There is a dire shortage of on-call specialists
- There is a need for improving hospital efficiency and patient flow
- The Joint Commission should put into place strong standards about ED crowding, boarding, and diversion
- There is need for increased funding for emergency care.[11]

WHAT ARE THE REAL CAUSES?

In 2003, Asplin and colleagues[12] used a consensus of experts to develop an "input," "throughput," and "output" model for ED patient flow. They concluded that the most frequently cited reason for ED overcrowding is the inability to move admitted patients from the ED to inpatient beds. The investigators believe that the causes and consequences of ED boarding of inpatients is the most important area for immediate research and operational changes to alleviate ED overcrowding and ambulance diversion. Solberg and colleagues[13] published the consensus of a panel of 74 national experts assessing 113 measures of ED and hospital workflow. They scored and chose 38 outcomes that may be useful in understanding, monitoring, and managing overcrowding. The output measures of ED boarding time, boarding burden, and hospital occupancy rate carried the highest weight.

Schull and colleagues[14] similarly concluded that admitted patients are the important determinants of ambulance diversion. By quantitative analysis, they determined that ambulance diversion increased with the number of patients boarding in the ED and with the boarding time, which is defined as the time from admission order to departure from the ED to a hospital bed. ED throughput time increased 18 minutes when there was an increase in inpatient occupancy of 10% and was significantly prolonged when occupancy exceeded a threshold of 90%. Rathlev and colleagues[15] showed that length of stay (LOS) was associated with hospital occupancy, hospital admissions in the ED, and elective surgical volume. With respect to diversion, the correlation with the number of ED boarders is substantially higher than the correlation with ED volume minus boarders and with ED throughput time.[16] Forster and colleagues[17] showed a strong association between increased hospital occupancy and ED throughput time for admitted patients. These findings emphasize the contribution of the "output" of admitted patients from the ED to overcrowding. Solutions must incorporate strategies to increase inpatient bed capacity either by increasing the number of staffed beds or by improving the efficiency of the admissions and discharge processes.

There is still the widespread belief among many that overcrowding is caused by EDs being overwhelmed with nonurgent patients. Research strongly contradicts this. Schull and colleagues[18] showed that low-complexity patients are associated with a negligible increase in ED LOS. Sprivulis and colleagues[19] demonstrated that ambulance diversion is not associated with low acuity patients.

As might be expected, overcrowding research that demonstrates adverse outcomes is limited by the lack of randomized controlled trials. Studies have been mostly single-institution, observational cohort studies and some with data pooled from multiple EDs. The clinical impact of overcrowding must be further defined and measured to generate the impetus for further change. Still, there is increasing data strongly suggesting higher risk of mortality and morbidity, preventable medical errors, poor pain control, and decreased patient satisfaction.

Bernstein and colleagues[20] found a weak association ($P = .03$) between high overcrowding conditions and a composite measure of the number of patients returning to the ED within 72 hours, the number of corrections of ED radiograph interpretations, and the number of quality improvement cases. The time to thrombolysis for patients with acute myocardial infarction was prolonged by 5.8 minutes (95% confidence interval 2.7–9.0) during high overcrowding conditions compared with that of no overcrowding.[21] The clinical significance of delaying thrombolysis by 5.8 minutes is unclear, and adverse effects on patient outcomes were not established. The results are nonetheless important because they clearly establish a direct link between overcrowding and delays in critical interventions in a cohort of more than 3000 patients. In another study, Schull and colleagues[22] showed that an increase in overcrowding in the ED was associated with a substantial increase in the emergency medical services system response and ambulance transport time for patients with chest pain.

There is further growing evidence of the association between ED crowding and delays in timely patient care, an increasingly common allegation in malpractice claims. Crowding is less likely to affect patients who are typically identified as critically ill early in the ED, such as patients with major trauma, life-threatening status asthmatics, or acute ST elevation myocardial infarction. Presentations with multiple-step processes of care, atypical presentations, and those for which developed protocols to speed care do not exist are more likely to be affected by ED crowding.[23] Studies have demonstrated clinically significant delays in the delivery of antibiotics for patients with community-acquired pneumonia and other infections.[23–25]

Prolonged ED LOS has been associated with a higher risk of death in patients admitted to intensive care units (ICUs) from the ED.[26] A number of studies, although not matched cohort studies, have suggested higher patient mortality risk with prolonged ED LOS.[27,28] A retrospective review linking ED crowding and boarding found a high risk of adverse events and errors.[29] Numerous studies show that ED crowding is associated with delays in analgesic therapy for patients with severe pain.[30,31]

SOLUTIONS

There is certainly not one silver bullet for solving ED crowding. But significant gains can be made by applying operational management principles in the ED and throughout the hospital to the inpatient, throughput, and outpatient model. Key factors are listed in **Box 1** with particular emphasis on senior leadership support, ED and hospital respected clinician champions, and consistency with strategy and other systems.

Fig. 1 is a simple approach to focus of efforts. Certainly, changes that are easy to implement and have a high impact should be made to happen quickly. Examples of these changes in the author's institution were the creation of an empowered inpatient bed czar, ED administrative attendings on call, and a small increase in ED attending coverage. In many cases, departments will start with easy-to-accomplish low-impact efforts. This has the benefit of seeing that early and visible success can occur. Hopefully, this can lead to more buy in for important efforts that are more difficult to implement.

Box 1
Key factors

- Senior leadership support
- Respected clinician champions
- Early and visible successes
- Support and reward for change
- Consistency with strategy and other systems (alignment)
  - Information
  - Reward
  - Evaluation

DIRECTED SOLUTIONS

Input

Many jurisdictions have in place city- or region-wide diversion policies that have either minimized or, by rule, eliminated diversion. San Diego and Sacramento have shown that formal coordinated diversion policies and guidelines can significantly reduce ambulance diversion.[32,33] Effects of limiting input of patients have not been shown to significantly affect overcrowding and diversion.[34,35] Despite the significant media focus placed on the potential benefits of redirecting nonurgent ED patients, these patients have not been shown to significantly affect ED LOS or crowding.[18]

Throughput

Applying operational management technology has shown success in ED throughput. Chan and colleagues[36] demonstrated significant decrease in the number of patients who left without being seen, waiting times, and ED LOSs, with the institution of rapid entry and accelerated care at triage. Gorelick and colleagues[37] showed a 15-minute overall decreased LOS after implementing an in-room registration process in a pediatric ED. Lee-Lewandrowski and colleagues[38] showed a decreased LOS after implementation of a point-of-care satellite laboratory as part of the ED.

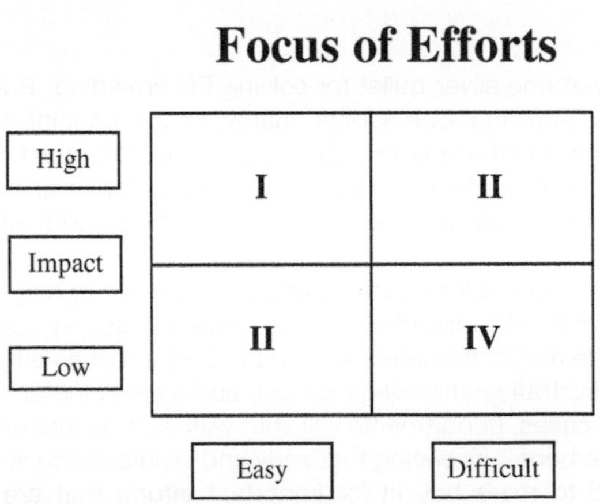

Fig. 1. *Courtesy of* M. Charns, DBA, Boston, MA.

Quinn and colleagues[39] showed the obvious but nonetheless important point that eliminating preadmission admitting-physician evaluation and need for all diagnostic testing improved ED LOS and ambulance diversion. This is especially applicable to the many institutions that still have medical residents come to evaluate patients for appropriateness for admission.

ED expansion, although certainly important for many reasons, including patient and staff satisfaction, has not been shown to decrease ambulance diversion or LOS.[40] Likewise, significant increases in ED nurse and physician staffing is usually neither an option nor a solution. Still, adequate staffing levels are essential. A study in California showed that lower staffing levels predisposed patients to longer wait times for care.[41] Another study showed that a permanent increase in the number of physicians during a busy shift reduced the LOS by 35 minutes.[42]

Many other areas have shown benefit or promise in improving throughput, including electronic medical records with laboratory, radiology, and old record interfaces; partnering with laboratory and radiology to expedite testing (eg, recent literature shows many patients do not need oral contrast for abdominal CT); frequent visitor task forces; and walkie talkies for communication with patient transporters.

In addition, ED physician and nursing leadership should develop systems to minimize medication, specimen labeling, and other errors.

Output

The evidence is extremely strong that the biggest contribution to ED crowding and ambulance diversion is the inability to get admitted patients, especially those who are critically ill, out of the ED. No significant success will occur without hospital leadership making this a priority. Although ED admissions in many centers are looked at as less profitable than others, the financial benefit of ED admissions is significant. The Agency for Healthcare Research and Quality showed that 55% of 29.3 million hospitalizations in 2003 began in the ED. Only 6.2% of admissions from the ED were uninsured, although Medicare and Medicaid accounted for 66%.[43] Bayley and colleagues[44] and McConnell and colleagues[45] showed in separate studies that diversion meant loss of hospital revenue. There will be some institutions with a large number of profitable elective admissions, where no obvious financial disincentive exists for boarding patients.[46] Efforts to decrease overcrowding and ambulance diversion must still exist and should be focused on patient safety and quality, improved access to care, and new models of reimbursement.

There is no question of the importance of hospital efforts to increase bed capacity. McConnell and colleagues[47] demonstrated that increased ICU capacity decreased ambulance diversion. Intuitively, this should also bring lower mortality risks based on past studies. Schneider and colleagues[48] showed that additional services for inpatients awaiting beds brought greatest subjective relief of overcrowding. Kelen and colleagues'[49] showed that an ED-managed acute care unit had a significant effect on decreasing overcrowding and ambulance diversion.

Programs aimed at improving hospital efficiency are essential. Litvak and colleagues[50] have promulgated the concept of controlling “artificial variability” by smoothing the admission of elective surgical and nonsurgical cases throughout the week. One study demonstrated an association between the number of daily elective surgical cases performed in the operating room and mean throughput time in the ED.[51]

Hospitalists have been shown to be important in handling increased hospital admissions with reduced LOS.[52] In addition, an active bed-management process with hospitalists and other bed czars have improved ED throughput and reduced ambulance diversion.[53]

Additional opportunity exists for each hospital to examine their entire discharge process with focus on early rounding, electronic notification of housekeeping, arrangement of early rides for patients, and multiple other areas of constant process improvement.

In addition, patient satisfaction can be improved, and the likelihood of litigation probably reduced by ED and hospital efforts directed at patient-centered care. This includes appearance of the department, respectful behavior, and explanation for wait times. Patient's perception of wait time, rather than actual time waiting to be seen by a physician, was the source of dissatisfaction. A study of 2300 patients showed that patients were dissatisfied when not told about prolonged wait times.[54] Finally, multiple studies have shown that dedicated hospital leadership–driven programs and multifaceted intervention programs can significantly decrease diversion and reduce LOS.[55–57] These interventions include more physicians, improved ancillary services, early warning systems, changes in hospital policy, and active bed management.

REFERENCES

1. Derlet RW, Richard JR. Frequent overcrowding in U.S. Emergency Departments. Acad Emerg Med 2001;8:151–5.
2. Asplin BR, Magid DS. If you want to fix crowding, start by fixing your hospital. Ann Emerg Med 2007;. 01.012.
3. American hospital association hospital statistics. Chicago 1999; Available at: www.healthforum.com.
4. Burt CW, McCaig LF. Trends in hospital emergency department utilization. United States 1992–99. Vital Health Stat 2001;2013:1–34.
5. Pitts SR, Niska RW, Xu J, et al. National hospital ambulatory medical care survey. 2006 emergency department summary. Natl Health Stat Report 2008;7:1–38.
6. Health Care Financing Administration, The Emergency Medical Treatment and Active Labor Act, as established under the Consolidated Omnibus Reconciliation Act (Cobra) of 1985. C42USC 1395 dd, Federal Register 59 (1994). p. 32086–127.
7. Adams J, Biros M. The endangered safety net: establishing a measure of control. Acad Emerg Med 2001;8:1013–5.
8. US Senate Committee on Finance, National Study of Hospital Emergency Departments Based Upon General Accounting Office (GAO) Survey of 689 US Hospitals 1992.
9. Tye L. Officials offer little hope for emergency room diversion. Boston Globe. November 19, 2000; Metro/Region section, A12.
10. United States General Accounting Office, Report to the ranking minority member committee on finance, US Senate. Hospital emergency departments, crowded conditions vary among hospitals and communities (2003) March.
11. Lewin ME, Altman S, editors. America's health care safety net, intact but endangered, Institute of Medicine. Washington, DC: National Academy Press; 2000.
12. Asplin BR, Magid DJ, Rhodes KV, et al. A conceptual model of emergency department crowding. Ann Emerg Med 2003;42:173–80.
13. Solberg LI, Asplin BR, Weinick RM, et al. Emergency department crowding: consensus development of potential measures. Ann Emerg Med 2003;42: 824–34.
14. Schull MJ, Lazier K, Vermuelen M, et al. Emergency department contributors to ambulance diversion. A quantitative analysis. Ann Emerg Med 2003;41:467–76.
15. Rathlev NK, Chessare J, Olshaker J, et al. The probability of ambulance diversion as a function of inpatient occupancy. Ann Emerg Med 2004;44(Suppl):S29.

16. Litvak E, McManus ML, Cooper A. Root cause analysis of emergency department crowding and ambulance diversion in Massachusetts. Report submitted by Boston University Program for the Management of Variability in Health Care Delivery under a grant from the Massachusetts Department of Public Health.
17. Forster A, Stiell I, Wells G, et al. The effect of hospital occupancy on emergency department length of stay and patient disposition. Acad Emerg Med 2003;10: 127–33.
18. Schull MS, Kiss A, Szalai JP. The effect of low complexity patients on emergency department waiting times. Ann Emerg Med 2007;49:257–64.
19. Sprivulis P, Grainger S, Nagree Y. Ambulance diversion is not associated with low acuity patients attending Perth metropolitan emergency departments. Emerg Med Australas 2005;17:11–5.
20. Bernstein SL, Berghese V, Leung W, et al. Development and validation of new index to measure emergency department crowding. Acad Emerg Med 2003; 10:938–42.
21. Schull MJ, Vermeulen M, Slaughter G, et al. Emergency department crowding and thrombolysis in acute myocardial infarction. Ann Emerg Med 2004;44:577–85.
22. Schull MJ, Morrison LJ, Vermuelen M, et al. Emergency Department overcrowding and ambulance transport delays, for patients with chest pain. Can Med Assoc J 2003;168:277–83.
23. Pines JM, Localio AR, Hollander JE, et al. The impact of emergency department crowding measures on time to antibiotics for patients with community-acquired pneumonia. Ann Emerg Med 2007;50:510–6.
24. Fee C, Weber EJ, Maak CA, et al. Effect of emergency department crowding on time to antibiotics in patients admitted with community-acquired pneumonia. Ann Emerg Med 2007;50:501–9.
25. Pines JM, Hollander JE, Localio AR, et al. The association between emergency department crowding and hospital performance on antibiotic timing for pneumonia and percutaneous intervention for myocardial infarction. Acad Emerg Med 2006;13:873–8.
26. Chalfin DB, Trzeciak S, Likourezos A, et al. Impact of delayed transfer of critically ill patients from the emergency department to the intensive care unit. Crit Care Med 2007;35:1477–83.
27. Richardson DR. Increase in patient mortality at 10 days associated with emergency department crowding. Med J Aust 2006;184:213–6.
28. Sprivulis PC, Da Silva JA, Jacobs IG, et al. The association between hospital overcrowding and mortality among patients admitted via Western Australian emergency departments. Med J Aust 2006;184:208–12.
29. Liu SW, Thomas SH, Gordon JA, et al. Frequency of adverse events and errors among patients boarding in the emergency department. Acad Emerg Med 2005;12:49b–50b.
30. Pines JM, Hollander JE. Emergency department crowding is associated with poor pain care for patients with severe pain. Ann Emerg Med 2008;51:1–5.
31. Hwang U, Richardson LD, Sonuyi TO, et al. The effect of emergency department crowding on the management of pain in older adults with hip fracture. J Am Geriatr Soc 2006;54:270–5.
32. Vilke GM, Castillo EM, Metz MA, et al. Community trial to decrease ambulance diversion hours: the San Diego county patient destination trial. Ann Emerg Med 2004;44:295–303.
33. Patel PB, Derlet RW, Vinson DR, et al. Ambulance diversion reduction: the Sacramento solution. Am J Emerg Med 2006;24:206–13.

34. Dent AW, Phillips GA, Chenhall AJ, et al. The heaviest repeat users of an inner city emergency department are not general practice patients. Emerg Med (Fremantle) 2003;15:322–9.
35. Afilalo J, Marinovich A, Afilalo M, et al. Nonurgent emergency department patient characteristics and barriers to primary care. Acad Emerg Med 2004; 11:1302–10.
36. Chan T, Killeen JP, Kelly P, et al. Impact of rapid entry and accelerated care at triage on reducing emergency department waiting times, length of stay, and rate of left without being seen. Ann Emerg Med 2005;46(6):491–7.
37. Gorelick MH, Yen K, Yun HJ. The effect of in room registration on emergency department length of stay. Ann Emerg Med 2005;45:128–33.
38. Lee-Lewandrowski E, Corboy D, Lewandrowski K, et al. Implementation of a point-of-care satellite laboratory in the emergency department of an academic medical center: impact on test turnaround time and patient emergency department length of stay. Arch Pathol Lab Med 2003;127:456–60.
39. Quinn JV, Mahadevan S, Eggers G, et al. Effect of implementing a rapid admission policy in the ED. Am J Emerg Med 2007;559–63.
40. Han JH, Zhou C, France DJ, et al. The effect of emergency department expansion on emergency department overcrowding. Acad Emerg Med 2007;14:338–43.
41. Lambe S, Washington DL, Fink A, et al. Waiting times in California's emergency departments. Ann Emerg Med 2003;41:35–44.
42. Bucheli B, Martina B. Reduced length of stay in medical emergency department patients: a prospective controlled study on emergency physician staffing. Eur J Emerg Med 2004;11:29–34.
43. Agency for Healthcare Research and Quality. Center for Delivery, Organization and Markets, Healthcare Cost and Utilization Project. Nationwide Inpatient Sample 2005. Available at: http://www.ahrq.gov. Accessed July 23, 2008.
44. Bayley MD, Schwartz JS, Shofer FS, et al. The financial burden on emergency department congestion and hospital crowding for chest pain patients awaiting admission. Ann Emerg Med 2005;45:110–7.
45. McConnell KJ, Richards CF, Daya M, et al. Ambulance diversion and lost hospital revenues. Ann Emerg Med 2006;48:702–10.
46. Handel DA, McConnell KJ. The financial impact of ambulance diversion on inpatient hospital revenues and profits. Acad Emerg Med 2009;16:29–33.
47. McConnell KJ, Richards CF, Daya M, et al. Effect of increased ICU capacity on emergency department length of stay and ambulance diversion. Ann Emerg Med 2005;45:471–8.
48. Schneider S, Zwemer F, Doniger A, et al. New York: a decade of emergency department overcrowding. Acad Emerg Med 2001;8:1044–50.
49. Kelen G, Scheulen D, Hill P. Effect of emergency department managed acute care unit on ED overcrowding and emergency medical services diversion. Acad Emerg Med 2001;8:1095–100.
50. Litvak E, Long MC, Cooper AB, et al. Emergency department diversion: causes and solutions. Acad Emerg Med 2001;8:1108–10.
51. Rathlev NK, Chessare J, Olshaker J, et al. Effect of the surgical schedule on daily emergency department throughput time. Ann Emerg Med 2004; 44(4 Suppl):S29.
52. Wachter RM, Goldman L. The hospitalist movement 5 years later. JAMA 2002; 287(4):487–94.
53. Howell E, Bersma E, Kravet S, et al. Active bed management by hospitalist and emergency department throughout. Ann Intern Med 2008;149:804–10.

54. Sun BC, Adams J, Orav EJ, et al. Determinants of patient satisfaction and willingness to return with emergency care. Ann Emerg Med 2000;35:426–34.
55. Lagoe RJ, Kohlbrenner JC, Hall LD, et al. Reducing ambulance diversion: a multi-hospital approach. Prehosp Emerg Care 2003;7:99–108.
56. Cardin S, Afilalo M, Lang E, et al. Intervention to decrease emergency department crowding: does it have an effect on return visits and hospital readmissions? Ann Emerg Med 2003;41:173–85.
57. Salazar A, Corbella X, Sanchez JL, et al. How to manage the ED crisis when hospital and/or ED capacity is reaching its limits: Report about the implementation of particular interventions during the Christmas crisis. Eur J Emerg Med 2002;9:79–80.

Risk Management for the Emergency Physician: Competency and Decision-Making Capacity, Informed Consent, and Refusal of Care Against Medical Advice

Brendan G. Magauran Jr, MD, MBA[a,b,*]

KEYWORDS

- Competency • Informed consent • Refusal of care
- Against medical advice • Risk management
- Substitute judgment

In the busy world of an emergency physician (EP), many patients are cared for simultaneously and numerous decisions are made on a continuing basis. Prioritizing patients and tasks based on severity of illness necessarily means that patients with lesser illness must wait. Regardless, the EP formulates a plan of care for each patient in the emergency department (ED), integrally involving the patient in the plan. Each plan also takes into account risk management on behalf of both the patient and EP. In any discussion on risk management in the ED setting, the concept of informed consent is central to mitigating risk for the EP and patient. Assuming that the patient is competent to make autonomous health care decisions, the EP has a duty to explain the patient's medical condition and treatment options in understandable terms. The associated risks and benefits of treatment options (including doing nothing) should also be communicated. This process allows the patient to choose a treatment option

[a] Department of Emergency Medicine, Boston Medical Center, Boston University School of Medicine, Dowling 1 South, 1 Boston Medical Center Place, Boston, MA 02118, USA
[b] Emergency Department, Boston Medical Center, Boston University School of Medicine, Dowling 1 South, 1 Boston Medical Center Place, Boston, MA 02118, USA
* Department of Emergency Medicine, Boston Medical Center, Boston University School of Medicine, Dowling 1 South, 1 Boston Medical Center Place, Boston, MA 02118.
E-mail address: magauran@bu.edu

Emerg Med Clin N Am 27 (2009) 605–614
doi:10.1016/j.emc.2009.08.001
emed.theclinics.com

that best fits the individual patient's goals and values, even if this treatment option is not what the EP is recommending.

Certainly, the majority of encounters between an EP and an ED patient can be enormously satisfying for both patient and physician. Emergency medical conditions that are promptly diagnosed and treated represent the ideal in emergency care. There are times, however, that this ideal is not possible, particularly when there is disagreement between the physician and patient concerning the proposed care plan. This article focuses on the minority of times that the EP and patient do not agree about the treatment option being chosen by the patient. Attention is placed on the risk management issues relevant to the patient's unexpected treatment choice. There can be many reasons why agreement is difficult and there can be significant risk placed on the EP depending on the specific reason for disagreement. Issues include capacity (either transient or permanent), substitute judgment for incapacitated patients, informed consent to treatment, the right to refuse care, and the decision to leave the ED against medical advice. Emphasis is placed on determining a patient's competency or capability of making clinical decisions, with particular focus on the EP deciding that patient competency requires a formal evaluation. The EP should have a strategy for assessing clinical decision-making capability and an understanding of what circumstances should act as a trigger for considering such an assessment. Attention to documentation issues around informed consent, common barriers to consent (minors, language, substance abuse, legal directives including guardianship, living wills, advance directives, etc), refusal of care, and ED discharge against medical advice (AMA) are examined.

COMPETENCE AND MEDICAL DECISION MAKING

For the EP, determining if a patient is competent to make clinical decisions relevant to a proposed care plan can be quite complex. Competency, in the medical setting, is a distinct entity from competency in the judicial setting. In the medical arena, competency to make medical decisions is used interchangeably with the word capacity in order to steer clear of the legal connotations associated with competency. For the majority of ED patients, capacity is a nonissue. There are, however, certain patients where capacity is a potential or even likely issue. Patients with cognitive deficits such as early Alzheimer disease, after stroke, psychiatric patients (schizophrenia, bipolar disorder, or disorders associated with psychosis and altered reality testing), substance abuse (particularly withdrawal states associated with altered mentation and overdose conditions associated with depressed levels of consciousness and mentation). There are two basic premises to capacity in the medical setting. The first premise is that patients understand best what is uniquely right for them. A patient's decision will maximize what works for their self-interest. The second premise is that the decision is autonomous.[1] In a report from the President's Commission for the Study of Ethical Problems in Medicine[2] from 1982, clinical decision-making capacity included three specific elements: the patient has a set of values and goals, the patient is able to understand and communicate information, and the patient is able to reason and deliberate about the choice being made by the patient. Applebaum[3] incorporates these elements in a chart on legally relevant criteria for decision-making capacity (**Table 1**).[1]

Patients with cognitive impairment increase the risk of a claim against the physician because the consent to treatment by these patients is considered invalid. A patient who is not capable of giving informed consent should not be relied on to make decisions about the care plan being considered. Under such circumstances, the physician must seek substituted judgment. A health care proxy serves this purpose, but the majority of patients do not have a health care proxy form filled out and available for the EP to read and verify.

CAPACITY ASSESSMENT

Assessment of capacity is done simultaneously with clinical assessment in most cases. Unless a patient is obviously impaired or incapable, or presents with a preexisting condition or chief complaint suggestive of cognitive impairment, the EP proceeds with the clinical encounter as if the patient is competent.[4] During this process it occasionally becomes apparent that a patient may lack capacity to make clinical decisions autonomously. At this point, a formal assessment of capacity should be performed. This assessment should be done with a translator, if necessary, and should include a mini-mental status examination and a neurologic examination. The mini-mental status examination correlates well with patients believed to be clinically incapable of deciding treatment options—at least in the inpatient setting.[5] All relevant information concerning potential diagnoses and treatment options should be given in understandable language; that is, presented at the level appropriate to the given patient so information is most likely to be understood. This information must include the risks and benefits of all treatment options including the option of no treatment. The information should be presented in a neutral manner without overstating or understating actual risks and benefits. Having been given the relevant information, the patient should be asked to tell the EP what it is that is understood. The patient should be able to paraphrase the relevant information indicating understanding of the medical condition, potential treatment options, and risks and benefits of the treatment options. Any misimpressions can be corrected. The patient should also state the reasoning behind the treatment option chosen. This process now ties together the criteria necessary for determining capacity in medical decision making: appreciation of current medical condition, understanding of treatment options, and ability to communicate the decision for the patient's treatment of choice. It is important to note that this process makes no determination on the outcome of the process. The focus is on the deliberative process necessary to make an autonomous decision. The real risk management issue for the EP centers more on the outcome of the process, particularly when a patient makes an unexpected choice that is very risky and is not the expected choice. It is generally at this point that the EP realizes that the patient may not be competent to make the treatment decision and, therefore, it is necessary to evaluate competency.

The need to assess competency is inversely proportionate to the degree of patient agreement with medical opinion on preferred treatment option. The more a patient agrees with the expected choice of treatment option, the less the need to screen for competency is perceived by the EP. Depending on the risk of the treatment option chosen, the greater the perceived need to screen for competency. Essentially, the patient who chooses an option that carries significantly higher risk and is an unexpected treatment choice, the greater the need to explore the patient's competency in making such a decision. There is disagreement about the relationship of a risky treatment option choice to the capability to make such a decision by the patient. Wear[4] and Wicclair[6] believe that the assessment of a patient's capability to make an informed treatment decision can be decoupled from the patient's final treatment decision. There is a theory of sliding-scale capacity that links the treatment decision rationale to the process used to reach the final treatment decision.[1,7–9] In essence, this theory holds patients who choose a riskier treatment option to a higher standard

Table 1
Legally relevant criteria for decision-making capacity and approaches to assessment of the patient

Criterion	Patient's Task	Physician's Assessment Approach	Questions for Clinical Assessment[a]	Comments
Communicate a choice	Clearly indicate preferred treatment option	Ask patient to indicate a treatment choice	Have you decided whether to follow your doctor's [or my] recommendation for treatment? Can you tell me what that decision is? [If no decision] What is making it hard for you to decide?	Frequent reversals of choice because of psychiatric or neurologic conditions may indicate lack of capacity
Understand the relevant information	Grasp the fundamental meaning of information communicated by physician	Encourage patient to paraphrase disclosed information regarding medical condition and treatment	Please tell me in your own words what your doctor [or I] told you about: The problem with your health now The recommended treatment The possible benefits and risks (or discomforts) of the treatment Any alternative treatments and their risks and benefits The risk and benefits of no treatment	Information to be understood includes nature of patient's condition, nature and purpose of proposed treatment, possible benefits and risks of that treatment, and alternative approaches (including no treatment) and their benefits and risks

Appreciate the situation and its consequences	Acknowledge medical condition and likely consequences of treatment options	Ask patient to describe views of medical condition, proposed treatment, and likely outcomes	What do you believe is wrong with your health now? Do you believe that you need some kind of treatment? What is treatment likely to do for you? What makes you believe it will have that effect? What do you believe will happen if you are not treated? Why do you think your doctor has [or I have] recommended this treatment?	Court have recognized that patients who do not acknowledge their illnesses (often referred to as "lack of insight") cannot make valid decisions about treatment Delusions or pathologic levels of distortion or denial are the most common causes of impairment
Reason about treatment options	Engage in rational process of manipulating the relevant information	Ask patient to compare treatment options and consequences and to offer reasons for selection of option	How did you decide to accept or reject the recommended treatment? What makes [chosen option] better than [alternative option]?	This criterion focuses on the process by which a decision is reached, not the outcome of the patient's choice, since patients have the right to make "unreasonable" choices

[a] Questions are *adapted from* Grisso and Applebaum.[1] Patients' responses to these questions need not be verbal.

of competency by requiring the patient to demonstrate greater clarity in explaining the rationale behind the choice of the higher risk treatment option.[10] From a practical standpoint and a risk management vantage point, coupling of the decision and treatment choice is important to the EP. Capable patients may choose options that are not consistent with what the EP considers the expected treatment choice. This unexpected treatment choice may be questioned in the future, particularly if an adverse event occurs or if the treatment choice is ineffective and there is a perception that another treatment choice would have been significantly better. It is in precisely these situations that documentation of a capability assessment coupled with a documented explanation of the patient rationale for the treatment choice highlighting the understanding of the risks and benefits of such a choice becomes extremely important. A further explanation of attempts to correct any misinterpretations will also serve to demonstrate that a capable patient made an autonomous decision based on maximizing the patient's best self-interest despite the fact that the choice was not the expected choice for the EP or, for that matter, a majority of individuals facing a similar decision.

INFORMED CONSENT

When a patient decides to refuse care or to leave the ED AMA, it is a most unsatisfactory choice for the EP. The EP's duty to protect a patient from harm is now cast in stark opposition to the duty to respect a patient's autonomy. An unexpected treatment choice on the part of a patient results in the EP assessing patient competence or capability to make clinical decisions. The principle of informed consent is paramount in providing the patient the necessary information required to make an informed choice from available treatment options. In emergency medicine, informed consent is not absolute. Life-threatening situations necessitating emergency intervention to prevent death or serious bodily harm are generally accepted as exceptions to this principle under the premise that preserving life is in accord with the duty of the EP to prevent harm to a patient and that the patient would choose life as a treatment option over certain death. In a General Accounting Office report from 1993 on the type of care provided in EDs across the United States, it was estimated that 49% of all ED visits were nonurgent based on discharge diagnoses.[11] Using discharge diagnosis is a poor proxy for determination of the urgency or emergency of ED visits as the presenting chief complaint may well represent a possible life-threatening condition or emergency medical condition that will not be discovered to be emergent or nonacute until a medical screening examination is performed.

Informed consent, like competency, is a term with legal and medical connotations. The EP has a duty to disclose the relevant clinical information to the patient so that the capable patient can understand treatment options and make an autonomous decision that maximizes the patient's best interest. As discussed before, each patient has a unique set of values and goals by which each treatment option's risks and benefits are heavily weighted. Whereas the EP is uniquely suited to understand the emergency treatment options and associated risks and benefits, the lack of a longstanding relationship with the patient makes it difficult for the EP to customize treatment alternatives in light of the patient's goals and values. In terms of risk management, it is important to understand that the patient's autonomy in determining the correct treatment option based on individual values and goals is the only control the patient has in the ED setting. The choice of setting and provider is by necessity not under patient control. Autonomy is then confined to treatment options that the patient can weigh in light of individual goals and values.

In the medical setting, informed consent has three main features: patient capacity to make the treatment decision, sufficient relative information that is understandable in terms of current condition and treatment options with corresponding risks and benefits, and the ability to voluntarily consent to the perceived treatment option that best fits the patient's values and goals without coercion.[12] Capacity has been discussed in detail earlier. Sufficient relative information necessary for informed consent in the legal arena has two competing standards. The first standard is from the perspective of the average qualified EP. This local professional standard requires the EP to disclose information that the average qualified physician would disclose under similar circumstances. This standard is not patient centered; therefore, the second standard requires the EP to disclose the relevant information that an average reasonable patient would require to make an informed treatment decision. This standard does not tailor the information to particular needs of a patient who does not neatly fit into the average patient category. For the practicing EP, this lack of clarity about the legal requirement of relevant information disclosure may retrospectively present risk management issues based on local legal jurisdictions and standards. The practice of the patient signing the consent to treatment form in most EDs gives blanket consent to all treatment options. To mitigate risk associated with potentially risky treatment options or procedures in the ED, it would be wise for the EP to simultaneously document the associated consent process. Voluntary consent to treatment is the third element of valid informed consent for the patient. Involuntary consent using manipulation, coercion, or duress to persuade a patient to consent to a treatment option is not morally or legally binding. Persuasion in the form of EP recommendation is permissible because it is usual and customary that the EP provides guidance concerning particular courses of action in a rational discussion.[12]

Special Considerations

Informed consent is extremely important in emergency medicine. Under life-threatening situations, however, there is an exception to the doctrine of informed consent. The American College of Emergency Physicians publishes a code of ethics. Ladd,[13] a philosopher, argues that the ED presents several ethical challenges to patients concerning autonomous decision making. Patients do not generally choose the hospital or the physician. Emergency medical service ambulances transport patients to the closest facility if the medics believe a life-threatening medical condition exists. The patient does not choose the EP on duty. Real choice for the ED patient lies, ironically, with the informed consent doctrine. This is ironic because the ED culture is one of saving life even if heroic measures are required. Unless a patient has a documented living will that specifically requests no heroic life support, heroic measures will be undertaken because of the underlying belief that life-sustaining treatments would be preferred by patients.[12,13]

Ladd[13] also argues that operational efficiency may come into conflict with patient autonomy. All EPs are aware of how an argument can be framed to suit a specific choice or desired option. Documentation of treatment options devoid of manipulation or coercion is important in demonstrating that the patient's choice of treatment is autonomous and not the result of being under duress. Recognizing that a physician's recommendation usually carries significant weight, it is reasonable for the EP or patient's family to use this recommendation as a tool to persuade the patient as long as the patient's ultimate decision is not made out of capitulation. The American Medical Association code of ethics states, "Patients should receive guidance from their physicians as to the optimal course of action."[14]

There are circumstances when an EP may want to treat a patient even though informed consent is not easily obtained. Situations involving patients (1) that are minors, (2) speak a language other than the language spoken by the EP, (3) with strong religious beliefs that do not sanction medical care or disallow certain medical practices (Jehovah's Witness and blood transfusions, Church of Scientology and medicine in general), (4) in active substance abuse or substance withdrawal states, (5) with altered mental status, with psychiatric illness with a psychotic mental state, and (6) presenting with depressed mental status or altered mental status as a chief complaint. In all such cases, the capability to make medical decisions should be assessed. Patients found to be incapable of consenting to medical care decisions require substitute judgment.

SUBSTITUTE JUDGMENT

The duty of the EP to a patient does not change if the patient is deemed incapable of making medical decisions. The patient's judgment is substituted by another person (usually a relative) for making medical decisions that reflect the values and goals of the patient. A power of attorney (POA) is a legal document that specifically names a responsible person, authorized by the patient and recognized by law, to make medical and legal decisions for an incapacitated patient. The POA may be separated into legal and medical documents as an individual may wish to have different people named for legal and health care decisions. An advance directive refers to specific instructions for anticipated medical conditions such as a do-not-resuscitate order or a do-not-intubate order. The environment in the ED generally requires patients to make decisions over a relatively short time. Patients that are obviously incapacitated and are being transported to the ED from a nursing home, generally have advance directives that accompany the paperwork from the nursing home. The next of kin is listed with contact information so that the EP may discuss treatment options with family, most often to confirm the patient wishes stated in the advanced directive.

Patients that experience a material change in their physical and mental condition so that they are now acutely incapable of medical decision-making present a unique challenge to the EP. The EP wishes to respect the autonomy of the patient and the patient's right to determine treatment options in line with their values and goals, while acting in the patient's best interest to protect the patient from harm. In situations such as this, there is an exemption to informed consent. The physician is expected to render life-sustaining treatment.

REFUSAL OF CARE

Competent patients can refuse care. This can be an admission, a procedure, or even a test. Because the choice may be unexpected, it is reasonable for the EP to consider competency before agreeing with a request to refuse care. As part of a good risk management strategy, it is worth examining the communication between the patient and EP. Establishing trust by introducing one's self, sitting, listening, not interrupting, asking open-ended questions, using understandable language, and making empathetic statements helps to mitigate communication issues and minimizes or prevents conflicts.

Despite an EP's good communication skills, a competent patient may still refuse care. Attempts to negotiate an acceptable compromise may potentially buy time for further patient reflection. Another option at the disposal of the EP is use of the family (or substitute) to help the patient fully appreciate the risks and benefits associated with treatment options. Ethics consults are another option in the general hospital setting, but are rarely used in the ED given the time constraints for decision-making. In the inpatient setting, psychiatry consultations are more commonplace for evaluating competency, and can be used in the ED particularly for patients with mental illness or substance abuse issues. As a last resort, legal consultation with the hospital attorney may be obtained in cases of life- or limb-threatening decisions or, particularly, for decisions by caregivers or substitutes.

DISCHARGING AGAINST AMA

Discharging patients AMA is a tool employed by the EP to document a patient's decision to leave the hospital despite the physician's recommendation for admission for further treatment. The medical literature is sparse concerning this topic in emergency medicine. A study looking at the rate of AMA discharges from a general medicine service estimates the rate to be 1% to 2% of all discharges.[15] Factors associated with AMA discharge include male gender, younger age, substance abuse, Medicaid, and being uninsured.[15] In a retrospective cohort analysis of ED patients over two 6-month periods in consecutive years, a significant number of patients discharged AMA were found to have significant pathology (17.5%).[16] The principle diagnostic diagnoses in the AMA group were cardiovascular disease, undifferentiated abdominal pain, respiratory illness, and cellulitis. In the patient group discharged AMA with cardiovascular complaints, 75% reported that their symptoms had improved or abated and the patients would not be returning for care. In a study by Pope and colleagues[17] examining missed diagnoses of acute cardiac ischemia in the ED, it was estimated that 2.1% of patients with acute myocardial infarction were discharged and that 2.3% of patients with acute cardiac ischemia were discharged. It makes sense that some of these patients could fall into the AMA discharge category even though this was not actually looked at in the study. Patients being discharged from the hospital, AMA or in regular fashion, present a risk management issue for the EP. Documentation that a patient being discharged AMA is competent to make such a decision is helpful, but documentation of capability to make medical decisions coupled with a discussion of the risks and benefits associated with such a decision is more helpful. In a review of four medical malpractice cases brought to suit over AMA discharges, documentation of AMA discharge was helpful, but the plaintiff's inability to prove negligence was the deciding factor.[18]

REFERENCES

1. Grisso T, Applebaum PS. Assessing competence to consent to treatment: a guide for physicians and other health professionals. New York: Oxford University Press; 1998.
2. President's Commission for the Study of Ethical Problems in Medicine and Biomedical and Behavioral Research The ethical and legal implications of informed consent in the patient-practitioner relationship. Making health care decisions, vol. 1, Report. Washington, DC: US Government Printing Office; 1982.
3. Applebaum PS. Assessment of patients' competence to consent to treatment. N Engl J Med 2007;357:1834.
4. Wear S. Informed consent: patient autonomy and clinical beneficence within health care. 2nd edition. Washington, DC: Georgetown University Press; 1998.
5. Raymont V, Bingley W, Buchanan A, et al. Prevalence of mental incapacity in medical inpatients and associated risk factors: cross-sectional study. Lancet 2004;364:1421–7.
6. Wicclair MR. Patient decision-making capacity and risk. Bioethics 1991;5:91–104.

7. Drane JF. Competency to give an informed consent. JAMA 1984;252:925–7.
8. Roth LH, Meisel A, Lidz CA. Tests of competency to consent to treatment. Am J Psychiatry 1977;134:279–84.
9. Holyrod B, Shalit M, Kalisen G, et al. Prehospital patients refusing care. Ann Emerg Med 1988;17:957–63.
10. Simon JR. Refusal of care: the physician-patient relationship and decisionmaking capacity. Ann Emerg Med 2007;50(4):456–61.
11. Young GP, Wagner MB, Kellerman AL, et al. Ambulatory visits to hospital emergency departments. JAMA 1996;276:460–5.
12. Moskop JC. Informed consent in the emergency department. Emerg Med Clin North Am 1999;17(2):327-40.
13. Ladd RE. Patients without choices: the ethics of decision-making in emergency medicine. J Emerg Med 1985;3:149–56.
14. Principles of Medical Ethics. AMA website. Available at: http://www.ama-assn.org/ad-com/polfind/Hlth-Ethics.pdf. Accessed April 8, 2009.
15. Alfandre DJ. “I'm going home”: discharge against medical advice. Mayo Clin Proc 2009;84(3):255–60.
16. Jerrard DA, Chasm R. Patients leaving against medical advice from the emergency department: How many of them actually return to continue their evaluation and what are the reasons the others do not? Ann Emerg Med 2004;44(4):S130–1.
17. Pope HJ, Aufderheide TP, Ruthazer R, et al. Missed diagnosis of acute cardiac ischemia in the emergency department. N Engl J Med 2000;342(16):1163–70.
18. Devitt PJ, Devitt AC, Dewan M. An examination of whether discharging patients against medical advice protects physicians for malpractice charges. Psychiatr Serv 2000;51(7):899–902.

Evaluation of Physician Competency and Clinical Performance in Emergency Medicine

William E. Baker, MD[a,b,*]

KEYWORDS

- Emergency medicine • Benchmarking • Quality of healthcare
- Quality indicators • Quality assurance

Measurement of physician competency and clinical performance has been an ongoing yet elusive goal for many years. Attempts to measure mastery of medical knowledge and clinical competency have long been integral to medical school and postgraduate training program assessments. The task of assessing the performance of practicing physicians involves perhaps even greater challenges. The evaluation of health care provided by individual physicians is not a new concept. However, it is gaining greater momentum as a crucial component in the movement to improve overall health care safety and quality. Emergency medicine is an active participant in this movement. The objectives of this article are to:

1. Provide a background history of assessing health care quality
2. Present an overview of current interest and importance of measuring physician competency and performance, including requirements related to certifying bodies and those integral to pay-for-performance programs
3. Describe some of the current methods of evaluating the practice performance of emergency physicians, including peer review and use of health care quality measures
4. Discuss the state of the literature as it pertains to health care quality and individual emergency physician performance

Information gathered for this article includes that obtained through searches of *MEDLINE*, Google, and Google Scholar. Relevant Web sites scrutinized for pertinent

[a] Department of Emergency Medicine, Boston University School of Medicine, Boston, MA, USA
[b] Department of Emergency Medicine, Boston Medical Center, Dowling 1 South, 1 Boston Medical Center Place, Boston, MA 02118, USA
* Department of Emergency Medicine, Boston Medical Center, Dowling 1 South, 1 Boston Medical Center Place, Boston, MA 02118.
E-mail address: wbaker@bu.edu

Emerg Med Clin N Am 27 (2009) 615–626
doi:10.1016/j.emc.2009.07.010
emed.theclinics.com

information also include those of the American Board of Emergency Medicine (ABEM), the American Board of Medical Specialties (ABMS), the National Quality Forum (NQF), the Ambulatory Care Quality Alliance, the Centers for Medicare and Medicaid Services (CMS), and the Joint Commission. The Joint Commission's hospital accreditation standards were also reviewed.

HISTORY AND CURRENT INTEREST IN PHYSICIAN PERFORMANCE

Ernest Amory Codman, a Boston surgeon, is credited as the pioneer of physician performance measurement and quality improvement. His book, *A Study in Hospital Efficiency: as Demonstrated by the Case Report of the First Five Years of a Private Hospital*, was originally published at his own expense in 1918[1] and describes the outcomes of all patients at his hospital over a 5-year period. The book was subsequently republished in 1996 by the Joint Commission[2] with a contemporary foreword, recollections, and introduction. Codman was a strong proponent of examining the end result of treatment and also advocated for transparency in performance measurement. His principles are remarkably consistent with those that form the foundation of contemporary directions in performance assessment. Dr Codman argued that it was important not only to measure performance, but also to disclose such results to others, including to patients. He also recognized that in his day, his ideas were considered, in his own words, "eccentric." He stated in the first three of nine proposals for hospitals seeking to ensure improvement, that they:

1. Must find out what their results are
2. Must analyze their results, to find their strong and weak points
3. Must compare their results with those of other hospitals

Codman had the bold foresight to state: "Such opinions will not be eccentric a few years hence."[2]

Since the Institute of Medicine first released its reports "*To Err Is Human: Building a Safer Health System*[3] and *Crossing the Quality Chasm: A New Health System for the 21st Century*,"[4] quality and safety in medicine have received unprecedented focus. One component of maintaining and improving quality in medicine involves measurement of practitioner clinical performance. Assessing and grading of the performance of practicing physicians are of interest to a wide range of entities. The Joint Commission requires that hospitals assess and monitor performance of practitioners with hospital medical staff privileges. The emergency physician is, except in rare unique circumstances, a hospital-based provider. Thus, a large portion of the practice evaluation is intertwined with hospital practitioner performance assessment requirements. Other interested parties include state medical licensure bodies, third-party payers (including the federal government), and professional certifying bodies. The ABEM mission statement indicates that a component of the board's role is to ensure the quality of the practice of emergency medicine. The process of ensuring such quality includes evaluating the performance of emergency physicians.[5]

BOARD CERTIFICATION AND PERFORMANCE EVALUATION

The ABMS assists specialty boards with the development and use of standards for the certification and ongoing evaluation of physicians. The ABMS considers board certification as demonstrating a physician's "exceptional expertise in a particular specialty and/or subspecialty of medical practice."[6] The ABMS is also committed to the concept of lifelong learning and competency in a specialty. Maintenance of certification requires ongoing measurement of six core competencies using a four-part process. The process components are:

Professional standing
Lifelong learning and self-assessment
Assessment of cognitive expertise
Assessment of practice performance[7]

In 1999, the Accreditation Council for Graduate Medical Education (ACGME) endorsed the concept of residents obtaining competencies in six general areas.[8] The six areas are:

Patient care
Medical/clinical knowledge
Practice-based learning and improvement
Interpersonal and communication skills
Professionalism
Systems-based practice

These six competencies are also integrated into the Joint Commission's requirements and recommendations as pertaining to practitioner credentialing and performance evaluation and will be discussed below. A detailed description of these competencies may be found on the ACGME Web site.[9]

ABMS describes practice performance assessment in general terms and requires that physicians be evaluated in their clinical practice and that such evaluation be based on specialty-specific standards of care. ABEM bases all of its in-training and competency assessment examinations on *The Model of the Clinical Practice of Emergency Medicine* (*EM Model*).[10] The *EM Model*, in combination with the six general competencies, forms the framework on which to base assessment of emergency physician performance and competency. Performance should be compared with that of the physician's peers and with national benchmarks. Additionally, ABMS recommends that physicians employ best evidence or consensus recommendations to improve care.[11] The ABEM, as an ABMS member board, endorses assessment of practice performance and such assessment is a component of the ABEM's Emergency Medicine Continuous Certification program. The program has not been fully implemented as of the publication of this article. Current information from ABEM indicates that such evaluation will be based on participation in existing practice improvement programs (the programs will not be designed or dictated by ABEM). Physicians will have to attest to their participation in an acceptable performance improvement program, but will not be required to submit actual practice data to ABEM. The anticipated implementation date of this component of the program will be 2010.[12]

PEER REVIEW

Medical peer review has been a longstanding tool for the evaluation of physician performance and is still employed today as a component of a comprehensive physician performance evaluation program. Medical peer review in simple terms is the process by which physicians evaluate the quality of work by colleagues. The activity involves the formal or informal assessment of a physician's qualifications, professional knowledge, and performance (including clinical outcomes related to a physician's care). Peer review may be performed by another individual physician or group of practitioners, either from the same specialty or via a multidisciplinary group. Goals of such assessment may include assessment of qualifications, medical knowledge, technical skills, and interpersonal skills, as well as medical outcomes. The Joint Commission on Accreditation of Hospitals, now officially called the Joint Commission, was formed in 1951. Shortly after its formation, the Joint Commission required peer review as a component of the process by which hospitals gained accreditation. To date, the Joint Commission is highly influential in setting standards by which practitioners are measured and peer review remains an important component of that process. The Joint Commission's practitioner practice evaluation requirements have evolved beyond peer review and will be discussed separately.

Peer review has, over the years, gained at least some acceptance by both medical and legal authorities as a means of self-regulation and improving overall health care. Government encourages medical peer review through protective legislation. The Health Care Quality Improvement Act of 1986 (HCQI), enacted by the federal government, argues the need for effective peer review as well as protection for physicians participating in peer review. The wording of this legislation is optimistic regarding the effectiveness of peer review as a performance-improvement tool. As stated in Title 42, Chapter 117, Subsection 11101,[13] Congress found that:

1. The increasing occurrence of medical malpractice and the need to improve the quality of medical care have become nationwide problems that warrant greater efforts than those that can be undertaken by any individual State
2. There is a national need to restrict the ability of incompetent physicians to move from State to State without disclosure or discovery of the physician's previous damaging or incompetent performance
3. This nationwide problem can be remedied through effective professional peer review
4. The threat of private money damage liability under Federal laws, including treble damage liability under Federal antitrust law, unreasonably discourages physicians from participating in effective professional peer review
5. There is an overriding national need to provide incentive and protection for physicians engaging in effective professional peer review

The act grants immunity to peer review participants. HCQI also legislated the creation of the National Practitioner Data Bank (NPDB). This clearinghouse of peer review information coupled with reporting requirements provides health care organizations access to practitioner information independent of that provided by that provider. Thus, a physician whose clinical privileges were limited at a hospital in one state cannot simply move to another hospital in another state and escape disclosure of such information to that hospital. HCQI also requires reporting to the NPDB of instances where a physician surrenders hospital privileges rather than undergo formal peer review investigation.

In addition to federal protections, all states afford some type of protections for the peer review process. These protections vary considerably from state to state, but generally fall into three categories: immunity from lawsuits for participating in the process, protection from discovery of peer review information, and the requirement that participants maintain confidentiality of peer review information and findings. Peer review programs vary considerably, as do the statutes that protect peer review (from state to state), and indeed may vary with a given situation. Additionally, although federal government encourages peer review, federal protections of peer review and their courts' interpretations of peer review privileges may vary from that of a state.[14]

A plethora of entities require peer review and the government encourages such participation through legislated protections. These protections are somewhat unusual from a legal perspective and also not without controversy regarding their justification as well as effectiveness. The protections afforded peer review are not consistent with general laws on privileges and immunities. Although protections vary and are not absolute, peer review laws deprive an individual full access to the judicial process through limiting access normally afforded to litigants. Some authorities question the effectiveness of peer review in achieving its intended goals. A 1995 report by the Office of the Inspector General (OIG)[15] expressed such concerns. This report found that in the first 3 years of the reporting requirements, hospitals reported 3154 practitioners to the NPDB. During that same time period, state medical boards took disciplinary actions against about 8000 physicians. Failure of hospitals to report to the NPDB suggests that adequate peer review may not be performed and, more likely, such peer review is simply not being reported as required. It is certain that a component of underreporting is related to failure to report some reviewed cases. A 2005 OIG report[16] revealed that numerous Health and Human Services cases were not reported by the federal government as required. In an often-cited 1999 legal study, Scheutzow[17] examined the peer review protections afforded by the federal government and individual states and compared these protections with peer review reports. The study found that the presence and strength of a state's protections were not associated with reporting to the NPDB. States with stronger penalties for failure to report had provided significantly more reports to the NPDB than those that did not have strong punitive legislation. A variety of reasons are postulated for why physicians and hospitals may be reluctant to participate in peer review. Participants may fear that legal protections are inadequate and they may also fear nonlegal repercussions. There are also no uniform criteria for peer review. Regardless, peer review is increasingly recognized as inadequate as the sole means for regulating practitioner performance and promoting safety and quality in health care. Some investigators[14,17] feel the costs outweigh the benefits.

THE JOINT COMMISSION AND PHYSICIAN PERFORMANCE EVALUATION

The Joint Commission accredits and certifies health care organizations with the goal of improving safety and quality of care provided to the public. Toward that goal, the Joint Commission provides hospitals with specific guidance through standards outlined in the medical staff sections of the accreditation requirements manuals. The hospital's medical staff is responsible for granting practitioners privileges to provide health care within that hospital, thus, in effect, determining the scope of an emergency physician's practice. Coupled with this requirement is a mandate that the hospital has a process for determining the practitioner's competency in the requested privileges and assessing the quality of care provided by these practitioners. This process must include ongoing evaluation of the competency of the practitioners.[18] Hospitals are saddled with the responsibility of maintaining a reliable and consistent process for evaluating the credentials of a practitioner specific to the privileges requested, including the practitioner's current competency to perform the requested privileges. Recommendations that such competency include assessment of proficiency in the six areas of "General Competencies," which, like ABMS and ABEM, the Joint Commission adapted from the ACGME.[19]

Assessment of practitioner competency involves two forms of evaluation, "focused professional practice evaluation" (FPPE) and "ongoing professional practice evaluation" (OPPE), each of which are covered in detail by separate Joint Commission standards.[20,21] FPPE involves evaluation of privilege-specific competency of practitioners without previous performance evaluation of that specific privilege at that hospital. Emergency physicians newly appointed to a hospital would be required to undergo an FPPE. Additionally, emergency physicians who request a new privilege would be required to undergo FPPE of their practice specific to that privilege. FPPEs may also be used when questions arise regarding the competency of a currently credentialed practitioner.[21] OPPEs are employed as tools to assist hospitals in deciding to maintain, modify, or revoke a practitioner's existing privilege. While many emergency physicians might erroneously perceive OPPE as only pertinent to them at the time of reappointment, OPPE is designed to be an "ongoing" process. Information from a practitioner's OPPE can be employed by the medical staff to modify or revoke existing privileges before the time of renewal.[20]

PRACTICE EVALUATION METRICS: CURRENT STATE AND CHALLENGES

There are a number of major challenges to the development and implementation of an effective physician clinical performance evaluation program. In an effort to move beyond the limitations of traditional peer review, those striving for more objective measures of health care quality and safety are turning toward comparative quality analysis or benchmarking. Benchmarking is the "method of measuring performance against established standards of best practice."[22] A prerequisite to successful benchmarking is defining quality health care on a measurable level. There is no widely accepted, comprehensive set of validated evidence-based metrics upon which to base such a program. In 2002, an Academic Emergency Medicine consensus conference was devoted to defining quality of care in emergency medicine. Proceedings of this conference were published in a *Special Consensus Issue* devoted entirely to this subject.[23] A cornerstone of measuring the quality of care provided is determining the yardstick for quality. The Academic Emergency Medicine consensus defined medical quality as "the care health professionals would want to receive if they got sick."[24] However, developing metrics to actually measure quality and, more specifically, practitioner clinical performance, has proven a daunting task.

In *Evaluating the Quality of Medical Care*, published in 1966[25] and republished in 2005,[26] Donabedian discussed three approaches to measuring quality in medicine: structure, outcomes measures, and process measures. Structure pertains to the environment of care. That is, things that are in place before the patient encounter. An effective, high-quality structure is crucial to providing quality health care, but it is challenging to correlate measurement of structural aspects of care to individual practitioner performance. The latest (2008 and 2009) CMS Physician Quality Reporting Initiative (PQRI) measure list[27] does include a structural metric. The PQRI is a CMS-sponsored incentive payment program that rewards eligible practitioners who satisfactorily report data on specific quality measures, defined by the program, for covered services furnished to Medicare beneficiaries. The 2009 PQRI measure #124 examines whether the provider has adopted and is using health information technology, including a "certified/qualified" electronic health record.

Outcomes measures examine discrete end points in health care and often focus on mortality, morbidity, and quality of life. They have been employed by various organizations ranging from the Joint Commission to such organizations as the Quality Indicator Project. The Quality Indicator Project began over 20 years ago with a group of Maryland hospitals voluntarily participating in developing metrics, measuring data pertaining to those metrics within their institutions, and sharing that data amongst the group of hospitals with the goal of improving quality of care. Example metrics from the Quality Indicator Project include unscheduled returns to the emergency department and length of stay in the emergency department.[28] Outcomes measures are not entirely practical as a yardstick for practitioner performance. Rarely is a patient outcome related solely to an individual practitioner's performance; they almost always involve an entire segment of the health care process. Outcome measures are also impractical to use because they require risk adjustment to fairly compare individual performance and also require a larger sample size than process measures.[29]

Medical care process relates to what occurs to the patient during an emergency department visit. Donabedian[26] specifically focuses on process at the level of the physician-patient interaction. He proposes that it is important to measure whether "good" care has been provided. He outlines broad categories of process, including "appropriateness, completeness and redundancy of information obtained through clinical history, physical examination and diagnostic testing; justification of diagnosis and therapy; technical competence in the performance of diagnostic and therapeutic procedures..."[26] More than 40 years ago, Donabedian realized the challenges involved in measuring process and remarked that such evaluation requires important attention to the standards employed. Because medical process evaluation examines whether medical care is properly practiced, it is a more effective tool in assessing practitioner performance than outcomes measures.[26,29]

The Joint Commission provides some general guidance regarding practice. Examples of criteria to employ in OPPE include both outcomes and process measures, examples being requests for tests and procedures and data on morbidity and mortality. Suggested methods of acquiring performance data include periodic chart review and direct observation and monitoring of diagnostic and treatment techniques.[20] Although the Joint Commission does not provide guidance on specific practitioner performance metrics in the medical staff standards, the *Specifications Manual for National Hospital Inpatient Quality Measures (Specifications Manual)*[27] contains a few measures pertinent to individual practitioner performance and a few that are relevant to emergency physicians. This manual is a result of collaboration on the part of the CMS and The Joint Commission to develop a uniform set of national hospital quality measures. Some of these measures overlap with those of the PQRI. An example of such a measure common to both is "Aspirin at arrival for acute myocardial infarction."[30]

The CMS is highly influential in promoting metrics for practice evaluation as part of the PQRI. This initiative came out of the 2006 Tax Relief and Health Act,[31] which required the establishment of a physician quality reporting system containing a pay-for-performance program. The CMS employs a list of quality measures derived through a consensus-based process. The measures are updated yearly and are available on line.[27] The CMS turns to such organizations as the NQF and the Ambulatory Care Quality Alliance[32] for consensus measures. Both endorse a set of emergency medicine measures and both outline a process for evaluating measures. The NQF process for development of the National Voluntary Consensus Standards for Emergency Care[33] includes involvement and recommendations from a variety of representatives. NQF membership is diverse and includes a heterogeneous group of health care stakeholders, including public health agencies, hospital systems, individual hospitals, professional societies, pharmaceutical companies, and health care consulting firms. The American College of Emergency Physicians is a member of NQF.[33] Recommendations are further developed through the NQF's formal Consensus Development Process.[34] The NQF measure evaluation criteria include such categories as measure importance, scientific acceptability of measure properties, usability, and feasibility.[35] The list of measures is dynamic and modified with additions and deletions annually. For instance, "Beta-Blocker at Time of Arrival for Acute Myocardial Infarction" is present on the 2007 PQRI list of measures. A 2007 update to 2004 guidelines on management of ST-elevation myocardial infarction[36] is more cautious about recommendations regarding beta-blockers in this setting and the measure was retired from the 2008 list.

The 2009 PQRI contains 153 measures in seven groups. The measure groups include diabetes, chronic kidney disease, preventive care, coronary artery bypass graft, rheumatoid arthritis, perioperative care, and back pain. However, only a portion of the listed PQRI measures is considered pertinent to emergency medicine and the focus is only on a small segment of the practice of emergency medicine. For instance, the *2007 PQRI Measure List*[37] contained 74 metrics and only 9 of them were considered pertinent to emergency medicine. A 2008 study by Glickman and colleagues[38] graded these 9 metrics according to whether they met specific criteria developed by the American College of Cardiology (ACC) and American Heart Association (AHA) Task Force on Performance Measures. This methodology was developed by the AHA/ACC for quantifying the quality of cardiovascular care.[39] Glickman found that 5 of the 9 metrics do not appear to meet all of the ACC/AHA criteria for measurement selection. He also found that several of the metrics already have such high levels of compliance on the national level as to raise doubts regarding their effectiveness as a quality improvement tool. Meanwhile, no national performance data pertains to the metric of electrocardiogram performed for nontraumatic chest pain (in patients over 40 years and older). The absence of published data is interesting because of the importance of the metric. It has been on the PQRI measure list every year since the program began. The strength of evidence supporting the measure and outcome differences (diagnosing acute ST-segment elevation myocardial infarction) is directly associated with adhering to the measure.[38]

RESEARCH IN EMERGENCY PHYSICIAN PERFORMANCE EVALUATION

Despite widespread requirements regarding the assessment of physician practice and competency, the emergence of voluntary pay-for-performance programs, and rising public interest, surprisingly little published by emergency medicine researchers in the medical peer reviewed literature has focused on performance evaluation. In a commentary published in 2006, Feldman[40] noted that a search of *MEDLINE* since 1966 yielded no reports of quality profiling at the level of the individual provider (specific to emergency medicine). A search by this author of *MEDLINE* (English language) from 1950 to the first week of March 2009, combining the MeSH (Medical Subject Headings of the National Institutes of Health) terms *benchmarking* (introduced in 1998) and *emergency medicine* yielded nine results. None of these articles was original research focusing on physician practice profiling, and there was only a single relevant review article, which was from Germany and published in an anesthesia journal.[41] A similar search combining *emergency medicine* and *outcome and process assessment (health care)* yielded 96 results. Only 1 of these results focused on profiling at the physician level and this article discussed pay for performance.[42] A search of the English-language literature from 2006 to the present combining MeSH terms *benchmarking* or *quality of health care* or *total quality management* or *quality indicators, health care* or *outcome and process assessment (health care)* with *emergency medicine* yielded 260 entries. Only 5[38,43–46] of these 260 articles were original research focusing on quality in emergency medicine and only 1 related to benchmarking emergency medicine physicians.[38] This author acknowledges that the described search overlooks some studies that are pertinent to the topic, but not mapped to the included MeSH headings. Regardless, there is considerable disparity between the large amount of work being done in the clinical setting to improve quality of care and to measure physician performance and that reported in the medical literature. Fortunately, momentum is building to stimulate and to perform high quality research in this area. Some recent research focused on critically appraising CMS measures for community-acquired pneumonia.[47] One brief report[48] focuses on CMS community-acquired pneumonia guidelines (on which measures are based) and their effect on physician prescribing patterns. The report identified a possible adverse effect of the guidelines, suggesting that, in a perceived effort to comply with the guidelines, physicians prescribe antibiotics to patients when they may not be necessary.

There is great need and opportunity for research in the area of quality in emergency medicine, including research focusing on individual physician performance. The interested reader is encouraged to review the Standards for Quality Improvement Reporting Excellence (SQUIRE) project guidelines.[49] SQUIRE aims to promote excellence in health care quality improvement literature so that articles are useable, easily discovered, and thus easily disseminated to a broader population. The SQUIRE guidelines provide an explicit framework for sharing the knowledge acquired by quality improvement efforts by examining those interventions closely, carefully, and in detail.

SUMMARY

Physician competency and clinical performance are critical components to delivery of high-quality and safe health care. Measurement of emergency physician competency and practice performance is becoming more important as a quality improvement strategy for certifying bodies and reimbursement programs. Peer review remains a component of this process, but benchmarking is evolving as a more appropriate and effective tool for this task. Emergency medicine would benefit from more research regarding measures that better reflect the scope and practice of emergency medicine. Great opportunities and challenges lie ahead for benchmarking the clinical performance of emergency medicine physicians.

REFERENCES

1. Codman EA. A study in hospital efficiency: as demonstrated by the case report of the first five years of a private hospital. Codman Hospital (Boston). Boston: Th. Todd Co; 1918.
2. Codman EA. A study in hospital efficiency: as demonstrated by the case report of the first five years of a private hospital. 1st edition. Oakbrook Terrace (IL): Joint Commission on Accreditation of Healthcare Organizations; 1996.
3. Kohn LT, Corrigan J, Donaldson MS, Institute of Medicine (U.S.), Committee on quality of health care in America. To err is human: building a safer health system. Washington, DC: National Academy Press; 1999.
4. Committee on Quality of Health Care in America of the Institute of Medicine. Crossing the quality chasm: a new health system for the 21st century. Washington, DC: National Academy Press; 2001.
5. American Board of Emergency Medicine (ABEM). What are ABEM's mission and purposes? ABEM; 2009. Available at: http://www.abem.org/PUBLIC/portal/alias__Rainbow/lang__en-US/tabID__3333/DesktopDefault.aspx#three. Accessed February 22, 2009.
6. American Board of Medical Specialties (ABMS). What board certification means. ABMS; 2008. Available at: http://www.abms.org/About_Board_Certification/means.aspx. Accessed March 9, 2009.

7. ABMS maintenance of certification. ABMS; 2008. Available at: http://www.abms.org/Maintenance_of_Certification/ABMS_MOC.aspx. Accessed March 9, 2009.
8. Accreditation Council for Graduate Medical Education (ACGME). Outcome project: general competencies; 1999. Available at: http://www.acgme.org/outcome/comp/compMin.asp. Accessed February 11, 2009.
9. Accreditation Council for Graduate Medical Education (ACGME). Outcome project: Common program requirements: general competencies. ACGME; 2007; Available at: http://www.acgme.org/outcome/comp/GeneralCompetencies-Standards21307.pdf. Accessed March 11, 2009.
10. Thomas HA, Beeson MS, Binder LS, et al. The 2005 Model of the clinical practice of emergency medicine: the 2007 update. Acad Emerg Med 2008;15(8):776–9.
11. American Board of Medical Specialties. (ABMS) MOC (Maintenance of Certification) competencies and criteria. ABMS; 2008. Available at: http://www.abms.org/Maintenance_of_Certification/MOC_competencies.aspx. Accessed March 9, 2009.
12. American Board of Emergency Medicine (ABEM). EMCC assessment of practice performance overview. ABEM; 2007 [updated 2007 May 11]. Available at: https://www.abem.org/public/portal/alias__Rainbow/lang__en-US/tabID__3802/DesktopDefault.aspx, http://www.abem.org/PUBLIC/portal/alias__Rainbow/lang__en-US/tabID__3422/DesktopDefault.aspx. Accessed March 9, 2009.
13. The public health and welfare, (Nov 14, 1986, 1986).
14. Fine DL. The medical peer review privilege in Massachusetts: a necessary quality control measure or an ineffective obstruction of equitable redress? Suffolk Univ Law Rev 2005;38(4):811–3.
15. Office of the Inspector General. Hospital reporting to the national practitioner data bank. In: Services DoHaH, editor. Washington, DC; 1995.
16. Office of the Inspector General. HHS agencies' compliance with the national practititioner data bank malpractice reporting policy, OEI-12-04-00310. In: Services DoHaH, editor. Washington, DC; 2005.
17. Scheutzow SO. State medical peer review: high cost but no benefit—is it time for a change? Am J Law Med 1999;25(1):7–60.
18. Joint Commission. Hospital accreditation requirements. MS.03.01.01[Internet] 2008; The Joint Commission E-dition v1.1.0.4. Available at: http://amp.jcrinc.com. Accessed March 15, 2009.
19. Joint Commission. Hospital accreditation requirements. MS.06.01.03[Internet] 2008; The Joint Commission E-dition v1.1.0.4. Available at: http://amp.jcrinc.com. Accessed March 15, 2009.
20. Joint Commission. Hospital accreditation requirements. MS.08.01.03[Internet] 2008; The Joint Commission E-dition v1.1.0.4. Available at: http://amp.jcrinc.com. Accessed March 15, 2009.
21. Joint Commission. Hospital accreditation requirements. MS.08.01.01[Internet] 2008; The Joint Commission E-dition v1.1.0.4. Available at: http://amp.jcrinc.com. Accessed March 21, 2009.
22. National library of medicine. Medical subject heading. 1998. Available at: http://www.ncbi.nlm.nih.gov/sites/entrez, http://www.nlm.nih.gov/cgi/mesh/2009/MB_cgi. Accessed March 10, 2009.
23. Various authors, Assuring quality in emergency care. Proceedings of the AEM 2002 Consensus Conference. Acad Emerg Med 2002;9(11):1063–212.
24. Cone DC, Nedza SM, Augustine JJ, et al. Quality in clinical practice. Acad Emerg Med 2002;9(11):1085–90.
25. Donabedian A. Evaluating the quality of medical care. Milbank Mem Fund Q 1966;44(3 Suppl):166–206.

26. Donabedian A. Evaluating the quality of medical care. 1966. Milbank Q 2005; 83(4):691–729.
27. Centers for Medicare & Medicaid Services. Physician quality reporting initiative, measures/codes. 2009. Available at: http://www.cms.hhs.gov/PQRI/15_MeasuresCodes.asp#TopOfPage. Accessed March 15, 2009.
28. Quality Indicator Project. Acute care indicators. Maryland Hospital Association; 2009. Available at: http://www.qiproject.org/pdf/Acute_Care_Indicators.pdf. Accessed March 15, 2009.
29. Graff L, Stevens C, Spaite D, et al. Measuring and improving quality in emergency medicine. Acad Emerg Med 2002;9(11):1091–107.
30. Joint Commission and Centers for Medicare & Medicaid Services. The specifications manual for national hospital quality measures, version 2.5b. 2008. Available at: http://www.jointcommission.org/performancemeasurement/performancemeasurement/current+nhqm+manual.htm, http://qualitynet.org/dcs/ContentServer?c=Page&pagename=QnetPublic%2FPage%2FQnetTier3&cid=1221491528970. Accessed March 15, 2009.
31. Tax Relief and Health Care Act, Pub. L. No. Division B, Title I Medicare improved quality and provider payments (Dec 8, 2006, 2006).
32. Ambulatory Care Quality Alliance (AQA). Performance measurement workgroup, AQA; 2005. Available at: http://www.aqaalliance.org/performancewg.htm. Accessed March 20, 2009.
33. National Quality Forum (NQF). National voluntary consensus standards for emergency care. Available at: http://www.qualityforum.org/projects/ongoing/emergency/. Accessed March 15, 2009.
34. National Quality Forum (NQF). National Quality Forum members. NQF; 2008. Available at: http://www.qualityforum.org/pdf/list_of_members.pdf. Accessed June 29, 2009.
35. National Quality Forum (NQF) 2008. Measure evaluation criteria. NQF. Available at:http://www.qualityforum.org/about/leadership/measure_evaluation.asp. Accessed March 15, 2009.
36. Antman EM, Hand M, Armstrong PW, et al. 2007 Focused update of the ACC/AHA 2004 Guidelines for the Management of Patients with ST-Elevation Myocardial Infarction: a report of the American College of Cardiology/American Heart Association Task Force on Practice Guidelines: developed in collaboration with the Canadian Cardiovascular Society endorsed by the American Academy of Family Physicians: 2007 Writing Group to review new evidence and update the ACC/AHA 2004 Guidelines for the management of patients with ST-elevation myocardial infarction, writing on behalf of the 2004 Writing Committee. Circulation 2008;117(2):296–329.
37. Centers for Medicare & Medicaid Services. 2007 physician quality reporting initiative (PQRI) physician quality measures. 2007. Available at: http://www.cms.hhs.gov/PQRI/33_2007_PQRI_Program.asp#TopOfPage. Accessed March 15, 2009.
38. Glickman SW, Schulman KA, Peterson ED, et al. Evidence-based perspectives on pay for performance and quality of patient care and outcomes in emergency medicine. Ann Emerg Med 2008;51(5):622–31.
39. Spertus JA, Eagle KA, Krumholz HM, et al. American College of Cardiology and American Heart Association methodology for the selection and creation of performance measures for quantifying the quality of cardiovascular care. Circulation 2005;111(13):1703–12.
40. Feldman JA. Quality-of-care measures in emergency medicine: When will they come? What will they look like? Acad Emerg Med 2006;13(9):980–2.

41. Francis RCE, Spies CD, Kerner T. Quality management and benchmarking in emergency medicine. Curr Opin Anaesthesiol 2008;21(2):233–9.
42. Sikka R. Pay for performance in emergency medicine. Ann Emerg Med 2007; 49(6):756–61.
43. Fee C, Weber EJ. Identification of 90% of patients ultimately diagnosed with community-acquired pneumonia within four hours of emergency department arrival may not be feasible. Ann Emerg Med 2007;49(5):553–9.
44. Griffey RT, Bohan JS. Healthcare provider complaints to the emergency department: a preliminary report on a new quality improvement instrument. Qual Saf Health Care 2006;15(5):344–6.
45. Pham JC, Kelen GD, Pronovost PJ. National study on the quality of emergency department care in the treatment of acute myocardial infarction and pneumonia. Acad Emerg Med 2007;14(10):856–63.
46. Wright SW, Trott A, Lindsell CJ, et al. Evidence-based emergency medicine. Creating a system to facilitate translation of evidence into standardized clinical practice: a preliminary report. Ann Emerg Med 2008;51(1):80–6, 86, e81–8.
47. Yu KT, Wyer PC. Evidence-based emergency medicine/critically appraised topic. Evidence behind the 4-hour rule for initiation of antibiotic therapy in community-acquired pneumonia. Ann Emerg Med 2008;51(5):651–62, 662, e651–2.
48. Nicks BA, Manthey DE, Fitch MT. The Centers for Medicare and Medicaid Services (CMS) community-acquired pneumonia core measures lead to unnecessary antibiotic administration by emergency physicians. Acad Emerg Med 2009;16(2):184–7.
49. Davidoff F, Batalden P, Stevens D, et al. Publication guidelines for improvement studies in health care: evolution of the SQUIRE Project. Ann Intern Med 2008; 149(9):670–6.

Triage, EMTALA, Consultations, and Prehospital Medical Control

Paul A. Testa, MD, JD, MPH[a,*], Maureen Gang, MD[a,b]

KEYWORDS

• Triage • EMTALA • Stabilize • Transfer • On-call
• Medical control • EMS

The Emergency Medical Treatment and Active Labor Act (EMTALA, or the Act,)[1] although on its face narrow in scope and brief in language, serves as a near universal prelude to every patient interaction emergency medicine physicians have within an emergency department (ED). It is not the Act itself that suggests such breadth. Rather, in its brevity it brought forth such expanse. The resulting efforts by courts, regulators, physicians, and the multitudes that intercede between them to interpret, comply, and enforce the Act have spawned voluminous regulations, opinions, and treatises.[2] Likewise, the provision of timely and appropriate medical care to patients presenting to the ED is a tenet of emergency medicine. The process of triage is often the first evaluative examination of a patient, but it is not uncommon for the emergency physician to have stewarded the care of a patient before arrival by remote medical control of prehospital emergency services. Each of these functions (medical control of prehospital emergency services, triage, and the undertaking of obligations under EMTALA) raise issues of liability and capability that need be explored in the context of patient care within every ED.

TRIAGE: THE EMERGENCY SEVERITY INDEX

As EDs have become increasingly crowded, there is significant risk that seriously ill patients may not be seen in a timely fashion. Patients pending evaluation may become discouraged by long wait times, and leave the ED without assessment of their complaints. Such scenarios may impact negatively on patient outcomes. The

[a] Department of Emergency Medicine, New York University School of Medicine, Bellevue Hospital Center, 462 First Avenue, OBV A342, New York, NY 10016, USA
[b] Emergency Department, Tisch Hospital, NYU Langone Medical Center, 560 First Avenue, New York, NY 10016, USA
* Corresponding author.
E-mail address: paul.testa@nyumc.org (P.A. Testa).

Emerg Med Clin N Am 27 (2009) 627–640
doi:10.1016/j.emc.2009.07.011 emed.theclinics.com
0733-8627/09/$ – see front matter

challenge to the triage nurse is to identify patients requiring more immediate intervention from those who can better afford to wait for medical assessment.

The emergency severity index was developed in 1998 and since then has had multiple revisions.[3] Endorsed by both the Emergency Nurses Associations and the American College of Emergency Physicians, the emergency severity index is a five-level triage tool that stratifies patients into groups based on both clinical symptoms and signs, and consideration of resources needed for patient evaluation and stabilization. Patients triaged into acuity category 1 (most urgent) are those who require significant departmental resources (staff, procedures, medications, laboratories, radiographs) for stabilization, whereas those placed in acuity class 5 (least urgent) require minimal treatment interventions.

The emergency severity index has been shown to be highly reproducible, with good interrater and intrarater reliability, although data are not as supportive for the pediatric infant population.[4] It has been shown accurately to represent the true acuity of the patient, with those assigned a lower acuity rarely requiring hospital admission. For those older than 65, the tool has been shown to correlate well with need for hospitalization, resource use, and 1-year survival.[5] With proper application, such consistency encourages EMTALA compliance, ensuring that patients presenting with similar medical complaints and conditions are assigned the requisite medical screening examination (MSE) in order of their potential for a life-threatening emergency medical condition in a nondiscriminatory manner.

The EMTALA mandate that hospitals consistently treat patients with similar medical complaints in a comparable manner may be tested when surge capacity is reached for patient care. During the swine flu epidemic of April and May 2009, EDs in New York reported registering up to three times the number of patients usually evaluated on a daily basis. Although these patients were triaged in the ED facilities, the MSEs were completed by licensed health care providers in sites other than the main EDs. Although not tested, it is believed that as long as the patients are evaluated within the hospital facility, the hospital remains EMTALA compliant.

EMTALA: DUTIES AND LIABILITIES

EMTALA effectively creates two sets of duties: the medical screening of nearly all patients, and duties pertaining to stabilization and transfer or acceptance of a patient with an emergency medical condition.[6,7]

The MSE

It is the obligation of all practicing emergency medicine physicians to, "maintain knowledge of and compliance with major federal and state regulations that affect the practice of emergency medicine, such as the Emergency Medical Treatment and Active Labor Act,"[8] which states:

> *In the case of a hospital that has a hospital emergency department, if any individual ... comes to the emergency department and a request is made ... for examination or treatment for a medical condition, the hospital must provide for an appropriate medical screening examination within the capability of the hospital's emergency department, including ancillary services routinely available to the emergency department, to determine whether or not an emergency medical condition exists*[9]

A duty is owed to any individual who "comes to the ED" and requests treatment, to provide for an appropriate MSE to determine whether or not an emergency medical condition exists.[10] The outcome of the MSE is binary: does or does not an emergency medical condition exist.[11]

The purpose of the Act is to protect patients with a medical emergency from discharge or transfer from an ED without a proper screening examination and stabilization of their condition because of economic concerns.[12] "A participating hospital may not delay provision of an appropriate medical screening examination ... or further medical examination and treatment required [by the Act] to inquire about the individual's method of payment or insurance status."[13]

Courts are well settled that by intent and design, EMTALA was set forth to discourage hospitals from patient dumping, failing to provide medical screening, or transferring or discharging patients based on patient's financial status.[14] The MSE requirement is a duty not to discriminate.[15] Although EMTALA applies to all patients rather than solely indigent patients, courts have settled the vagueness of the phrase "appropriate medical screening" to be that screening a hospital would have offered to any paying patient.[16] Provisions of EMTALA are not purely for the benefit of uninsured persons; EMTALA applies to any and all patients.[17]

EMTALA does not define "appropriate medical screening." All presenting patients are entitled to receive medical screening calculated to identify critical medical conditions. This screening must be similar to that which is provided for any other patient with similar complaints.[12] Under the Act, the only acceptable way to assess for an emergency medical condition is by conducting an appropriate MSE.[18] It need be made clear that triage is not a MSE but rather triage serves only to control the order in which patients are seen based on the nature of their presentation. The determination of the existence of an emergency medical condition cannot be made by the triage of patients.

It is generally accepted that a MSE must contain, at a minimum, the following[19]:

- Maintenance of and entry into a log, including disposition
- Triage record
- Ongoing vital signs
- Physical examination
- esting used and results obtained
- If on-call consultants were involved in the evaluation
- Documentation of all such data listed

Failing to uniformly follow screening procedures supports finding of EMTALA liability for disparate treatment by a hospital.[20] A plaintiff must allege that he or she went to the ED seeking treatment, and that he or she was not screened in the same way all others are screened.[21]

Hospitals are required to apply uniform screening procedures to all individuals coming to the ED.[22] In its own Policy Statement on the matter, the American College of Emergency Physicians states[23]:

- Emergency departments should have a standardized process to ensure that patients presenting for medical care receive an appropriate MSE by a qualified medical person
- The examiner should be designated by hospital bylaws, rules, and regulations
- Appropriate medical treatment should be provided for emergency medical conditions, as is required by the EMTALA

The MSE must be done so as to be reasonably likely to diagnose critical medical conditions. The Act does not create a federal medical malpractice claim.[24] Faulty screening alone does not violate the Act, whereas nonuniform screening does.[25,26]

The appropriateness of an MSE is usually not judged by its diagnostic accuracy, but rather by its equitable implementation as compared with other patients with similar symptoms.[27] Evidence that a hospital did not follow its own screening procedures supports finding of EMTALA liability for disparate treatment.[20]

The Act and subsequent interpretation recognizes and allows for the specifics of an MSE to vary in accordance with unique capabilities of specific hospitals but not for specific patients.[22] The Act also allows reasonable registration procedures in the ED as long as they do not result in a delay in performing the screening examination or treatment.[28]

Potential Issues Related to the MSE

The requirements of the Act apply to dedicated EDs.[29] A dedicated ED is one that is licensed by the state as an ED, offered to the public as an ED, or provided one third of its visits on an urgent basis without requiring a previously scheduled appointment over the previous year.[30] The Act is generally considered to cover most hospital property.[31] EMTALA applies when a person requesting evaluation or care enters the campus with few exceptions. The term "hospital property" means the entire main hospital campus, including parking lots, sidewalks, and driveways of hospital departments, including a buffer of outdoor space within 250 yards of the hospital.[32]

The Act specifies the MSE may only be performed by a physician or "qualified medical personnel" who must be approved as qualified by the medical staff in accordance with a hospital's medical staff bylaws or the medical staff rules and regulations.[33] An individual functioning as qualified medical personnel must be acting within the scope of his or her license. There must be a job description for their role with established qualifications and competencies, and the formal designation as qualified medical personnel needs to be within their personnel records. The hospital must maintain a written protocol defining the authorized functions and setting forth when a patient is considered beyond the nonphysician, qualified medical personnel's' scope of practice.[34] With this requirement, the Act essentially allows a hospital to deem certain patients too ill to be screened by anyone other than a physician.

All patients presenting to the dedicated ED seeking treatment must be recorded in a patient log that archives presentation and disposition. The log must indicate whether these individuals refuse treatment, were denied treatment, were treated, were admitted, were stabilized, were transferred, or were discharged.[35]

It is the position of the American College of Emergency Physicians, under the Act, that a minor must be examined and stabilized, or if needed, transferred to another hospital for emergency care without prior consent being obtained from a guardian. If no emergency medical condition is identified during the MSE, then efforts should be made to obtain consent for care.[36] Prior to that determination, the MSE is not to be delayed.

The duties arising from the Act end when the patient is formally admitted to the hospital,[37] even if those formally admitted patients never leave the dedicated ED ("boarded patients") for an inpatient bed elsewhere in the hospital. As defined, such patients are determined to be inpatients, and the duties contained within the Act no longer apply.[38] A hospital cannot evade its obligations under the Act,[10] however, by admitting the patient without intent to treat but rather to discharge or transfer without stabilization.[39]

Stabilizing and Transfer Under EMTALA

Courts, relying on the legislative history of the statute, have held that Congress did not intend to provide a guarantee of the result of ED treatment,[40] only compliance with the twin duties of the MSE, and subsequently stabilization and possible transfer. It is the clinical determination of the finding of an emergency medical condition that triggers the duty, under the Act, to stabilize and potentially transfer. The Act reads:

> *If any individual ... comes to a hospital and the hospital determines that the individual has an emergency medical condition, the hospital must provide either:*
> *(A) within the staff and facilities available at the hospital, for such further medical examination and such treatment as may be required to stabilize the medical condition, or*
> *(B) for transfer of the individual to another medical facility*[41]
> *(if you do not have the capacity to stabilize the emergency medical condition at your facility).*

An "emergency medical condition" is such a condition that for which the absence of immediate medical attention could reasonably be expected to result in placing the health of the individual in serious jeopardy, serious impairment to bodily functions, or serious dysfunction of any bodily organ or part.[29] Severe pain and active labor fall within this definition.

"To stabilize" a patient with an emergency medical condition means, "to assure, within reasonable medical probability, that no material deterioration of the condition is to result from or occur during the transfer of the individual[.]"[42] Once a patient has been stabilized there are no further obligations under the Act. Likewise, the duty to stabilize a patient does not arise until an emergency medical condition is detected.[43]

The statutory definition of "stabilize" is one of a flexible standard of reasonableness that is dependent on context.[44] The standard is one of stabilization, not recovery or cure[45] much less alleviation of an emergency condition.[46] If determined to have been stabilized, an incorrect diagnosis does not give rise to liability under the Act.[47,48]

If the patient cannot be stabilized by the emergency physician, there are two options under the Act: consult the appropriate specialist from the hospital's mandatory on-call panel for stabilizing treatment; or, if no specialist is available or the facilities inadequate, transfer the patient to a facility that can provide stabilizing care.[18] "Transfer" includes moving the patient to an outside facility or their discharge.[49] The Act's obligations must be read together, and for a hospital to be liable under requirements pertaining to stabilization and transfer, an emergency medical condition must have been predetermined to exist.[50]

A patient determined by a MSE to have an emergency medical condition cannot be transferred until stabilized unless[51]

- *a physician... has signed a certification that, the medical benefits reasonably expected from the provision of appropriate medical treatment at another facility outweigh the increased risks ... from effecting transfer, or*
- *if a physician is not physically present ... a qualified medical person ... has signed a certification ... after a physician in consultation with the person, has made[the similar] the determination;*
  ...and the transfer is an "appropriate transfer"

Essentially, an appropriate transfer is one in which the receiving facility has available space and qualified personnel for the treatment of the individual, and has agreed to accept transfer of the individual and to provide appropriate medical treatment.[52] It only need be shown that the transfer was inappropriate under the terms of the Act, not that there was inappropriate motive for the transfer.[53]

In considering transfer of the stable versus the unstable patient, under the Act, if the patient can be stabilized at the hospital where the patient presents, then the patient cannot be transferred, excluding a patient request for transfer. When a patient cannot be stabilized under the terms of the Act because of lack of capability or capacity, the emergency physician may secure an "appropriate transfer" if the risk-benefit analysis weighs in favor of the transfer and is in the patient's best interest. This is a permissive option under the statute and is short of an affirmative duty transfer, which has been ruled by at least one court not to exist.[54]

Specialized Facilities and a Duty to Transfer

It is well established that a hospital may also be fined under the Act for its failure to accept an appropriate transfer if it has the staff and equipment to treat the patient.[29] Furthermore, specialized facilities retain special obligations[55]:

> *A participating hospital that has specialized capabilities or facilities (such as burn units, shock-trauma units, neonatal intensive care units, or (with respect to rural areas) regional referral centers ... shall not refuse to accept an appropriate transfer of an individual who requires such specialized capabilities if the hospital has the capacity to treat the individual.*

This obligation is independent of whether or not the receiving hospital has a dedicated ED. This is often referred to colloquially as the "reverse dumping" provision of the Act.[56]

Recent changes to the Transfer Law made final in 2009 clarify the "specialized care" transfer acceptance requirements as applied to inpatients.[57] Once an individual is admitted in good faith, the admitting hospital has satisfied its obligation under the Act with respect to that individual, even if the individual remains unstable.[58] A hospital with specialized capabilities does not have an EMTALA obligation to accept an appropriate transfer of that admitted individual. Specifically, §489.24(f)(2) states, "The provisions of this paragraph (f) do not apply to an individual who has been admitted to a referring hospital under the provisions of paragraph (d)(2)(i) of this section." The Interpretive Guidelines for §489.24(f) clearly state that a recipient hospital's obligations do not extend to inpatients of another hospital. A specialized hospital cannot be cited for violating EMTALA if it refuses to accept the transfer of an inpatient from a referring hospital.[59] A specialized hospital may accept in transfer inpatients that require evaluation or treatment that is not available at the referring hospital.

It is the position of Centers for Medicare and Medicaid Services, however, that this rule does not apply to patients who are protected under EMTALA, such as those placed in observation status rather than admitted as inpatients. These patients are deemed outpatients even if they occupy a bed overnight.[59]

SPECIALTY CONSULTATIONS UNDER EMTALA

Hospitals are required to maintain a list of on-call physicians for "duty after the initial examination to provide treatment necessary to stabilize an individual with an emergency medical condition."[60] The on-call list requirement is not part of EMTALA but rather is found within the general provider agreement requirement for a hospital's participation in the Medicare program.[61] The on-call list requirement applies not only to hospitals with dedicated EDs, but to all hospitals subject to EMTALA requirements to accept appropriate transfers.[62] The on-call list should be composed so as to[63]

> *...provide services to the meet the needs of their community in accordance with the resources they have available ... [and] ... to provide adequate specialty on-call*

coverage consistent with the services provided at the hospital and the resources the hospital has available.

EMTALA incorporates the on-call list by extending the second duty of stabilization to on-call specialty physicians. Specifically[64]

If ... a physician determines that the individual requires the services of ... the on-call physician and the on-call physician fails or refuses to appear within a reasonable period of time, and the physician orders the transfer of the individual because the physician determines that without the services of the on-call physician the benefits of transfer outweigh the risks of transfer, the physician authorizing the transfer shall not be subject to a penalty ... However, the previous sentence shall not apply to the hospital or to the on-call physician who failed or refused to appear.

EMTALA provides the enforcement mechanism, "against both a physician and a hospital when a physician who is on the hospital's on-call list fails or refuses to appear within a reasonable period of time."[59] If a physician is on a hospital's on-call list, has been requested by the treating physician to appear at the hospital, and fails or refuses to appear within a reasonable period of time "...then the hospital and the on-call physician may be subject to sanctions for violation of the EMTALA statutory requirements."[59] That does not mean EMTALA precludes a treating physician in an ED from consulting with a physician who is on the on-call list, although the consultant may not be physically present in the ED.

It can be reasonably suggested that there lacks a broad understanding of the full scope of the responsibilities of on-call physicians under EMTALA.[65] Not infrequently an on-call physician, despite a request, refuses to appear as obligated under the Act.[66] When a patient is transferred to another hospital as a result of the failure or refusal of an on-call physician to respond, the Act requires that the on-call physician's name be reported to the receiving facility. The receiving facility then must report any suspicion of a violation.[67] If the transferring emergency medicine physician, in such a circumstance, undertakes reasonable efforts to gain the appearance of the on-call physician who is failing or refusing physically to come to the ED, the on-call physician and the hospital, not the emergency physician, is liable under the Act.[64] What constitutes reasonable efforts on the part of the emergency staff to secure the appearance of an on-call physician varies with the circumstances.[68] The emergency medicine physician's effort is compared retrospectively with the standard of care for ED physicians similarly situated. Such efforts as contacting the on-call physician's department chair or the hospital's chief of staff so as to produce the on-call physician are often suggested to be the sort of effort the emergency physician should undertake before affecting transfer.[18]

Neither the Act nor its Interpretive Guidelines set forth what is a reasonable response time for on-call physicians to appear in an ED. Rather, the Interpretive Guidelines state[69]

...expected response time should be stated in minutes in the hospitals policies. Terms such as "reasonable" or "prompt" are not enforceable by the hospital and therefore inappropriate in defining physician's response time.

There is an obvious risk created by a hospital setting a "30-minute" rule in its medical staff bylaws, because a failure to appear with the predetermined time by the on-call physician if only by minutes could be construed as an EMTALA violation by both the on-call physician and the hospital.

It has been held that an on-call physician owes a legal duty to patients in the ED despite never directly treating the patients.[70] The duty is to provide to hospital personnel reasonable notice along with the name of one's replacement if one is the on-call physician but unable to fulfill on-call obligations. This is not recognition of a physician-patient relationship but rather a finding of general negligence by an on-call physician in addition to a violation under EMTALA.

Like so much of the Act, concise language masks a complex sharing of obligations and duty, which has led to a large body of case law and regulations, in the absence of clarity of enforcing guidance. Despite such a mandate, there has historically been tremendous difficulty maintaining on-call specialty physician coverage for EDs.[71] An effort was made in 2003 to make on-call requirements more flexible in the hopes of facilitating greater on-call participation. The 2003 rules permit on-call physicians to schedule some elective surgery during the time they are on call and permitting simultaneous on-call duties.[72]

Many hospitals have starting offering payment to physicians for taking call responsibilities, something the Act does not explicitly preclude. One statewide survey found 43% of hospitals pay a per diem stipend to at least a single specialty, and 31% of hospitals guarantee pay for uninsured patients treated while on-call.[73] On a national level, a survey done by the American College of Emergency Physicians found 36% of respondents to be paying a per diem stipend for on-call coverage.[74] Although permissible, the practice of per diem stipends alters none of the Act's obligations for a hospital or on-call physician including arranging back up if the on-call physician is unable to come to the ED, and the same standard applied with regard to reasonable response time.[75]

Similarly, hospitals may enter into a contract with a physician group so as to secure on-call coverage. Although that is permissible under the Act, only a physician, not a group, may be listed on the on-call list. The State Operating Manual explicitly states that, "[p]hysician group names are not acceptable for identifying the on-call physician. Individual physician names are to be identified on the list."[76]

In 2009, additional changes were implemented that permit participation in formal community call plans among geographically grouped hospitals.[77] A community call plan substantively requires[78]

- A clear delineation of on-call coverage responsibilities, when each hospital is responsible for on-call coverage (for a specific time period, or for a specific service)
- A description of the specific geographic area to which the plan applies
- Assurances that any local and regional emergency medical system protocol formally includes information on community on-call arrangements
- A statement specifying that even if an individual arrives at a hospital that is not designated as the on-call hospital, that hospital still has an obligation to provide a MSE and stabilizing treatment within its capability, and that hospitals participating in the community call plan must abide by the regulations governing appropriate transfers

Participation in a community call plan in no way abridges the duties owed a presenting patient under EMTALA.[79] Given the newness of this option, there is little explicit guidance for implementation beyond the Interpretive Guidelines for §489.20(r)(2) and §489.24(j),[75] which clearly state "...hospitals participating in the community call plan are not relieved of their recipient hospital obligations to accept appropriate transfers from hospitals not participating in the plan."

Hospitals must fulfill all duties under the Act pertaining to transfer of patient irrespective of participating in a formal community call plan. As evidenced by the pressure for these stepwise efforts, including payment for on-call responsibilities, contracting with physician groups and community call plans, one of the most pressing challenges to the provision of patient care under the Act is ensuring appropriate, responsive on-call specialty care for the ED.

MEDICAL CONTROL: THE LIABILITY OF EMERGENCY PHYSICIANS WHEN MANAGING PREHOSPITAL PATIENTS

The role of emergency physicians in prehospital medical control, both hospital-based and by emergency medical service telemetry centers, continues to expand with implementation of standards of expedited intervention for such conditions as stroke or myocardial ischemia. Prehospital medical control is a well-established responsibility for many emergency physicians.[80] Prehospital medical control by a physician is mandated for EMS in nearly all states. As such, medical control physicians provide treatment guidance without on-scene presence in both real-time and crafting treatment algorithms for on-location providers.[81] There is, nonetheless, scant literature reviewing civil court action relating to risk management and professional liability of medical control by emergency physicians.

With near uniformity, the few published reviews of cases against emergency medical services note a surprisingly small percentage of all cases that actually name the physician providing remote medical control as a codefendant.[82,83] More commonly, hospitals, police departments, or officers and governmental entities are codefendants with an emergency medical system (EMS.) In one review of 86 cases brought against EMSs, only four listed physicians who had direct involvement with the treatment rendered.[82] Another similar review of 76 cases brought against EMSs found physicians named as codefendants in only three of the cases, with one of those cases caused by a motor vehicle accident involving ambulance transport, not direct patient care.[83]

A frequent demand placed on the medical control emergency physician is determination of when a prehospital patient has capacity to refuse care from or transport by emergency medical services. Emergency medical service providers frequently encounter patients with low acuity or who do not consent to transport. Although the basic determination of capacity is one similar to that conducted within an ED, there is the profound limitation with the physician not being on-scene. Furthermore, one may argue the invasion of the personal liberty in transport against consent compared with treatment of the same is a smaller harm and as such might be seen in a more permissive light. Weighing patient autonomy with what is often an assessment-by-proxy of capacity remains a legal and ethical challenge to physicians providing medical control.[84] Although attempts have been made to implement decision tools for these scenarios, the assessment of capacity at a distance is fraught with the potential of the withdrawal of care from a compromised patient.[85] A duty to treat while transporting a patient with an active medical condition and the incapacity to make a decision is well supported.[84] When in doubt, the emergency physician should authorize patient transfer to the hospital.

Varying between jurisdictions is the issue of whether EMTALA attaches and may be violated by a physician providing remote medical control and directing an ambulance with an incoming patient away from their own ED.[86] Some courts when interpreting EMTALA require either a patient's physical presence in the ED, or at least the hospital's premises, before EMTALA and the duties therein are imposed.[87] Others, however, more broadly interpret the EMTALA's use of the phrase "comes to the ED."[88] Similarly, the Department of Health and Human Services by way of Centers for Medicare and Medicaid Services interprets that statutory phrase broadly to include not just the ED itself, but all hospital property (sidewalks, outlying facilities, and ambulances) so that once a patient seeking medical treatment presents at any facility or vehicle owned or operated by the hospital, they have "come to" the ED.[89,90,91]

Appellate courts have rarely recognized claims of common-law negligence arising from remote medical control and communications by emergency medicine physicians of in-field EMS staff.[80] This is logical under common-law; because no duty is defined, no abrogation can be found to support a cause for negligence. One review of published cases identified only eight reported cases. Although all eight named a hospital, EMS company, or EMS field staff, only three named the emergency medicine physician acting as medical control and none found against said physician. Only one of the cases involved actual medical advice. Rather, the bulk of these few cases turn on a duty of due care determined to be a duty not to unreasonably transport.[80] The reported cases serve to further limit this duty in consideration of treatment capability of the involved hospital and the patient's consent.

Despite often-raised concerns of liability and litigation by physicians functioning as medical control there remains little published review of actual civil litigation against such physicians.[83] Recognized and established sovereign immunity, emergency medical care immunity, and Good Samaritan immunity have been relied on to intercede between the medical control agent and the civil court system.[82] The scope of these protections varies widely from jurisdiction to jurisdiction. Additionally, acts determined to be grossly negligent, raised as civil rights violations or charged under criminal code, are not sheltered by such immunities.[82]

One cannot infer, from the near absence of reported legal cases, an absence of legal risk. Remote medical control by emergency medicine physicians of EMS providers clearly raises the risk of personal legal liability. If past reported claims inform the future of potential risk, the bulk of such risk comes from decisions pertaining to diversion and hospital bypass, not medical advice or remote stewardship of care. Recognizing biases in claims reported, the emergency medicine physician has faced and will continue to face legal liability arising from transport issues and medical judgment.

SUMMARY

Medical control of prehospital emergency services, triage in the ED, and the dual duties within EMTALA challenge emergency medicine physicians with both statutory obligations and liabilities. Each independently may seem to present a definable boundary of liability for the practitioner. Under EMTALA, the sequential duties of the MSE and subsequent stabilization or transfer are confounded by the potential for tremendous sanction for a mechanistic violation. Nevertheless, the true obligation is to provide appropriate care to all who present to the ED and not simply weigh the totality of risk to the emergency medicine physician.

REFERENCES

1. 42 USCS § 1395dd.
2. Lee. An EMTALA primer: the impact of changes in the emergency medicine landscape on EMTALA compliance and enforcement. 13 Ann Health L 145, Winter 2004.
3. Gilboy N, Tanabe P, Travers DA, et al. Emergency severity index, version 4: implementation handbook, agency for healthcare research and quality. Rockville (MD): AHRQ; 2005. Publication No. 05-0046-2.

4. Hinrichs J, et al. 324-C Research Paper Presentation III: changing your practice 7. Emergency severity index intra-and inter-rater reliability in an infant sample: a pilot quality study. J Emerg Nurs 2005;31(5):427.
5. Baumann M, Strout T. Triage of geriatric patients in the emergency department: validity and survival with the emergency severity index. Ann Emerg Med 2007; 49(2):234–40.
6. Magruder v Jasper County Hosp. 243 F Supp 2d 886 (2003, ND Ind).
7. Moy MM. EMTALA answer book. University of Chicago (IL); 2009.
8. American College of Emergency Physicians Policy Statements: emergency physician rights and responsibilities. Ann Emerg Med 2008;52:187–8.
9. 42 USCS § 1395dd (a).
10. Moses v Providence Hosp. & Med. Ctrs., Inc, (2009, 6th Cir.) 561 F.3d 573.
11. Thornton v Sw. Detroit Hosp., (1990, 6th Cir.) 895 F.2d 1131, 1134.
12. Harry v Marchant, (2001, CA11 Fla) 237 F3d 1315, 14 FLW Fed C 326, vacated, reh, en banc, gr (2001, CA11 Fla) 259 F3d 1310, 14 FLW Fed C 1061 and en banc, reinstated, in part, mod, in part (2002, CA11 Fla) 291 F3d 767, 15 FLW Fed C 590.
13. 42 USCS § 1395dd (h).
14. Burton v William Beaumont Hosp. (2005, ED Mich) 373 F Supp 2d 707.
15. Bitterman RA. EMTALA and the ethical delivery of hospital emergency services. Emerg Med Clin North Am 2006;24:557–77.
16. Cleland v Bronson Health Care Group (1990, CA6 Mich) 917 F2d 266, reh den, en banc (1990, CA6).
17. Arrington v Wong 237 F3d 1066 (2001, CA9 Hawaii).
18. Perth HA. The Emergency Medical Treatment and Active Labor Act (EMTALA): guidelines for compliance. Emerg Med Clin North Am 2004;22:225–40.
19. Moy MM. EMTALA answer book. University of Chicago. 2009 edition. Illinois: Aspen Publishing; 2009. p.1–7.
20. Battle v Memorial Hosp. (2000, CA5 Miss) 228 F3d 544, 54 Fed Rules Evid Serv 1364, 47 FR Serv 3d 1073, reh den, reh, en banc, den (2000, CA5 Miss) 237 F3d 633.
21. Brenord v Catholic Med. Ctr. of Brooklyn & Queens, Inc. (2001, ED NY) 133 F Supp 2d 179.
22. Phillips v Hillcrest Med. Ctr. (2001, CA10 Okla) 244 F3d 790, 2001 Colo J C A R 1643, cert den (2002) 535 US 905, 152 L Ed 2d 142, 122 S Ct 1203 and reh den (2002) 535 US 1043, 152 L Ed 2d 666, 122 S Ct 1811.
23. American College of Emergency Physicians Policy Statements: medical screening of emergency department patients. Ann Emerg Med 2006;48:510.
24. Colon v Hosp. Dr. Pila (2004, DC Puerto Rico) 330 F Supp 2d 38.
25. Correa v Hospital San Francisco (1995, CA1 Puerto Rico) 69 F3d 1184, 33 FR Serv 3d 884, cert den (1996) 517 US 1136, 134 L Ed 2d 547, 116 S Ct 1423 and (criticized in Broughton v St. John Health Sys. (2003, ED Mich) 246 F Supp 2d 764).
26. Cohen B. Disentangling EMTALA from Medical Malpractice: Revising EMTALA's Screening Standard To Differentiate Between Ordinary Negligence and Discriminatory Denials of Care. 82 Tul. L. Rev. 645–92 (December, 2007).
27. Marshall v East Carroll Parish Hosp. Serv. Dist. (1998, CA5 La) 134 F3d 319, 40 FR Serv 3d 181.
28. US Department of Health and Human Services, Centers for Medicare and Medicaid Services, Medicare Program Clarifying policies related to the responsibilities of Medicare-participating hospitals in treating individuals with emergency medical conditions: final rule. 68 Federal Register 53222 (2003).

29. Teshome G, Closson FT. Emergency medical treatment and labor act: the basics and other medicolegal concerns. Pediatr Clin North Am 2006;53(1):139–55.
30. CFR 489.24(b).
31. Strickler J. EMTALA: the basics Jona's healthcare law, ethics, and regulation. 2006;8(3):77–81, 78.
32. US Department Health and Human Services, Centers for Medicare and Medicaid Services. Medicare Medicaid state operations manual, app. V interpretive guidelines – responsibilities of Medicare participating hospitals in emergency cases Tag A406 rev. March 6, 2009.
33. USCS § 1395dd (9a).
34. Cfr CH. IV Section 489.24.
35. US Department Health and Human Services, Centers for Medicare and Medicaid Services. Medicare Medicaid state operations manual, app. V interpretive guidelines – responsibilities of Medicare participating hospitals in emergency cases, part i – investigative procedures.
36. Bitterman RA. The medical screening examination requirement. In: Bitterman RA, editor. Providing emergency care under federal law: EMTALA: with new supplement. Dallas (TX): American College of Emergency Physicians; 2000. p. 25.
37. 42 C.F.R. §489.24(a); 68 Fed. Reg. 53,221–53264 (Sept. 9, 2003).
38. Bitterman RA. EMTALA ends once patient is admitted to the hospital. ED legal letter. Nov 1, 2008 pNA.
39. Bryant v Adventist Health System/West (2002, CA9 Cal) 289 F3d 1162.
40. Cleland v. Bronson Health Care Group, Inc., (1990, 6th Cir.) 917 F.2d 266.
41. 42 USCS § 1395dd (b).
42. USCS §1395dd(e)(3)(A).
43. Jackson v E. Bay Hosp. (2001, CA9 Cal) 246 F3d 1248.
44. Cherukuri v Shalala (1999, CA6) 175 F3d 446, 1999 FED App 160P.
45. Thornton v Southwest Detroit Hosp. (1990, CA6 Mich) 895 F2d 1131, 104 ALR Fed 157
46. Brooker v Desert Hosp. Corp. (1991, CA9 Cal) 947 F2d 412, 91 CDOS 8381, 91
47. Fisher by Fisher v New York Health & Hosps. Corp. (1998, ED NY) 989 F Supp 444.
48. Gundavaram H. Recent Developments in Health Law: American Journal of Law & Medicine and Harvard Law & Health Care Society: EMTALA: Screening Can Satisfy EMTALA, Despite Misdiagnosis; 31 J.L. Med. & Ethics 169 (2003).
49. 42 USCS §1395dd(e)(4).
50. Broughton v St. John Health Sys. (2003, ED Mich) 246 F Supp 2d 764.
51. 42 USCS § 1395dd (c).
52. 42 U.S.C. §1395dd (c)(2).
53. Roberts v. Galen of Virginia (1999) 525 US 249, 142 L Ed 2d 648, 119 S Ct 685, 59 Soc Sec Rep Serv 513, 99 CDOS 379, 99 Daily Journal DAR 425, 1999 Colo J C A R 286, on remand, remanded (1999, CA6 Ky) 187 F3d 637.
54. Preston V. Tenet Healthsystem Mem'l Med Ctr. (E.D. La. 2006) 463 F. Supp. 2d 583.
55. 42 U.S.C. §1395dd (g).
56. Iscan E. Note: EMTALA's oft-overlooked reverse dumping provision and the implications for transferee hospital liability following St. Anthony hospital; 82 Wash. U.L.Q. 1201-1223 (Fall, 2004). St. Anthony Hospital v US Department of Health and Human Services (10th Cir. 2002) 309 F.3d 680.
57. Bitterman RA. Transferring patients: EMTALA rule to apply to those needing more care. ED Legal Letter. June 1, 2008 pNA.

58. Center for Medicaid and State Operations/Survey and Certification Group. Inpatient Prospective Payment System (IPPS) 2009 final rule revisions to Emergency Medical Treatment and Labor Act (EMTALA) regulations, Ref: S&C-09–26, March 6, 2009. p. 4.
59. Center for Medicaid and State Operations/Survey and Certification Group. Inpatient Prospective Payment System (IPPS) 2009 Final Rule Revisions to Emergency Medical Treatment and Labor Act (EMTALA) Regulations, Ref: S&C-09-26, March 6, 2009 Interpreting Guidelines. p. 11, 12, 21, 22.
60. 42 USCS § 1395cc (a)(1)(I)(iii).
61. 42 USCS §§ 1395 et seq.
62. Center for Medicaid and State Operations/Survey and Certification Group. Inpatient Prospective Payment System (IPPS) 2009 Final Rule Revisions to Emergency Medical Treatment and Labor Act (EMTALA) Regulations, Ref: S&C-09-26, March 6, 2009. p. 6; Interpretive Guidelines §489.20(r)(2) and §489.24(j).
63. 73 Fed. Reg. 48662 (August 19, 2008)
64. 42 USCS § 1395dd (d)(1)(C)
65. Cone DC, Alexander V, Myint W. EMTALA knowledge among on-call specialists at an academic medical center. J Emerg Med 2006;30(4):444–6.
66. Johnson LA, Taylor TB, Lev R. The emergency department on-call backup crisis: finding remedies for a serious public health problem. Ann Emerg Med 2001; 37(5):495–9.
67. 42 USCS § 1395dd (c)(2)(C).
68. Know legal risks when consulting on-call specialists. ED Legal Letter. Feb 1, 2008 pNA.
69. US Department of Health and Human Services, Centers for Medicare and Medicaid Services, Medicare Medicaid state operations manual, app. V interpretive guidelines – responsibilities of Medicare participating hospitals in emergency cases tag A404 rev. March 6, 2009.
70. Miller v. Corrado (Mo. Ct. App. Dec. 14, 1999)14 S.W.3d 42.
71. Bitterman RA. Shortage of on-call specialists for your ED? Help may be on the way. ED Legal Letter. July 1, 2008 pNA.
72. 68 Fed. Reg. 53, 221-53264(Sept. 9, 2003); 42 CFR 489.24 effective Nov. 10, 2003.
73. McConnell JK, Johnson LA, Arab N, et al. The on-call crisis: a statewide assessment of the costs of providing on-call specialist coverage. Ann Emerg Med 2007; 49:727–33.
74. American College of Emergency Physicians. On-Call Specialist Coverage in U.S. Emergency Departments, American College of Emergency Physicians, Irving, TX (2006).
75. Moy MM. EMTALA answer book. Illinois: University of Chicago; 2009. Sec. 6–45.
76. US Department of Health and Human Services, Centers for Medicare and Medicaid Services, Medicare Medicaid State Operations Manual, app. V interpretive guidelines – responsibilities of Medicare participating hospitals in emergency cases Tag A-2404/C-2404.
77. 42 CFR.489.24(j)(2)(iii) ref. 42 CFR 489.20(r)(2).
78. FY 2009 IPPS Final Rule (CMS-1390-F); 73 Fed. Reg. 48434 (August 19, 2008).
79. 73 Fed. Reg. 48667(August 19, 2008).
80. Shanaberger CJ. Case law involving base-station contact. Prehospital Disaster Med 1995;10(2):75–80 [discussion: 81].
81. Benitez FL, Pepe PE. Role of the physician in prehospital management of trauma: North American perspective. Curr Opin Crit Care 2002;8(6):551–8.

82. Morgan DL, Trail WR, Trompler VA. Liability immunity as a legal defense for recent emergency medical services system litigation. Prehospital Disaster Med 1995; 10(2):82–90 85–88 [discussion: 90–91].
83. Morgan DL, Wainscott MP, Knowles HC. Emergency medical services liability litigation in the United States. 1987 to 1992. Prehospital Disaster Med 1994;9: 214–21.
84. Hoyt BT, Norton RL. Online medical control and initial refusal of care: Does it help to talk with patients?. Philadelphia. Acad Emerg Med 2001;8(7):725–30.
85. Stuhlmiller D, Cudnik M, Sundheim S, et al. Adequacy of online medical command communication and emergency medical services documentation of informed refusals. Philadelphia. Acad Emerg Med 2005;12(10):970.
86. Arrington v Wong, 237 F.3d 1066, 1070 (9th Cir. 2001).
87. Morales v Sociedad Espanola de Auxilio Mutuo y Beneficencia, 524 F.3d 54, 2008 US App. LEXIS 8390 (1st Cir. P.R., 2008).
88. C.F.R. § 489.24.
89. CFR Parts 413, 482, and 489 from Federal Register: September 9, 2003 (Volume 68, Number 174, page 53257).
90. Lopes V Kapiolani Med. Ctr., 410F. Supp. 2d 939 (D. Haw). 2005.
91. COMMENT: EMTALA: Perez V. Protecting patients first by not deferring to the final regulations, 4 Seton Hall Cir. Rev. 149(2007).

Critical Aspects of Emergency Department Documentation and Communication

Kenneth T. Yu, MD, MBA[a,*], Robert A. Green, MD, MPH[b]

KEYWORDS

- Documentation • Hand-off • Change of shift
- Discharge instructions • Follow-up
- Emergency department

The working environment of an emergency department (ED) is a unique, complex, and dynamic environment. This is reflected in the varying, often overwhelming volume of patients seen in busy emergency departments, as well as the range of acuity of clinical encounters.[1] In addition, an ED is an example of a multifaceted organization composed of complex social environments, where interruptions are frequent and disruptive.[2–5] Such busy environments, where decisions are made under time pressure and with incomplete information, have been considered conducive to error[6] and claims of malpractice.[7] Studies such as the Harvard Medical Practice Study reported that approximately 1.5% to 3.0% of observed adverse events occurred in emergency departments.[8] Most importantly, these studies found that emergency departments had the highest proportion of preventable errors.

Amidst the apparent chaos, documentation often suffers.[9] The ED chart serves as the sole means for the emergency provider to note the details of the care provided to the patient during a visit. Aside from provider and patient memory, it is the only lasting record of the ED visit. Thorough documentation by the physician certainly facilitates accurate billing. More importantly, it can inform primary or future health care providers about the ED evaluation and treatment, as well as protect the ED physician in the event of bad outcomes and litigation.

Every aspect of the ED providers' interactions with their patients and their sub sequent documentation and communication is a potential medico-legal risk. The

The authors have no conflicts of interest to report. There was no external funding for this work.

[a] Department of Emergency Medicine, New York Presbyterian Hospital/Weill Cornell Medical Center, 525 East 68th Street, Box 573, New York, NY 10065, USA
[b] Department of Emergency Medicine, New York Presbyterian Hospital/Columbia University Medical Center, 622 West 168th Street, Suite 137, New York, NY 10032, USA
* Corresponding author.
E-mail address: kty9001@med.cornell.edu (K.T. Yu)

Emerg Med Clin N Am 27 (2009) 641–654
doi:10.1016/j.emc.2009.07.008
0733-8627/09/$ – see front matter. Published by Elsevier Inc.

management of critically ill patients will often be scrutinized after the fact, especially if there are poor outcomes. Documentation of the initial condition of the patient, timely and thorough examination and evaluation,[10] prompt resuscitation, and timing of specialty consults can be of special importance in cases of major trauma,[11] stroke, myocardial infarction,[12–15] and other emergent conditions. Excellent documentation may protect a physician from liability during a malpractice suit, whereas poor documentation, although not clearly tied to worse outcomes,[16–20] often leads to the commonly argued assertion, "if it wasn't documented, then it wasn't done," which only supports a plaintiff's case against a provider.

Aside from emergent conditions, there are a number of high-risk diagnoses that require careful documentation because of the potential for litigation resulting from missed diagnoses or bad outcomes. Some examples include pediatric fever, asthma, abdominal pain, hand injuries, intoxication, domestic violence, child abuse, and suicidal ideation. One can imagine the scrutiny that occurs after a case of missed appendicitis, a presumed intoxication that is actually an intracranial bleed, or a psychiatric patient who commits suicide after having been discharged from the ED. Proper documentation of a careful history, physical examination, and the physician's thought process regarding worst-case scenario diagnoses may help protect the provider to some degree.

Another aspect of documentation is the important concept of patient reassessment. Many charts now contain a check-box next to the statement "Patient improved." However, this broad statement is not nearly as powerful as having recorded serial sets of vital signs, pain assessments, and focused reexaminations of the patient. Timed reassessment notes are especially important for patients who are discharged from the ED after a prolonged stay, as physicians need to document improvement and appropriateness for discharge. Pediatrics is particularly high stakes because providers often must rely on general appearance and vital signs as opposed to subjective descriptions of improvement in young children.

Documentation that is inconsistent with actions taken in the ED can also put the provider at increased medico-legal risk. For example, a triage complaint of chest pain that is not addressed by the physician owing to later denial of chest pain should be explained in the physician note with at least an acknowledgment of the discrepancy. In teaching institutions, inconsistencies may also occur between a resident and attending diagnosis. A resident documenting an impression of "stroke" while the attending physician's impression is "atypical migraine" requires an explanation of the attending's thought process. Lack of consistency in documentation may invite scrutiny later on.

Other important areas of ED documentation include procedure notes (eg, neurovascular status before and after a closed reduction of a fracture), event notes (eg, a fall while in the ED), adverse reactions to medications, determinations of capacity, refusal of medical care, notes detailing safety for discharge, various discussions with patients, and details pertaining to the physician thought process. Concise notes documenting these key issues are good medical practice, and they may help to limit a physician's potential liability.

Although documentation is obviously quite important, the ED provider's primary goal is providing timely, compassionate, and excellent quality care to all patients. Oftentimes this occurs in the setting of severe crowding, boarding of admitted patients, and continuously arriving sick patients. This dualism, providing the safest and highest quality care with the constant potential for medico-legal risk, is a complex dynamic. This is the issue that we address in this article. After starting with a discussion of the various types of ED documentation currently in use, we highlight the important documentation aspects of two critical transitions in the ED—patient hand-offs and discharges.

TYPES OF ED CHARTS

Several types of ED charts have been developed over time, including free-text charts, preformatted generic charts, preformatted complaint-specific charts, and dictated and transcribed charts. Each chart type exists in paper and electronic forms, and each is associated with several advantages and disadvantages.

The oldest form of documentation is the free-text paper chart. Traditionally, it is simply a blank space to allow the physician to document the entire note, from chief complaint all the way to final disposition. The main advantage of the free-text paper chart is the ability of the provider to tailor the note to a specific problem area, using the space as needed. For example, the bulk of the space may be used to describe a detailed examination of the hand in evaluating a penetrating hand injury. Disadvantages include a longer time needed to complete a free-text chart, potential illegibility, and potential omission of important parts of the history or physical examination because of the lack of prompts available in other chart types.

With paper versions of the free-text chart, an advantage is the ability to edit or complete a note later on. Generally, time-stamps preclude this with electronic charting. Time-stamps and this editing ability can both be seen as a medico-legal advantage (eg, completing documentation after the fact of an examination actually performed earlier) or disadvantage (eg, retrospectively editing a chart after a bad outcome). Electronic records have the advantage of being accessible from any networked computer, whereas paper charts may be inaccessible (eg, with the patient at CT scan) or missing from time to time. However, access to electronic records is subject to inadequate numbers of computer terminals, network outages, and software glitches whereas paper records are not.

More recently, preformatted generic charts were introduced to improve physician documentation. For example, if a dedicated space was labeled for vital signs, a provider may be more likely to record the vital signs. A 2001 study[21] concluded that overall ED physician documentation was improved with the use of a structured, preformatted chart. Improved documentation is certainly a billing and medico-legal advantage, because of prompting for key elements of the encounter such as vital signs, descriptors of the history of present illness, important components of the examination, pertinent negatives, pain-scale documentation, and reassessment notes, to name a few. Another advantage is that these charts require less time to complete because of the use of labels and check-boxes. The main disadvantage of this chart type is the ambiguity associated with some of the wording; for example, phrases such as "motor WNL" may be listed under the neurologic examination. The exact meaning of this phrase is open to interpretation when the box next to it is checked off.

Disadvantages of paper versions of the preformatted generic chart include potential space constraints. For example, a provider may not have enough space to elaborate on a specific examination element that is critical to the case (eg, a detailed hand examination). In addition, many charts do not leave room to detail serial examinations and reassessments, patient improvement or deterioration, physician thought process, and modification of initial differential and treatment plan based on new information or change in patient condition. These elements of the provider note may be very helpful in the event of bad outcomes. Electronic versions may allow easier customization as to the use of space compared with paper versions. Previously discussed time-stamp and editing issues are still applicable here.

Preformatted complaint-specific charts provide further ability to customize a provider's documentation. For example, very different items need to be documented for a chest pain encounter, as opposed to an ankle injury visit. Complaint-specific charts typically list key elements to check off as positive or negative and often remind the physician to document why the patient is unlikely to have worst-case scenario diagnoses (eg, "no evidence of swelling or redness to the neck" for a toothache/facial pain encounter). A 1992 prospective study by Humphreys and colleagues[22] compared preformatted charts to blank charts in evaluating gynecologic complaints in the ED and concluded that documentation of the history, examination, and laboratory tests was significantly more complete on programmed charts (although outcome and patient satisfaction were not affected). The authors also concluded that patients more accurately recalled their diagnoses and were more satisfied with the physicians' explanations of their diagnoses. Wrenn and colleagues[23] further supported these findings in 1993, concluding that structured complaint-specific ED forms improve documentation and may improve communication, reimbursement, and medico-legal risk. Marill and colleagues[24] confirmed this reimbursement improvement and added the advantage of physician satisfaction when they compared the T-System of paper templates (Emergency Services Consultants, Irving, TX) with undirected written documentation. Other studies have also shown documentation improvements in areas such as asthma,[25] head injury,[26] and poisonings.[27]

Numerous electronic versions of complaint-specific charts have also been developed,[28] and they carry the same advantages and disadvantages discussed previously. The goal of these software packages is to allow quick electronic documentation of a patient encounter while capturing important medico-legal and billing elements of the visit using a variety of templates and prompts. For example, a robust list of pertinent positives and negatives for the history and physical examination would be displayed so the physician could select or cross off these items. The program could also help generate an appropriate differential diagnosis list, reminding the provider of worst-case scenarios that must be considered, given the current findings.

Electronic Medical Records (EMRs) and Computerized Order Entry Systems (CPOE) have a significant advantage as well. With increasing sophisticated use of Clinical Decision Support (CDS), medical errors can be mitigated. For example, with proper use, allergy information entered at triage can detect medication ordering errors made by providers hours later. Oftentimes, clinicians forget to check allergies before either writing orders in the ED or when writing prescriptions upon discharge. Alerts can come close to eradicating these types of errors. The use of CDS can be enormously helpful in avoiding other errors as well. Some examples include warnings when writing orders for low molecular weight heparin—alerting the practitioner that the creatinine clearance is less than 30 mg/dL and offer the option of using unfractioned heparin. Some electronic medical records have risk management modules that help the practitioner consider diagnoses that are rare; for example, certain symptoms combined with height and weight may prompt a message to consider Marfan syndrome and aortic dissection.

The introduction of electronic medical records brings with it its own risks of new potential errors as well. The use of drop-down menus and the need for quickness of data entry into these systems can result in mishaps. For example, when writing prescriptions on discharge, a wrong medication can be chosen from a long list of similarly sounding medications in a drop down list. This has led to the "look twice, click once" admonition when using EMRs. Electronic medical record systems need to be examined closely for attention to these types of details. The use of tall-man lettering (highlighting differences between similar sounding drugs), generic versus brand name integration, and checking for drug-drug interactions are all important features when evaluating a system for the ED.

The big divide within the emergency medicine EMR discussion is the use of specialized software designed and used only within EDs versus the enterprise-wide solutions that are used throughout hospitals including EDs. The specialized products for the ED have made great strides with ease of use, risk management tools, and acceptance in ED settings; however, hospital administrators often prefer, for good reasons, to have the entire enterprise on one system. The downsides and benefits of both are beyond the scope of this article, but there are valid arguments on both sides of this discussion. Having one integrated system, for example, enables simpler and more effective medication reconciliation among all the outpatient providers, the ED, and the inpatient visit. The lack of sophisticated features specific to the ED, however, typically seen in these systems, is a downside to these enterprise-wide systems, one that will likely be resolved within the next decade.

The final ED documentation type is the dictated and transcribed chart. Instead of writing or typing the details of an encounter, a provider verbally records the details of the visit via telephone, and shortly thereafter, a medical transcriptionist types the documentation for the physician. A retrospective study by Cole and Counselman[29] compared transcribed and handwritten ED charts of chest pain patients and concluded that transcribed charts contained more complete documentation. In addition, a prospective study from San Francisco[30] concluded that a dictation system decreases documentation time, improves legibility, increases provider efficiency, and improves physician satisfaction. Another study[31] later confirmed the improvement in provider efficiency and reduced documentation error rates using a dictation system. Clearly, the benefits must outweigh the additional cost of the transcription service. The obvious disadvantage of dictation and transcription is misinterpretation of the recorded dictation by the transcriptionist, which can result in errors in the typed medical record. Transcription can also be somewhat confusing in academic centers where there are numerous providers (eg, residents and attendings) taking care of a patient.

There is no perfect ED medical record, but there are certainly distinct advantages and disadvantages to each documentation type.

HAND-OFFS AND CHANGES OF SHIFT

"First, do no harm." Although medical errors have existed since before Hippocrates, the true magnitude of adverse events in health care was brought to the forefront of public debate after the Institute of Medicine (IOM) reported in 1999 that approximately 98,000 deaths per year were attributable to errors in hospitals.[32] Emergency departments were characterized as complex, tightly coupled systems intrinsically prone to accidents. In a subsequent report,[33] great importance was given to the concept of "seamless" health care as the means of improving patient safety. Seamless health care calls for interdependent people and technologies to function as a unified whole. This concept is highly significant at the points of information transfer such as clinician hand-offs, where patient safety is at risk of being compromised.[33]

The Joint Commission has published data on communication errors indicating that approximately 65% of reported sentinel events involve issues with communication.[34] Hand-offs in emergency medicine involve communication between both nurses and physicians at changes of shift, hand-offs with admitting teams, and those between nurses and physicians. These hand-offs, given the nature of emergency medicine, occur innumerable times a day in even moderately busy departments and therefore are usually concise. The potential for loss of significant information is obvious. These "nodes of interface"[35] provide for a significant opportunity for the degradation of important information and potential for opportunities for negative clinical outcomes. Various additional factors, such as an increasingly complicated patient population and reductions in resident duty hours have added pressure to the hand-off process within the ED. These factors are significant causes of concern in the management of risk within any critical care environment, especially the ED.[35]

Hand-offs and changes of shift are similar nodes of interface, thus they will be dealt with together for the purposes of this manuscript. Hand-off communication is a central tenet of the Joint Commission's National Patient Safety Goals.[36] Every hospital, by now, should have in place a structured method of communication to decrease the chance of error during the process of hand-off communication.

The second National Patient Safety Goal, 2E, specifically addresses the importance of the hand-off process and in section E specifies the elements of performance. These include (1) ensuring a process for effective hand-off communication that includes interactive communication that allows for the opportunity for questioning between the giver and receiver of patient information; (2) up-to-date information regarding the patient's condition, care, treatment, medications, services, and any recent or anticipated changes; (3) a method to verify the received information; (4) an opportunity for the receiver of the hand-off information to review relevant patient historical data; and (5) the limitations of interruptions during hand-off communication.

Variations in communication skills, styles, and time constraints between both physicians and nurses can contribute to a breakdown in effective communication, which can lead to adverse outcomes for patients.[37] Many hospitals have chosen to use the SBAR (Situation, Background, Assessment, and Recommendation) form of hand-off communication. This method is particularly useful in the ED setting. SBAR is an easy-to-remember technique that provides for consistent, structured communication between members of the health care team during a critical situation.[38]

A structured tool such as SBAR can standardize the approach and decrease variability in communication between providers. This applies to both ED and inpatient recipients of information. SBAR or another standardized approach can keep the process concise yet ensure that the critical information is transmitted in a reliable fashion. Oftentimes, SBAR forms or small cards are created to be used as prompts for the process. Several EDs have created SBAR nursing FAX report forms, one of which is available on the Institute for Healthcare Improvement (IHI) Web site[39] for download. This tool ensures that the critical information needed is handed off in a consistent manner when patients are transported from the ED to an inpatient unit.

Similarly, a written prompt for use during physician hand-off can improve the consistency of physician-to-physician hand-off at changes of shift. An example of a verbal SBAR hand-off would be as follows:

- **Situation:** This is an 85-year-old male who presented to the ED 5 hours ago with abdominal pain and vomiting for 1 day. He is currently undergoing evaluation and is presently at CT scan. His vitals signs are stable, with a blood pressure of 140/90, pulse of 90, normal respiratory rate, and oxygen saturation of 98% on room air.
- **Background:** He has a history of smoking, hypertension, myocardial infarction, and no previous abdominal conditions. He takes metoprolol for high blood pressure, aspirin, and zolpidem for sleep.
- **Assessment:** His examination revealed mild right upper quadrant as well as mid-abdominal tenderness. Our impression was possible cholecystitis, and

less likely, aortic aneurysm or diverticulitis. Bedside sonogram done in the ED was unrevealing.

- **Recommendation:** Review CT scan results, reexamine, likely admit for observation.

Using a structured sign-out/hand-off tool can increase the efficiency and effectiveness of the hand-off process. In an analysis by Arora and colleagues,[40] 25 incidents of communication failures were examined. These cases were resident cases that involved the omission of medications, pending examinations, studies ordered, or active issues. The use of a structured format can help with organization and cognitive thought processes to include items that are active and important for the ongoing care of the patient.

DISCHARGE INSTRUCTIONS AND FOLLOW-UP

The other critical transition for ED patients occurs at discharge. When a patient is deemed safe for discharge from the ED, the provider must ensure that the patient receives good instructions, both verbally and in printed form. Patients may often have difficulty remembering multipart instructions given only verbally. In addition, Roberts[41] suggests brightly colored paper to help patients not lose their instructions. These printed instructions should explain the diagnosis (or diagnoses) given, what was done in the ED, the name of the ED provider, specific instructions regarding activity and medications, what to expect going forward, with whom and when to follow up, and the symptoms for which to seek medical treatment or return to the ED. If there are test results still pending, the patient should be directed as to how and when to obtain these results.[41] All of these items are important for effective treatment, continuity of care, and patient comprehension. Asking patients to repeat the instructions given may help confirm their understanding.[41] If the patient may not comprehend the instructions, they must be relayed to a responsible party (eg, parents of a child, nursing home staff for a patient with dementia).

The risk of not communicating these key components of the discharge instructions has obvious implications on patient satisfaction and outcomes. ED physicians should beware of cases such as an incidentally found lung nodule where outpatient CT scan and primary care surveillance would be recommended but where the discussion was not properly documented. Malpractice may be claimed years later if the patient developed lung cancer and had forgotten to mention the nodule to their primary doctor. Lack of documentation of such follow-up recommendations probably does not sit well with a sympathetic jury, whereas solid documentation may be protective of the ED provider.

Too often, patients leave the ED thinking "they said I was fine," which, in many cases, is not the actual discharge diagnosis. Numerous studies have demonstrated that patients (and parents of pediatric patients) frequently do not understand their discharge instructions.[42–46] Patients who do not understand their instructions clearly may have difficulty carrying them out. One pediatric ED study showed that only 63% of patient guardians obtained prescribed medications after discharge.[47] Another concluded that dissatisfaction with discharge instructions independently correlated with nonfilling of prescriptions.[48,49] The effect of insurance status on prescription filling remains controversial.[50,51]

Ideally, the language used in discharge instructions should be written at a level that can be understood by the patient. Sometimes, patients cannot actually read the printed instructions because of illiteracy;[45,52,53] one University of Virginia ED study concluded that hospital and commercially generated patient education materials ranged from 8th to 13th grade level, whereas more than 40% of their ED patients could not read at the 8th grade level.[53] Other studies report similar findings, with Davis and colleagues[54] noting a gap of more than 5 years between patient reading levels and the comprehension levels required by written patient materials.[55,56] Patients who speak other languages and not English should be able to converse with the help of a translator because comprehension deficits are well demonstrated in non–English-speaking ED patients.[43] Many computer-generated instructions can be printed in Spanish or other languages. At other times, handwritten instructions can be simply illegible to the patient, and clearly this can negatively affect comprehension and compliance with instructions.

Most recently, Engel and colleagues[57] interviewed ED patients immediately after discharge and found that 78% of patients demonstrated deficient comprehension of ED discharge instructions, with 34% of the deficiencies involving understanding of post-ED care. These findings are in line with those reported in earlier studies from Missouri[45] and New York.[58] In the latter study, only 42% of patients were able to name their diagnosis, and only 37% could state the purpose of the medications prescribed to them. To make matters worse, most patients who had deficiencies of comprehension did not realize it, reporting inappropriately high confidence in their recall. These deficiencies are present immediately after discharge and do not account for memory attrition that may occur over longer periods of time (eg, when patients see their primary doctor the following week).

Comprehension and retention of discharge instructions can be improved by strategies including the physician spending more time explaining the diagnosis and instructions to the patient,[46] simplifying the language used in discharge instructions,[59] using standardized instructions,[60] using diagnosis-specific information sheets,[61] and even including illustrations.[62] Older pre-printed discharge instructions such as those for head trauma precautions have given way to more complete explanations of the diagnosis, what to watch out for, what to expect, and when to follow up.[41]

Follow-up with a primary care provider or specialist is another essential component of a discharge plan and instructions. Despite being given ED referrals, patients often do not follow up with a doctor, commonly because of appointment availability or insurance issues. According to a major study by Asplin and colleagues[63] in 2005, patients with private insurance failed to obtain a follow-up appointment 36% of the time with appointments being refused by the clinic 40% of the time, most commonly because the clinics were not accepting new patients. Not surprisingly, Medicaid patients fared worse, failing to obtain a follow-up appointment 66% of the time with appointments being refused 80% of the time, most commonly because the clinics did not accept Medicaid. One pediatric study[47] showed that only 60% of patient guardians complied with follow-up instructions to see a physician. Again, privately insured patients fared better than those without private insurance (77% compared with 47% compliance with follow-up). Some studies have reported better compliance with referrals among females, adults older than 40 years, children younger than 18 months, increased severity of complaints, referrals to private physicians, and having private insurance.[64,65]

Several studies have addressed ways to increase successful ED referrals. One study demonstrated that computerized discharge instructions improved patient compliance with follow-up appointments.[66] Perhaps this effect is attributable to the ED provider forgetting to write specific referral instructions on handwritten discharge papers, whereas they are programmed to appear on computerized instructions. Numerous studies have demonstrated that making a follow-up appointment for the patient before discharge significantly improves follow-up compliance.[49,67–70] One Canadian study[69] came to the same conclusion and added that its free clinic appointments also increased compliance with referral. Barlas and colleagues[71] found increased compliance when free 48-hour ED follow-up was offered. Apparently, the more reminders and increased ease of obtaining an appointment results in improved compliance with referrals.

One other item relating to discharge instructions is the process of medication reconciliation, which is mandated by The Joint Commission as one of its 2009 National Patient Safety Goals.[36] The objective of this effort is to ensure that patients and their primary care providers always have an up-to-date list of their medications and that any provider who is making changes to the medication list should be reviewing the new list for any potentially dangerous situation such as drug interactions, drug allergies, and other issues. Of course, this process is difficult with patients who cannot remember their long list of medications. At other times, difficulties may arise because electronic databases may not include some medications that are foreign or experimental. This update of the patient's current medication list must be completed before discharge from the ED (or any other department), as medications are often stopped or started in the ED. A copy of this medication list should be given to the patient to bring to the primary care physician or next provider.

Sometimes, patients may not be discharged from the ED in the typical fashion. Patients that leave the ED without being seen, fail to complete an ED visit (leave after being evaluated), or sign out against medical advice (AMA) should ideally receive instructions, as well as have the interaction or conversation documented in the medical record. Bad outcomes after a patient leaves in this manner will inevitably result in scrutiny of the ED documentation. A plaintiff's attorney will certainly argue that the patient should have been seen and evaluated more quickly and clearly should have had the risks of leaving the ED better explained. Consequently, important items to document in these cases, when possible, include a thorough history and examination, severity of illness and risks, lack of danger to self or others, patient competency and capacity (including lack of intoxication), and patient understanding of the risks and benefits of and alternatives to leaving the ED.[72] Alfandre[73] estimated that between 1% and 2% of all medical admissions result in AMA discharge, and predictors include younger age, Medicaid or no insurance, male gender, and substance or alcohol abuse. In one UK study,[74] 50% of self-discharge patients were under the influence of drugs or alcohol. In terms of outcomes and risk, Lee and colleagues[75] found that chest pain patients who left the ED against medical advice were at higher risk for myocardial infarction than those who were discharged but at lower risk than those who were admitted.

When patients leave without the provider being aware of the departure (such as those who leave from the waiting room before being seen), this conversation and assessment may not be possible. However, patients who sign out against medical advice should be counseled regarding severity of illness and risks of leaving the ED, and they should receive discharge instructions as well as optimal medical treatment for their condition. Thorough documentation and discharging a patient against medical advice may partially protect the provider, but it does not prevent liability altogether, as demonstrated by several malpractice cases in the literature.[10,12–15,72]

PEARLS AND PITFALLS

Following is a brief list of key points to remember in the process of ED documentation and communication with patients.

1. High-risk diagnoses

   Recognize these conditions. Think about what could go wrong after the patient is discharged. Document clearly the rationale for why the condition is or is not something dangerous. Be conservative. Splinting a patient with minimal snuffbox tenderness in their dominant hand may be well worth the extra effort.

2. Reevaluations
   Serial examinations are very important. Detailing patient improvement is especially important for patients who are discharged home after a lengthy ED visit. Otherwise, the chart will reflect only the initial condition of the patient, which often is a patient who is less stable and more uncomfortable that the one who is being discharged home.
3. Thought process
   It is imperative to detail the physician thought process (differential diagnosis, probabilities, rationale for actions taken). Why was pulmonary embolism unlikely and not something to be ruled out with testing? Without a clear roadmap, a plaintiff's attorney can connect the dots (or data points on the chart) in the way that most benefits the case being made against the provider.
4. Patient discussions
   Documenting important conversations with the patient may help support a provider's actions and more accurately portray the patient's understanding of the diagnosis (or lack thereof). Rather than concluding "I was fine," a patient who verbalizes understanding that there is a remote possibility that atypical chest pain could represent angina may be more likely to return if worse and/or obtain an outpatient stress test.
5. Leaving AMA
   A patient who signs out AMA does not leave the ED physician without risk. Extremely careful documentation must accompany this disposition. Most importantly, a provider note must attest to the patient's capacity to make such a decision and to the patient's verbalized understanding of the risks of and alternatives to leaving AMA. Not fully explaining and detailing the specific risks might, in the eyes of a jury, have led to a patient making a decision without the proper information.
6. Patient hand-offs
   With the high volume of many EDs, the hand-off between providers is often the transition point where information is lost and from which bad outcomes result. The SBAR methodology is just one way to effectively communicate a patient's plan to an oncoming physician. Not properly transmitting an organized plan puts the patient (and the provider) at risk.
7. Discharge instructions and follow-up
   Patients are more likely to remember their diagnoses and carry out their discharge instructions if they are spelled out in detail and in printed form. Follow-up plans should be clearly specified (where, when), and the patient should be specifically told what to look out for and when to become concerned and return to the ED.

SUMMARY

The environment of the ED is unique. The arrival pattern of patients is not completely predictable, leading to great variations in provider-to-patient ratios. ED physicians are unfamiliar with new patients presenting to the ED. In contrast, familiarity with patients' known histories, personalities, and prior presentations helps their primary care providers place the patients' complaints in context. There is also no limitation to the spectrum of illness that any single provider in the ED will encounter.

These facts place the emergency physician in a position of increased vulnerability, as compared to some other specialties, with regard to patient adverse outcomes and potential litigation. The lack of an ongoing, caring relationship with the patient increases the risk of legal actions when things do go awry. This article has focused on the importance of clear documentation of events that occur in the ED. It is the opinion of the authors that documentation is critical and that in most circumstances it will help rather than hinder the defense of the care provided in the ED. This conclusion is not contingent on the type of documentation tool used in your department.

In addition to the imperative to document as completely as possible, the additional vulnerability to the emergency provider is the process of sign-out and hand-off communication. ED providers transfer care to other ED providers, inpatient providers, and, if discharged, to outpatient providers. All of the communication between providers within the ED and those within the continuum of care needs to be standardized to improve care. No longer are haphazard methods of communication acceptable. One example of a standardized hand-off approach was outlined in the article.

Finally, discharge instructions are critical both for patient safety and to protect the ED provider in the event of a liability action. Clear instructions to the patient, especially the importance of follow-up in a reasonable period of time and the indications to return immediately if worrisome symptoms occur, are paramount. Failure to clearly delineate these instructions is a disservice to our patients and puts unnecessary risk on the provider.

ACKNOWLEDGMENTS

Special thanks to Rahul Sharma, MD, MBA, for reviewing this manuscript.

REFERENCES

1. Kovacs G, Croskerry P. Clinical decision making: an emergency medicine perspective. Acad Emerg Med 1999;6:947–52.
2. Alvarez G, Coiera E. Interruptive communication patterns in the intensive care unit ward round. Int J Med Inform 2005;74:791–6.
3. Brixey J, Robinson D, Tang Z, et al. Interruptions in workflow for RNs in a level one trauma center. AMIA Annu Symp Proc 2005;86–90.
4. Laxmisan A, Hakimzada F, Sayan OR, et al. The multitasking clinician: decision-making and cognitive demand during and after team handoffs in emergency care. Int J Med Inform 2007;76(11–12):801–11.
5. Coiera E, Jayasuria R, Hardy J, et al. Communication loads on clinical staff in the emergency department. Med J Aust 2002;176:415–8.
6. Bertram D. Managing an emergency department: the effect of patient flow on physician performance. QRB Qual Rev Bull 1983;9:175–80.
7. Reason J. Human error. Cambridge, England: Cambridge University Press; 1990.
8. Leape L, Brennan T, Laird N, et al. The nature of adverse events in hospitalized patients. Results of the Harvard Medical Practice Study II. N Engl J Med 1991;324:377–84.
9. Schoenfeld P, Baker M. Documentation in the pediatric emergency department: a review of resuscitation cases. Ann Emerg Med 1991;20:641–3.
10. Traulhein J. Malpractice in the emergency department—a review of 200 cases. Ann Emerg Med 1984;13:709–11.
11. Palmer I, Baskett P, McCabe S. A new chart to assist with advanced trauma life support. J R Army Med Corps 1992;138:118–25.
12. Karcz A, Holbrook J, Auerbach B, et al. Preventability of malpractice claims in emergency medicine: a closed claims study. Ann Emerg Med 1990;19:865–73.

13. Rusnak R, Stair T, Hansen K, et al. Litigation against the emergency physician: common features in cases of missed myocardial infarction. Ann Emerg Med 1989;18:1029–34.
14. Karcz A, Korn R, Burke M, et al. Malpractice claims against emergency physicians in Massachusetts: 1975–1993. Am J Emerg Med 1996;14:341–5.
15. Karcz A, Holbrook J, Burke M, et al. Massachusetts emergency medicine closed malpractice claims: 1988–1990. Ann Emerg Med 1993;20:641–3.
16. Lyons T, Payne B. The relationship between physicians' medical recording performance to their medical care performance. Med Care 1974;12:463–9.
17. Murphy J, Jacobson S. Assessing the quality of emergency care: the medical record versus patients' outcomes. Ann Emerg Med 1984;13:158–65.
18. Fessel W, Brunt EV. Assessing quality of care from the medical record. N Engl J Med 1972;286:134–8.
19. Sanazaro P, Worth R. Concurrent quality assurance in hospital care. N Engl J Med 1974;298:1171–7.
20. Switz D. The problem-oriented medical record. Arch Intern Med 1976;136:1119–23.
21. O'Connor A, Finnel L, Reid J. Do preformatted charts improve doctors' documentation in a rural hospital emergency department? A prospective trial. N Z Med J 2001;114:443–4.
22. Humphreys T, Shofer F, Jacobson S, et al. Preformatted charts improve documentation in the emergency department. Ann Emerg Med 1992;21:534–40.
23. Wrenn K, Rodewald L, Lumb E, et al. The use of structured, complaint-specific patient encounter forms in the emergency department. Ann Emerg Med 1993;22:805–12.
24. Marill K, Gauharou E, Nelson B, et al. Prospective, randomized trial of template-assisted versus undirected written recording of physician records in the emergency department. Ann Emerg Med 1999;33:500–9.
25. Robinson S, Harrison B, Lambert M. Effect of a preprinted form on the management of acute asthma in an accident and emergency department. J Accid Emerg Med 1996;13:93–7.
26. Wallace S, Gullen R, Byrne P, et al. Use of a proforma for head injuries in the accident and emergency department. J Accid Emerg Med 1994;11:33–42.
27. Buckley N, White I, Dawson A, et al. Preformatted admission charts for poisoning admissions facilitate clinical assessment and research. Ann Emerg Med 1999;34:476–82.
28. Yamazaki S, Satomura Y, Suzuki T, et al. The concept of "template" assisted electronic medical record. Medinfo 1995;8:249–52.
29. Cole A, Counselman F. Comparison of transcribed and handwritten emergency department charts in the evaluation of chest pain. Ann Emerg Med 1995;25:445–50.
30. Witt D. Transcription services in the ED. Am J Emerg Med 1995;13:34–6.
31. Dawdy M, Munter D, Gilmore R. Correlation of patient entry rates and physician documentation errors in dictated and handwritten emergency treatment records. Am J Emerg Med 1997;15:115–7.
32. Kohn L, Corrigan J, Donaldson M. editors. To err is human: building a safer health system. Washington, DC: National Academies Press; 2000.
33. Crossing the quality chasm: a new health system for the 21st century. Washington, DC: Institute of Medicine (US), Committee on Quality of Health Care in America; 2001.

34. Improving America's hospitals: the Joint Commission's annual report on quality and safety, 2007. Oakbrook Terrace (IL): The Joint Commission; 2008.
35. Dunn W, Murphy J. The patient handoff. Chest 2008;134:9–12.
36. The Joint Commission - 2009. National patient safety goals: hospital program. Available at: http://www.jointcommission.org/PatientSafety/NationalPatientSafetyGoals/09_hap_npsgs.htm. Accessed February 24, 2009.
37. Arford P. Nurse-physician communication: an organizational accountability. Nurs Econ 2005;23:72–7.
38. Woodhall L, Vertacnik L, McLaughlin M. Implementation of the SBAR communication technique in a tertiary center. J Emerg Nurs 2008;34:314–7.
39. Institute for Healthcare Improvement. Available at: http://www.ihi.org. Accessed February 24, 2009.
40. Arora V, Johnson J, Lovinger D, et al. Communication failures in patient sign-out and suggestions for improvement: a critical incident analysis. Qual Saf Health Care 2005;14:401–7.
41. Roberts J. ED discharge instructions: another chance to help patients and prove your worth. Emerg Med News 2006;28:17–20.
42. Anonymous. Majority of emergency patients don't understand discharge instructions. ED Manag 2008;20:97–8.
43. Crane J. Patient comprehension of doctor-patient communication on discharge from the emergency department. J Emerg Med 1997;15:1–7.
44. Grover G, Berkowitz C, Lewis R. Parental recall after a visit to the emergency department. Clin Pediatr 1994;33:194–201.
45. Logan P, Schwab R. Patient understanding of emergency department discharge instructions. South Med J 1996;89:770–4.
46. Spandorfer J, Karras D, Hughes L, et al. Comprehension of discharge instructions by patients in an urban emergency department. Ann Emerg Med 1995;25:71–4.
47. Wang N, Kiernan M, Golzari M, et al. Characteristics of pediatric patients at risk of poor emergency department aftercare. Acad Emerg Med 2006;13:840–7.
48. Matsui D, Joubert G, Dykxhoorn S, et al. Compliance with prescription filling in the pediatric emergency department. Arch Pediatr Adolesc Med 2000;154:195–8.
49. Thomas E, Burstin H, O'Neill A, et al. Patient noncompliance with medical advice after the emergency department visit. Ann Emerg Med 1996;27:49–55.
50. Kajioka E, Itoman E, Li M, et al. Pediatric prescription pick-up rates after ED visits. Am J Emerg Med 2005;23:454–8.
51. Saunders C. Patient compliance in filling prescriptions after discharge from the emergency department. Am J Emerg Med 1987;5:283–6.
52. Jolly B, Scott J, Feied C, et al. Functional illiteracy among emergency department patients: a preliminary study. Ann Emerg Med 1993;22:573–8.
53. Powers R. Emergency department patient literacy and the readability of patient-directed materials. Ann Emerg Med 1988;17:124–6.
54. Davis T, Mayeaux E, Fredrickson D, et al. Reading ability of parents compared with reading level of pediatric patient education materials. Pediatrics 1994;93:460–8.
55. Gibbs R, Gibbs P, Henrich J. Patient understanding of commonly used medical vocabulary. J Fam Pract 1987;25:176–8.
56. Davis T, Crouch M, Wills G, et al. The gap between patient reading comprehension and the readability of patient education materials. J Fam Pract 1990;31:533–8.

57. Engel K, Heisler M, Smith D, et al. Patient comprehension of emergency department care and instructions: are patients aware of when they do not understand? Ann Emerg Med 2009;53:454–61.
58. Makaryus A, Friedman E. Patients' understanding of their treatment plans and diagnosis at discharge. Mayo Clin Proc 2005;80:991–4.
59. Jolly B, Scott J, Sanford S. Simplification of emergency department discharge instructions improves patient comprehension. Ann Emerg Med 1995;26:443–6.
60. Isaacman D, Purvis K, Gyuro J, et al. Standardized instructions: do they improve communication of discharge information from the emergency department? Pediatrics 1992;89:1204–8.
61. Waisman Y, Siegal N, Siegal G, et al. Role of diagnosis-specific information sheets in parents' understanding of emergency department discharge instructions. Eur J Emerg Med 2005;12:159–62.
62. Austin P, Matlack R, Dunn K, et al. Discharge instructions: do illustrations help our patients understand them? Ann Emerg Med 1995;25:317–20.
63. Asplin B, Rhodes K, Levy H, et al. Insurance status and access to urgent ambulatory care follow-up appointments. JAMA 2005;294:1248–54.
64. Fosarelli P, DeAngelis C, Kaszuba A. Compliance with follow-up appointments generated in a pediatric emergency room. Am J Prev Med 1985;1:23–9.
65. Vukmir R, Kremen R, Dehart D, et al. Compliance with emergency department patient referral. Am J Emerg Med 1992;10:413–7.
66. Vukmir R, Kremen R, Ellis G, et al. Compliance with emergency department referral: the effect of computerized discharge instructions. Ann Emerg Med 1993;22:819–23.
67. Kyriacou D, Handel D, Stein A, et al. Factors affecting outpatient follow-up compliance of emergency department referrals. J Gen Intern Med 2005;20: 938–42.
68. Magnusson A, Hedges J, Vanko M, et al. Follow-up compliance after emergency department evaluation. Ann Emerg Med 1993;22:560–7.
69. Murray M, LeBlanc C. Clinic follow-up from the emergency department: do patients show up? Ann Emerg Med 1996;27:56–8.
70. Zorc J, Scarfone R, Li Y, et al. Scheduled follow-up after a pediatric emergency department visit for asthma: a randomized trial. Pediatrics 2003;111:495–502.
71. Barlas D, Homan C, Rakowski J, et al. How well do patients obtain short-term follow-up after discharge from the emergency department? Ann Emerg Med 1999;34:610–4.
72. Devitt P, Devitt A, Dewan M. An examination of whether discharging patients against medical advice protects physicians from malpractice charges. Psychiatr Serv 2000;51:899–902.
73. Alfandre D. "I'm going home": discharges against medical advice. Mayo Clin Proc 2009;84:255–60.
74. Henson V, Vickery D. Patient self discharge from the emergency department: who is at risk? Emerg Med J 2005;22:499–501.
75. Lee T, Short L, Brand D, et al. Patients with acute chest pain who leave emergency departments against medical advice: prevalence, clinical characteristics, and natural history. J Gen Intern Med 1988;3:21–4.

Physical and Chemical Restraints

Victoria A. Coburn, MD, Mark B. Mycyk, MD*

KEYWORDS

- Physical restraint • Chemical restraint • Violence
- Safety • Sedation

Combative and violent patients are commonly encountered in the emergency department (ED).[1] These patients may be brought in by concerned family members, referred to the ED by other health professionals, or transported by police or emergency medical services (EMS) personnel for causing a public disturbance. These patients pose significant diagnostic and management challenges to the physicians, nurses, technicians, and other staff members who are trying to care for them. A combative patient's behavior can have numerous causes, including but not limited to psychiatric illness, substance abuse and withdrawal, traumatic injury, and metabolic disturbances. Emergency physicians are expected to manage an agitated patient's behavior safely, determine if a medical or traumatic cause is a contributor to the agitation, and arrange for appropriate disposition.[2] To differentiate between an organic and a functional cause for agitated or violent behavior, it is imperative to obtain a history and perform a complete physical examination on these patients, and, in some cases, order laboratory work and radiologic imaging. Unfortunately, agitated or violent behavior is itself an obstacle to that medical workup and puts the individual patient and all caregivers at risk of injury. When de-escalation strategies are ineffective in getting a violent patient to cooperate, the use of physical and chemical restraints needs to be considered. Once the decision is made to use restraints, it is important to follow hospital policy on patient monitoring and documentation. Hospital policies on restraints should be derived from the Joint Commission's Restraint and Seclusion Standards because the use of restraints is tracked by the Joint Commission.[3]

EPIDEMIOLOGY

Violence is prevalent in our society. According to the Centers for Disease Control and Prevention (CDC)'s National Institute for Occupational Safety and Health (NIOSH), nonfatal assaults occur in 8.3 per 10,000 health care workers yearly, whereas the rate of nonfatal assaults in private sector industries is 2 per 10,000.[4] Of all health

Department of Emergency Medicine, Boston University School of Medicine, Boston Medical Center, 1 Boston Medical Center Place, Dowling 1 South, Boston, MA 02118, USA
* Corresponding author.
E-mail address: mark.mycyk@bmc.org (M.B. Mycyk).

Emerg Med Clin N Am 27 (2009) 655–667
doi:10.1016/j.emc.2009.07.003 emed.theclinics.com

care areas examined, violence has been found to be more prevalent in EDs, waiting rooms, psychiatric wards, and geriatrics units. The ED environment, with high stress, fragmented communication, long waiting times, overcrowding, staff shortages, financial issues, and confusion, can provoke violence in predisposed individuals. Surprisingly, 50% of health care workers will be victims of physical violence during their career.[5] Studies suggest that working in an ED, with more than 50,000 patient visits per year and an average waiting time longer than 2 hours, puts health care workers at higher risk of injury from violent patients.[1,6]

PATHOPHYSIOLOGY

It is helpful for the emergency physician to be familiar with the characteristics that predispose patients to violent or aggressive behavior in the ED. Positive predictors of potential violent behavior are male gender, having a prior history of violence, arriving in the custody of the police, being a victim of violence, and having a history of alcohol or drug abuse.[7,8] Psychiatric illness (especially schizophrenia, personality disorders, mania, and psychotic depression) has also been identified as a significant risk for violent behavior in the ED.[7]

Schizophrenics can experience command auditory hallucinations instructing them to perform violent acts or have delusions that others are trying to harm them. These patients may be noncompliant with their medications, nonresponsive to treatment, or be using alcohol or drugs, which can lead to violent behavior.[7,9,10] Certain personality disorders, such as borderline and antisocial, are more prone to violent behavior because these patients have little remorse for their actions on staff. Patients with mania can also exhibit periods of violence and aggression during episodes of emotional lability.

Agitation can have an organic cause. The differential diagnosis is broad and includes delirium, dementia, traumatic brain injury, neurological disease, metabolic disturbance, infection, vascular or circulatory issues, renal or hepatic insufficiency, and endocrine dysfunction.[7] Intoxication or withdrawal from alcohol or any other recreational drug can lead to out-of-control behavior. Even with sedative abuse (alcohol, benzodiazepines) some patients may experience a "paradoxical disinhibition" (an increase in impulsivity due to a decrease in the frontal self-regulatory function).[7] It is important for the physician to differentiate between functional and organic causes for a patient's aggressive behavior and carefully rule out organic causes even in patients with a history of psychiatric illness or substance abuse problems. One must never assume out-of-control behavior is solely caused by psychiatric illness; all patients should have their blood glucose level checked on arrival and further diagnostic testing, such as serum and urine tests, cranial computer tomographic scan, and lumbar puncture, should be considered as clinically indicated. First time out-of-control behavior has a higher incidence of organic cause in patients older than 40 years with no known psychiatric history, patients with disorientation or hallucinations, and patients with abnormal vital signs.[11]

RECOGNIZING AND DE-ESCALATING THE VIOLENT PATIENT

EMS personnel are at a high risk of encountering violent patients: 14% of calls are precipitated by a violent act and violence occurs during 5% of their overall transports.[12,13] When EMS is transporting a violent patient to a hospital, ideally a call should be made to alert ED staff to prepare and mobilize appropriate resources.

Violence is not usually the initial response of a patient in the ED but is the result of increasing tension and frustration. In addition to the risks mentioned earlier, certain cues from the patient can predict the possibility of violent behavior. If these cues are noticed, a situation can be diffused before it escalates and gets out of control. The 3 phases of violence should be understood to initiate de-escalation before harm occurs or restraint procedures are used.[14]

Phase 1: Anxiety

Patients in this early phase are often loud, have pressured speech, and exhibit body movements the only purpose of which seems to be to expend energy: pacing, clenching fists, and constantly changing position on the stretcher). Because such features are frequently seen in anxious ED patients who do not have a propensity for violence, these cues are often ignored by staff and those prone to violence unfortunately escalate beyond this phase. To avoid progression to increasingly aggressive behavior, many of these patients could be appeased by simply being acknowledged by staff.[14] Establishing a rapport with the patient goes a long way. Patients should be treated with courtesy, respect, and empathy. Offering food and drink or warm blankets can be useful in establishing trust and rapport because it appeals to the most basic human needs.[15] Physicians should relay their concern for patients and assure them that they are in a safe environment.[16]

Phase 2: Defensiveness

In the second phase, patients are verbally abusive, using inappropriately profane language. Their behavior is irrational. Feeling that one is losing control of the situation is usually the underlying cause. Limits need to be set for patients in this phase with some choices offered. Limits should be simple, clear, enforceable, and consistent; the patient needs to know the consequences of choosing not to stay within these limits. Staff must be calm and professional but firm when interacting with patients. It is important to avoid countertransference. These patients can be difficult and cause the staff to become angry. If aggression continues or escalates, isolating the patient should be considered.[14] Seclusion can be helpful because extraneous stimulation in patients with hallucinations, paranoia, or agitation can intensify the psychosis.[7] Seclusion should not be used for patients needing continuous monitoring, such as suicidal or overdosed patients.

Phase 3: Physical Aggression

In the third phase, patients exhibit completely irrational and out-of-control behavior with threatening language or violent acts toward themselves, other patients, or staff. Verbal management techniques are ineffective with patients in this phase, so physical and chemical restraints are warranted. The decision to use restraints is never an easy one; it is important to remember that restraints for patients in this phase are meant for the safety of the patient, staff, and others, not for punishment.[14] The Joint Commission stresses that restraints should only be used as a last resort when less restrictive interventions are ineffective.[3]

PHYSICAL RESTRAINTS

Physical restraints should be considered when previous efforts to establish rapport and trust, to set limits, and to inform a patient of the consequences of not cooperating have failed. The decision to order physical restraints is difficult because complications can occur and their use can be perceived as coercion or punishment instead of a last resort to ensure safety.[17] Indications for restraining a patient include (1) preventing harm to oneself, (2) preventing harm to other patients, (3) preventing harm to caregivers and other staff, and (4) preventing serious disruption or damage to the environment.[18] Restraints can be helpful in allowing the physician to perform a medically indicated examination in a patient with altered mental status or when indicated medications need to be safely administered. Although restraining patients can be risky, appropriate use when needed may be less risky than not preventing the patient's out-of-control behavior, which can lead to delayed treatment of the patient or injury to the ED staff. Restraints should never be used for staff convenience.[17]

Every institution should have a detailed protocol for the use of restraints.[3] This protocol should identify the members of a restraint team and how to activate the team. All members of the restraint team should be appropriately trained and familiar with the restraining procedure. The team should have at least five members, including a designated leader who explains the process to the patient in clear language. This show of force alone can sometimes prompt better behavior from an aggressive patient. If possible, to prevent lawsuits, at least one member of the team should be a woman, especially when a woman is to be restrained. Before entering a patient's room and initiating the restraining procedure, all personal belongings that could potentially be used as a weapon or cause injury should be removed, including such apparently benign objects as necklaces, lanyards with IDs, stethoscopes around the neck, neckties, or hanging earrings.[18,19]

During the restraining procedure, the team leader maintains the safety of the patient's head while each of the other members takes control of a preassigned extremity. Each extremity should be controlled at the major joint (elbow, knee) and the restraint should be tied to the frame of the bed, not the handrails. All restraint positions carry certain risks, and careful monitoring of the restrained patient is essential. If aspiration is a risk, the patient should be restrained on the side, otherwise restraint in the supine position may facilitate the medical examination and be more comfortable for the patient. Sentinel event tracking by the Joint Commission indicates that restraining patients on their side reduces adverse restraint events.[3] Restraining a patient in the prone position predisposes them to suffocation.[20] If a patient is to be restrained in the prone position, the airway must remain unobstructed at all times and the expansion of the lungs must not be restricted by excessive pressure on the patient's back.[15,17] Restraining patients in the supine position predisposes them to aspiration. If a patient is to be restrained in the supine position, the head must be free to rotate to the side and, when possible, the head of the bed must be elevated.[3] If four-point restraints are used, the arms should be restrained so that one arm is up and one down. This position makes it difficult for the patient to generate enough force to overturn the stretcher. If two-point restraints are used, the contralateral arm and leg should be restrained. If additional restraint is needed, a sheet can be placed around the chest and tied to the stretcher, taking care that the sheet is not so tight that it prevents adequate chest expansion.[21]

Soft restraints can be used in semicooperative patients, but for patients who are combative and trying to escape, leather restraints are preferred. Soft restraints can tighten and cause circulatory compromise as a patient struggles, whereas leather restraints rarely compromise distal circulation but are more difficult to cut and remove in an emergency.[21] While restrained, patients should be under continuous observation and close monitoring. Change in position is important to prevent rhabdomyolysis, pressure sores, and paresthesias.

The treating physician should not be involved in the actual restraint process to preserve the doctor-patient relationship. However, a member of the medical team should be present during the restraining process to monitor the patient. The restraint procedure requires careful documentation by the physician and the nurse.[3] Physician documentation should cite that verbal techniques failed to calm the patient, the specific indication for the restraining procedure, the time the restraints were applied, the time-limited duration of the restraining procedure, the planned medical workup or treatment, and the patient's decision-making capacity. Nursing documentation should include frequent assessment of the patient's vital signs, general condition, and personal needs. Formal reassessment should occur every 15 minutes for signs of injury associated with application of restraints, measurement of vital signs, nutrition and hydration status, circulation, and range-of-motion of extremities, hygiene and elimination, physical and psychological status, patient comfort, and readiness for discontinuation of restraint. The patient must be reassessed by a physician at the end of predefined time limits. When clinically appropriate, restraints should be removed one at a time in 5-minute intervals until two are left. If the patient remains cooperative, the last two can be removed.

The Joint Commission provides up-to-date guidelines and standards for restraints and seclusion on their website.[3] These include:

(1) A physician or licensed practitioner must see and evaluate the patient within 1 hour of initiating intervention.
(2) Seclusion or restraint can only be used when clinically justified and after consideration of alternative treatment options.
(3) Seclusion and restraints must have time-limited orders: 4 hours for adults (older than 17 years), 2 hours for adolescents (9–17 years), 1 hour for patients younger than 9 years.
(4) Patients must have continuous monitoring with periodic evaluation with the intent to discontinue intervention at the earliest possible time.
(5) A face-to-face reevaluation must be performed before each renewal of initial time-limited orders.
(6) Clinical leadership (ie, the medical director) must be notified after 12 hours of continuous seclusion or restraint and every 24 hours thereafter.
(7) With the patient's informed consent, family should be notified promptly when seclusion or restraint is initiated.
(8) Debriefing with patient and staff should be performed after intervention has been discontinued.

Emergency physicians should be familiar with the risks associated with the use of physical restraints. In a survey covering a 10-year period from 50 states, 142 patient deaths occurred while in restraints, although many of these occurred outside of the ED setting.[17,22] The Joint Commission lists patient injury or death under restraint as one of the top 10 sentinel events in the ED.[3] There are many issues that can be the source or cause of patient injury or death. These issues include miscommunication among staff or between staff and patient, procedural noncompliance, inadequate patient assessment, and restraint of a patient in a room not under continuous observation by staff. During Joint Commission inspections, failure to document and practice safe use of restraints is one of the leading citations.[3]

Abrasions and bruising are the most common complications.[23] Positional asphyxia has been reported to occur if the patient is restrained in the prone or hobble position.[3,20] Death can also occur if the restraints are not applied properly or the patient is not carefully monitored.[24] Factors related to excited delirium, including acute intoxication, withdrawal, and untreated psychosis, are more likely to contribute to sudden death.[20] Protracted struggling against restraints can lead to hyperthermia, increased sympathetic tone with vasoconstriction, and lactic acid release from prolonged isotonic muscle contractions leading to metabolic acidosis. Cardiovascular collapse from this metabolic acidosis has been found in many restraint-associated deaths.[20] Any complications from the restraining procedure need to be documented fully.

Studies have evaluated various methods to improve compliance with the federal requirements listed earlier. A recent innovation is the use of computerized forcing functions that signal when a restraint order is expiring. One study locked physicians out from their computer system if a restraint order was not renewed or discontinued at a predetermined time. That same study demonstrated that the overall time patients spent in restraints decreased when the number of appropriately documented restraint orders per patient increased.[25] There is concern that physicians may be less likely to use physical restraints in settings with computerized forcing functions, and instead use more pharmacological restraints or other informal restraint methods that do not require an order, or completely bypass the computerized order entry system.[26] Careful, consistent, thorough, and standardized documentation , whether done on paper or in a computerized fashion, minimizes the risk of miscommunication, adverse events, and other complications from physical restraints.

CHEMICAL RESTRAINTS

Chemical or pharmaceutical restraints, called "rapid tranquilization" in older literature, should also be considered in conjunction with or in place of physical restraints. Physical restraints can be counterproductive because struggling against restraints may prevent obtaining a history or completing a thorough physical examination.[27] Chemical restraints can help gain better control of the agitated patient and allow evaluation and treatment. Complications associated with struggling against physical restraints, such as hyperthermia, dehydration, rhabdomyolysis, or lactic acidosis, can all be minimized with the early use of chemical sedation.[27]

Antipsychotics/Neuroleptics

Because so many patients with violent behavior in the ED have an underlying psychiatric illness, antipsychotic (neuroleptic) medications, either alone or with benzodiazepines, have been used most commonly in the ED setting. Antipsychotics have a high therapeutic index and a lack of addictive potential. This class of medication has a high affinity for the dopamine-2 receptor. Contraindications to these medications include an allergy to the class, Parkinson disease, and anticholinergic drug intoxication. Relative contraindications include pregnancy, lactation, and hypovolemia.

Haloperidol (Haldol), a butyrophenone antipsychotic, is easily given intramuscularly (IM) at doses of 2.5 to 10 mg. Repeat doses can be given at 30- to 60-minute intervals, but the desired effect is usually obtained within three doses. The half-life of haloperidol is 10 to 19 hours. Intravenous (IV) administration has not been approved by the US Food and Drug Administration (FDA), but it has been frequently given via this route. Extrapyramidal syndrome (EPS) is a potential side effect of haloperidol and, in rare cases, has been reported to occur days after administration, even after only one dose. Signs of EPS include akathisia and acute dystonia (torticollis, opisthotonos, or oculogyric crisis). Occurrence of EPS is easily treated with diphenhydramine (Benadryl) or benztropine (Cogentin).[28] Haloperidol can be safely given in the same syringe as lorazepam, thus facilitating administration, hastening onset of sedation, and resulting in fewer EPS episodes than when haloperidol is given alone.[29] Numerous studies have also shown the benefit of using haloperidol to treat aggressive methamphetamine-intoxicated patients.[30,31] Quickly sedating patients with methamphetamine intoxication is particularly important because so many are at risk for rhabdomyolysis, hypertensive crisis, cardiac ischemia, and cardiac dysrhythmias. It has been suggested that haloperidol's dopaminergic antagonism and antimuscarinic properties are neuroprotective in methamphetamine toxicity.[30,31]

Droperidol (Inapsine), also a butyrophenone, used to be one of the most commonly used chemical sedatives in EDs. Routine use has significantly diminished since the FDA issued a black box warning in 2001 about droperidol because of a potential risk for prolongation of the QT interval and resultant torsades de pointes in high doses (QT prolongation has been caused by haloperidol at doses greater than 50 mg IV, but it has no FDA black box warning).[32] Studies have demonstrated that droperidol results in faster control of the patient, shorter duration of effect (half-life = 2 hours), more consistent sedation, and a smaller incidence of EPS when compared with haloperidol, so its use in the ED setting seems ideal.[33] Today, if a clinician prefers to use droperidol, a pretreatment electrocardiogram should be obtained, but in the agitated, combative patient, doing so is obviously quite a challenge and the infrequent use of droperidol not surprising. Continued cardiac monitoring after administration is also recommended.[34]

Neuroleptic malignant syndrome (NMS) is an idiosyncratic adverse effect that can occurs in 1% of patients receiving antipsychotics. NMS is recognized by autonomic instability, hyperthermia, altered mental status, and muscle rigidity. Creatine phosphokinase levels may be elevated.[35] Treatment is supportive, with aggressive cooling measures and cessation of all neuroleptics. In some cases dantrolene is indicated for treatment of extreme muscle rigidity.

Second generation antipsychotic medications, more commonly called "atypical antipsychotics," are newer agents common in outpatient psychiatry and recently incorporated into the ED setting for the treatment of violent patients.[36] Risperidone, olanzapine, and ziprasidone are the most commonly used atypical antipsychotics in the ED. Atypical antipsychotics inhibit dopamine-2 and serotonin receptors and thus provide more tranquilization and less sedation. An important benefit of these atypical antipsychotics is the lower incidence of EPS from the serotonergic activity.[36]

Risperidone (Risperdal) may be given IM or orally by elixir or a recently available disintegrating tablet. Studies have shown risperidone to be as effective as IM haloperidol and less sedating than in the acute treatment of psychosis.[37] Convincing an out-of-control patient to take risperidone orally can be challenging, but onset is rapid with the orally dissolving tablets, so this option is safer and potentially more convenient for nursing staff.

Olanzapine (Zyprexa), available IM or in orally dissolving tablets, has been found to be comparable in efficacy to either lorazepam or haloperidol in many well-controlled studies assessing its use for the treatment of agitated elderly patients with Alzheimer disease, bipolar patients with mania, and schizophrenic patients in acute agitation.[38,39] Occurrence of dystonia and akathisia are less common than with haloperidol.[40,41] Mild hypotension is a common side effect and olanzapine has significant anticholinergic properties, which could exacerbate an agitated patient who overdosed on an anticholinergic agent such as diphenhydramine or jimsonweed.

Ziprasidone (Geodon) has been approved by the FDA for the treatment of acute agitation in patients with schizophrenia and bipolar patients with mania. Studies have shown IM ziprasidone to be superior to haloperidol and occurrence of EPS less common.[42,43] The peak plasma concentration of the IM formulation is achieved in 30 to 45 minutes (8 hours for oral formulation). Importantly, ziprasidone was found to prolong the QTc by 20 milliseconds and therefore is not indicted for patients with pre-existing QTc prolongation.[44,45]

Benzodiazepines

Lorazepam (Ativan) is one of the more frequently used benzodiazepines for the treatment of agitation in the ED setting. It is a favorable medication because of its rapid onset, lack of active metabolites, effectiveness in patients intoxicated with a sympathomimetic agent such as cocaine, and availability in oral, IM, and IV formulations. Of all the benzodiazepines, it is the one most reliably absorbed when administered IM, so it is especially useful in the agitated patient without IV access.[46–48] It has a half-life of 10 to 20 hours. It is also particularly useful in patients with alcohol dependence or cirrhosis because its inactivation is preserved in the setting of liver disease.[49] Most common side effects include sedation, confusion, nausea, and ataxia. Patients must be closely monitored for respiratory depression. It is a class D agent in pregnancy and should also be avoiding in lactating women. As mentioned earlier, studies by Battaglia and colleagues[29] have shown that the sedative effect from the combination of lorazepam and haloperidol is superior to higher doses of either medication alone. In addition, occurrence of EPS is less common in those given lorazepam and haloperidol together compared with those given haloperidol alone.[29]

Midazolam (Versed) is a water-soluble short-acting benzodiazepine that can be administered IM or IV, has a rapid time to onset (18 minutes) and a time to arousal of 30 to 120 minutes (average 82 minutes). When administered IV, midazolam may result in significant hypotension, whereas IM it has little effect on the cardiopulmonary system.[50] One study revealed that midazolam had similar efficacy to haloperidol or lorazepam but was superior to both in that time to arousal was significantly lower.[51] A shorter time to arousal is a useful quality in the ED in that it allows these patients' evaluations to be completed more rapidly, allowing for faster determination of the appropriate disposition of the patient (**Table 1**).

Seclusion

For some patients, seclusion can be an alternative to restraint by allowing for some freedom of movement. However, even limited freedom of movement can be dangerous, especially for large adolescents and adults who can harm themselves and others with their strength, agitation, and free use of their extremities. Psychological harm can also be caused if the patient feels isolated or has a sense of rejection.[53] Rooms used for seclusion need to be safe, calm, and ideally have two exits. Walls need to be indestructible and solid. Furniture needs to be heavy and immovable. The color of the room needs to be calming and there needs to be windows with unbreakable glass to allow for monitoring. No free-standing objects should be in the room. Clear exits and panic buttons should also be present.[54] Continuous observation is required.

ASSAULT

Hospital staff can be victims of assault before a violence management team can be activated and the patient restrained. As noted earlier, 50% of health care workers will be a victim of work-place violence during their career.[5] A few recommendations can help minimize personal injury when facing a potentially violent patient. Do not face the patient head on; keep a sideward stance and try to keep a buffer zone of at least four body widths from the patient. Have your arms ready for self-protection. Try to appear calm and avoid sudden movements. Minimize direct eye contact and try to deflect any kicks or punches. If bitten, do not pull away but instead push into the patient and use the other hand to close their nares, causing them to reflexively open their mouth. Avoid arguing and do not lie, bargain, or make promises. Try to

Table 1
Comparison of antipsychotics and benzodiazepines

	Half-Life	Time to Onset	Disadvantages/ Advantages
Haloperidol	18 h	30–60 min (IV, IM)	EPS; NMS; can be given in same syringe with lorazepam
Droperidol	2.3 h	30 min	QT prolongation, torsades de pointes; NMS
Risperidone	Orally 20 h	Orally 1 h	Less sedating
Olanzapine	21–54 h	Orally 6 h/IM 15–45 min	Anticholinergic; useful in elderly, bipolar and schizophrenic patients
Ziprasidone	PO 7 h/IM 2–5 h	PO 6–8 h/IM 1 h	Less EPS; useful in bipolar and schizophrenia
Lorazepam	Adults 13 h, elderly 16 h, ESRD 32–70 h	Orally 30–60 min IV 5–20 min	Rapid onset; inactive metabolites even with liver disease
Midazolam	1–4 h (prolonged with cirrhosis, CHF, elderly, obesity	IM 15 min IV 1–5 min	Minimal cardiopulmonary effect with IM; hypotension with IV; short time to arousal

Abbreviations: CHF, congestive heart failure; ESRD, end-stage renal disease.
Data from Lexi-comp/Up to Date.[52] Available at: http://www.uptodate.com/home/clinicians. Accessed July 30, 2009.

control the natural instinct to shout which inadvertently reciprocates the violence.[15] Do not reach for any weapon the patient may be holding.[55]

PREVENTATIVE MEASURES AND PREPARATION FOR THE COMBATIVE PATIENT

Various environmental, administrative, and behavioral preventative measures can be implemented to help make the ED a safer environment.[56,57]

Certain environmental designs can strategically minimize violence in hospitals. Monitoring systems such as metal detectors and security cameras have been found to discourage aggressive behavior in the ED and other industries. Waiting rooms should be designed to accommodate and assist visitors and patients who may have a delay in service. The triage area, waiting rooms, and reception areas should have heavy furniture that cannot be lifted and used as weapons; glass should be shatterproof or bulletproof; nursing stations should be enclosed because nurses are often the first target of violence.[4] Uniformed security available 24 hours a day is one of the best ways to increase the safety of a department and hospital. Alarm systems and other ways of emergency signaling should be in place in all EDs. A panic button in patient rooms and hallways can be helpful. A verbal alarm system to get the attention of other staff, such as a code like "Dr. Armstrong to room 8," is another effective way to mobilize appropriate staff without upsetting other patients.[18]

Administrative controls to help reduce patient violence include designing staffing patterns to minimize patient waiting times and to prevent staff from working alone. Restricting the movement of the public throughout the hospital or various sections of the ED by card-controlled ID access has also been recommended.

Behavioral prevention strategies include continually educating and training all staff to recognize and manage violent events and assaults, resolve conflicts when dealing with patients, and maintain situational awareness. Patient searches are important to exclude weapons from the ED: studies have revealed that up to 10% of patients presenting to the ED carry some type of weapon. Searches can be performed either by having a policy that all patients undress and change into a gown or having a sign posted that all individuals entering the ED will be searched for weapons.[58]

Disposition

The violent patient may be considered for discharge if the patient is cooperative, demonstrates no evidence of intoxication, organic problems have been adequately excluded as the cause of a patient's agitation, other medical and psychiatric problems have been addressed, mental status is normal, and vitals signs are normal. Violent patients who elope before their evaluation is completed pose a significant risk to themselves and to others. Elopements can also be a legal risk to health care providers, so local authorities should be notified in such cases.

SUMMARY

As EDs continue to become more crowded, safely managing violent or aggressive patients will continue to be challenging. Appropriately trained personnel, adherence to protocol, careful attention to documentation, and good common sense will minimize complications and ensure safe use of physical or chemical restraints when indicated.

REFERENCES

1. Lavoie FW, Carter GL, Danzi DF, et al. Emergency department violence in United States teaching hospitals. Ann Emerg Med 1988;17(11):1227–33.
2. Martel M, Sterzinger A, Miner J, et al. Management of acute undifferentiated agitation in the emergency department: a randomized double-blind trial of droperidol, ziprasidone, and midazolam. Acad Emerg Med 2005;12(12):1167–72.
3. The Joint Commission. Available at: www.jointcommission.org/. Accessed April 2, 2009.
4. CDC. Department of Health and Human Services. Centers for Disease Control and Prevention. National Institute for Occupational Safety and Health. Available at: www.cdc.gov/niosh/docs/2002-101. Accessed March 15, 2009.
5. Mahoney BS. The extent, nature and response to victimization of emergency nurses in PA. J Emerg Nurs 1991;17(5):282–91.
6. McAneney CM, Shaw KN. Violence in the pediatric emergency department. Ann Emerg Med 1994;23(6):1248–51.
7. Citrome L, Volavka J. Violent patients in the emergency setting. Psychiatr Clin North Am 1999;22(4):789–801.
8. Tardiff K. Diagnosis and management of violent patients. In: Michels R, Cavener JD, Cooper AM, et al, editors. Psychiatry, vol. 3. Philadelphia: Lippincott-Raven; 1997. p. 1–17.

9. Regier DA, Farmer ME, Rae DS, et al. Comorbidity of mental disorders with alcohol and other drug abuse. Results from the Epidemiologic Catchment Area (ECA) Study. JAMA 1990;264(19):2511–8.
10. Swanson JW. Mental disorder, substance abuse and community violence: an epidemiological approach. In: Monahan J, Steadman HJ, editors. Violence and mental disorder: developments in risk assessment. Chicago (IL): University of Chicago Press; 1994. p. 101–36.
11. American Psychiatric Association. Practice guidelines for the treatment of patients with delirium. Am J Psychiatry 1999;156(5 Suppl):1–20.
12. Martel M, Miner J, Fringer R, et al. Discontinuation of droperidol for the control of acutely agitated out-of-hospital patients. Prehosp Emerg Care 2005;9(1):44–8.
13. Mock EF, Wrenn KD, Wright SW, et al. Prospective field study of violence in EMS calls. Ann Emerg Med 1998;32(1):33–6.
14. Nonviolent crisis intervention workbook. Brookfield (WI): National Crisis Prevention Institute; 1987.
15. Isaacs E. The Violent patient. In: Adams JG, Nadel E, DeBlieux P, et al, editors. Emergency medicine. 1st edition. Philadelphia: Saunders Elsevier; 2008. p. 2047–56.
16. Hill S, Petit J. The violent patient. Emerg Med Clin North Am 2000;18(2):301–15.
17. Annas GJ. The last resort–the use of physical restraints in medical emergencies. N Engl J Med 1999;341(18):1408–12.
18. Rice MM, More GP. Management of the violent patient: therapeutic and legal considerations. Emerg Med Clin North Am 1991;9(1):13–30.
19. Kuhn W. Violence in the emergency department: managing aggressive patients in a high-stress environment. Postgrad Med 1999;105(1):143–8.
20. Hick JL, Smith SW, Lynch MT. Metabolic acidosis in restraint associated cardiac arrest: a case series. Acad Emerg Med 1999;6(3):239–43.
21. Lavoie FW. Consent, involuntary treatment and the use of force in an urban emergency department. Ann Emerg Med 1992;21(1):25–32.
22. Kozub ML, Skidmore R. Seclusion and restraint: understanding recent changes. J Psychosoc Nurs Ment Health Serv 2001;39(3):24–31.
23. Zun LS. A prospective study of the complication rate of the use of patient restraint in the emergency department. J Emerg Med 2003;24(2):119–24.
24. Chan TC, Vilke GM, Neuman T, et al. Restraint position and positional asphyxia. Ann Emerg Med 1997;30(5):578–86.
25. Griffey RT, Wittels K, Gilboy N, et al. Use of computerized forcing function improves performance in ordering restraints. Ann Emerg Med 2009;53(4): 469–76.
26. Bisantz A, Wears R. Forcing functions: the need for restraint. Ann Emerg Med 2009;53(4):477–9.
27. Diaz JE. Chemical restraint. J Emerg Med 2000;19(3):289–91.
28. Currier GW, Trenton A. Pharmacologic treatment of psychotic agitation. CNS Drugs 2002;16(14):219–28.
29. Battaglia J, Moss S, Rush J, et al. Haloperidol, lorazepam or both for psychotic agitation? A multicenter, prospective, double blind, emergency department study. Am J Emerg Med 1997;15(4):335–40.
30. Kuribara H. Early post treatment with haloperidol retards induction of methamphetamine sensitization in mice. Eur J Pharmacol 1994;256(3):295–9.
31. Kuribara H. Inhibition of methamphetamine sensitization by post methamphetamine treatment with SCH 23390 or haloperidol. Psychopharmacology 1995; 199(1):34–8.

32. Kao LW, Kirk MA, Evers SJ, et al. Droperidol, QT prolongation and sudden death: what is the evidence? Ann Emerg Med 2003;41(4):546–58.
33. Chase PB, Biros MH. A retrospective review of the use and safety of droperidol in a large, high-risk, inner-city emergency department patient population. Acad Emerg Med 2002;9(12):1402–10.
34. Knott J, Taylor D, Castle D. Randomized clinical trial comparing intravenous midazolam and droperidol for sedation of the acutely agitated patient in the emergency department. Ann Emerg Med 2006;47(1):61–7.
35. Dubin WR, Weiss KJ. Emergency psychiatry. In: Michels R, Caverner JD, Cooper AM, et al, editors, Psychiatry, vol. 2. Philadelphia: Lippincott-Raven; 1997. p. 1–15.
36. Rund DA, Ewing JD, Mitzel K, et al. The use of intramuscular benzodiazepines and antipsychotic agents in the treatment of acute agitation or violence in the emergency department. J Emerg Med 2006;31(3):317–24.
37. Currier GW, Simpson GM. Risperidone liquid concentrate and oral lorazepam versus intramuscular haloperidol and intramuscular lorazepam for treatment of psychotic agitation. J Clin Psychiatry 2001;62(3):153–7.
38. Meehan KM, Wang H, David SR, et al. Comparison of rapidly acting intramuscular olanzapine, lorazepam and placebo: a double blind randomized study in acutely agitated patients with dementia. Neuropsychopharmacology 2002; 26(4):494–504.
39. Meehan K, Zhang F, David S, et al. A double blind, randomized comparison of the efficacy and safety of intramuscular injections of olanzapine, lorazepam or placebo in treating acutely agitated patients diagnosed with bipolar mania. J Clin Psychopharmacol 2001;21(4):389–97.
40. Breier A, Meehan K, Birkett M, et al. A double blind, placebo controlled dose response comparison of intramuscular olanzapine and haloperidol in the treatment of acute agitation in schizophrenia. Arch Gen Psychiatry 2002;59(5):441–8.
41. Wright P, Birkett M, David SR, et al. Double blind, placebo controlled comparison of intramuscular olanzapine and intramuscular haloperidol in the treatment of acute agitation in schizophrenia. Am J Psychiatry 2001;158(7):1149–51.
42. Brook S, Lucey JV, Gunn KP. Intramuscular ziprasidone compared with intramuscular haloperidol in the treatment of acute psychosis. J Clin Psychiatry 2000; 61(12):933–41.
43. Brook S. Intramuscular ziprasidone: Moving beyond the conventional in the treatment of acute agitation in schizophrenia. J Clin Psychiatry 2003;64(suppl 19): 13–8.
44. Bellnier TJ. Continuum of care: stabilizing the acutely agitated patient. Am J Health Syst Pharm 2002;59(17 Suppl 5):S12–8.
45. Goodnick PJ. Ziprasidone: Profile on safety. Expert Opin Pharmacother 2001; 2(1):1655–62.
46. Salzman C. Use of benzodiazepines to control disruptive behavior in inpatients. J Clin Psychiatry 1988;49(Suppl 12):13–5.
47. Greenblatt DJ, Divoll M, Harmatz JS, et al. Pharmacokinetic comparison of sublingual lorazepam with intravenous, intramuscular and oral lorazepam. J Pharm Sci 1982;71(2):248–52.
48. Greenblatt DJ, Shader RI, Franke K, et al. Pharmacokinetics and bioavailability of intravenous, intramuscular and oral lorazepam in humans. J Pharm Sci 1979; 68(1):57–63.
49. Tesar GE. The agitated patient, part II: pharmacologic treatment. Hosp Community Psychiatry 1993;44(4):627–9.

50. Gerecke M. Chemical structure and properties of midazolam compared with other benzodiazepines. Br J Clin Pharmacol 1983;16(Supp 1):11S–6S.
51. Nobay F, Simon B, Levitt A, et al. A prospective double-blind, randomized trial of midazolam versus haloperidol versus lorazepam in the chemical restraint of violent and severely agitated patients. Acad Emerg Med 2004;11(7):744–9.
52. LexiComp/Up-To-Date. Available at: http://www.uptodate.com/home/clinicals. Accessed July 30, 2009.
53. Masters KJ, Bellonci C, Bernet W, et al. Practice parameter for the prevention and management of aggressive behavior in child and adolescent psychiatric institutions with special reference to seclusion and restraint. J Am Acad Child Adolesc Psychiatry 2002;41(2):4S–25S.
54. Rankins RC, Hendey GW. Effect of a security system on violent incidents and hidden weapons in the emergency department. Ann Emerg Med 1999;33(6):676–9.
55. Fernandes CMB, Raboud JM, Christenson JM, et al. The effect of an education program on violence in the emergency department. Ann Emerg Med 2002;39(1):47–55.
56. Blanchard JC, Curtis KM. Violence in the emergency department. Emerg Med Clin North Am 1999;17(3):717–31.
57. Here's how to prevent assaults on staff. ED Manag 2001;13(6):66–9.
58. Mattox EA, Wright SW, Bracikowski AC. Metal detectors in the pediatric emergency department: patron attitudes and national prevalence. Pediatr Emerg Care 2000;16(3):163–5.

Evaluation of the Psychiatric Patient

Tara Raviprakash Sood, MD, Christopher M. Mcstay, MD*

KEYWORDS

• Medical clearance • Psychiatric clearance • Delirium
• Psychiatric emergencies • Involuntary hospitalization

Patients presenting to the emergency department (ED) with behavioral disturbances account for approximately 6% of all ED visits.[1] A psychiatric emergency is defined by the American Psychiatric Association as "an acute disturbance in thought, behavior, mood, or social relationship, which requires immediate intervention as defined by the patient, family, or social unit." Emergency physicians are often responsible for the initial assessment of these patients' psychiatric complaints, which might include homicidal and suicidal behavior and acute psychosis. Furthermore, the emergency physician might be asked to provide "medical clearance" before transfer to definitive psychiatric care. The purpose of the medical screening is to identify medical conditions that might be causing or contributing to the psychiatric emergency or that might be dangerous or inappropriate to treat in a psychiatric facility.[2] Appropriate treatment in the ED is essential to avoid morbidity and mortality resulting from misdiagnosis of medical conditions as psychiatric illnesses and from mismanagement of psychiatric illnesses.

FOCUSED MEDICAL ASSESSMENT

In 1979, Weissberg[3] described three scenarios in which the term "medically cleared" was applied to psychiatric patients: (1) no physical illness was found in the patient; (2) coexisting medical problems were determined not to be the primary cause of the acute psychiatric emergency; (3) an acute medical condition was stabilized and the patient deemed "clear" to be transferred to the care of psychiatry. The past and present use of the phrase "medically clear" is ambiguous and might be interpreted and applied differently by emergency physicians and psychiatrists. To the emergency physician, "medically clear" usually means the patient does not have any acute illness requiring emergent care. Chronic conditions, such as diabetes and hypertension, might require ongoing medical attention despite the patient having been "cleared." The accepting psychiatrist might interpret "medically clear" to mean the total absence of medical conditions that might require ongoing care. Because of ongoing variability

Department of Emergency Medicine, New York University, Bellevue Hospital Center, BCD 3rd Floor, 462 1st Avenue, New York, NY 10016, USA
* Corresponding author.
E-mail address: christopher.mcstay@nyumc.org (C.M. Mcstay).

Emerg Med Clin N Am 27 (2009) 669–683
doi:10.1016/j.emc.2009.07.005
emed.theclinics.com

of the process and definition of "medical clearance," the American College of Emergency Physicians recommends the label "focused medical assessment" to describe the process of excluding illness that needs acute care.[4] Some authors have suggested eliminating the term "medically clear" and replacing it with a comprehensive discharge note, which includes a history, physical examination, treatment plans for any medical diagnoses,[5] and other care instructions such as wound care.

The number of patients with psychiatric emergencies requiring medical assessments has increased over time. Larkin and colleagues[1] reported 53 million mental health–related ED visits from 1992 to 2001, an increase from 17.1 to 23.6 mental health patients per 1000 visits. Patients attempting suicide increased from 0.8 to 1.5 per 1000 patients.[6] One-third of those attempting suicide are ultimately admitted to the hospital, with 10% requiring admission to an intensive care unit setting.[7] Mental health–related visits represent a large patient population requiring specialized attention from the emergency physician and psychiatrist.

ED evaluations for mental health visits are often inconsistent and incomplete. Riba and Hale[8] reported these inconsistencies in their study of 137 ED patients with psychiatric symptoms. They reported that history of present illness was recorded at a rate of 33%, abnormal vital signs noted at a rate of 32%, and general appearance recorded at a rate of 64%. Furthermore, only 8% of the patients had a fully documented neurologic examination and 8% had no physical examination noted. Tintinalli and colleagues[5] reported similar inconsistencies and lack of assessment of patients with psychiatric complaints, including 20% of charts without a documented mental status examination. "Medically clear" was documented in 80% of patients in whom medical disease should have been identified.

Several studies have demonstrated high rates (up to 50%) of coexisting medical disease in patients who present with psychiatric emergencies.[9] Coexisting medical conditions may be primarily responsible for a patient's behavioral change or a contributing factor to it. Although some medical conditions may not require urgent intervention, they should be identified so that they might be included in the ongoing management of the patient.

The emergency physician's evaluation of the patient with psychiatric complaints plays an integral part in the patient's care. The level of medical care offered in a psychiatric ward can be insufficient to provide safe care for many patients with acute medical illness.. Furthermore, because of limitations at the receiving ward or facility, the emergency physician's medical evaluation may be the only one that the patient receives. Some of the contributing factors are:[2] (1) low ratio of staff to patients compared with medical wards; (2) lack of staff experience in recognizing, monitoring, and managing deterioration of medical conditions from stable to unstable; (3) possibility of bodily harm from other psychiatric patients; (4) inability of patients to fully participate in group therapy and other activities; and (5) increased risk of spreading infectious agents.

MEDICAL CONDITIONS WITH PSYCHIATRIC SYMPTOMS

With a thorough history and physical examination, the emergency physician aims to identify a possible organic cause for the patient's psychiatric symptoms. In 1981, Hall and colleagues[10,11] reported that 46% of the patients admitted to a psychiatric ward had an unrecognized medical illness that either caused or exacerbated their psychiatric illness. Five groups of patients are generally regarded to be at high risk of medical illness: the elderly; patients with a history of substance abuse; patients without a psychiatric history; patients with pre-existing medical disorders, and patients from a lower socioeconomic level.[2,12]

Delirium

Delirium is an acute state of confusion or disturbance of consciousness caused by a medical illness. Terms that have been used interchangeably with delirium include organic brain syndrome, acute confusional state, metabolic encephalopathy, and toxic encephalopathy. There are 4 key elements in the diagnosis of delirium: time course, disturbance of consciousness, change of cognition, and evidence of medical cause.[13] The change in mental status typically develops over a short period and fluctuates during the course of the day. Disturbance in consciousness is often indicated by a reduced awareness of the environment. Memory deficit, disorientation, and language disturbance are examples of changes in cognition. In general, patients presenting with disorientation are more commonly afflicted with medical illness than with psychiatric illness.[14] In contrast to delirium, patients presenting with dementia display a more gradual onset of symptoms, without fluctuation and without a corresponding alteration in consciousness. For older individuals, the emergency physician should have a high index of suspicion because the prevalence of delirium in elderly patients in the ED is approximately 10% (**Table 1**).[15]

The differential diagnosis of medical conditions presenting with behavioral symptoms is broad and includes infections, metabolic derangements, endocrine abnormalities, medications, substance abuse, and central nervous system (CNS) disorders.[16] Failure to recognize organic causes of behavioral disturbance could lead to delays in recognition and treatment, with associated morbidity and mortality.

Infections

Patients with an infection of the CNS can present with behavioral changes. Patients presenting with bacterial and viral meningitis often have an altered level of consciousness, irritability, or psychosis.[17] Herpes simplex encephalitis can affect the limbic system, which manifests as olfactory and gustatory hallucinations, anosmia, personality change, and/or psychotic behavior.[18,19] In the elderly, systemic infections, such as urinary tract infections and pneumonia, can present with confusion and depressed consciousness.

Table 1
Clinical factors that help differentiate delirium from psychiatric disease

Characteristic	Delirium	Psychiatric Illness
Age	<12 y or >40 y	13–40 y
Onset	Acute	Acute
Course	Fluctuation	Constant
Past medical history	Substance abuse, medical illness	Previous psychiatric history
Family history		Family history of psychiatric illness
Affect	Emotional lability	Flat affect
Vital signs	Usually abnormal	Usually normal
Orientation	Usually impaired	Rarely impaired
Attention	Impaired	Disorganized
Hallucinations	Primarily visual	Primarily auditory
Speech	Slow, incoherent, dysarthric	Usually coherent
Consciousness	Decreased	Alert

Data from Williams ER, Shepherd SM. Medical clearance of psychiatric patients. Emerg Med Clin North Am 2000;18:185–98.

Metabolic/Endocrine Abnormalities

Hypo- and hyperthyroidism are the most common endocrine abnormalities that cause psychiatric symptoms. Hypothyroidism frequently presents with dysphoria, affective lability, and emotional withdrawal, which can progress to delusion and hallucinations. Patients with hyperthyroidism can have anxiety, nervousness, and hyperactivity.[20]

Diabetes can also present with altered mental status or anxiety.[17] Hyperglycemia causes mental status changes ranging from lethargy to coma. Hypoglycemia may lead to acute anxiety, agitation, or psychosis, often associated with palpitations and tremulousness. Mental status can range from lethargy to coma.[17] In any patient with alteration in mental status, blood glucose level should be tested immediately. Prolonged hypoglycemia can lead to permanent neurologic damage, so delays in diagnosis and treatment must be avoided. Other endocrine disorders that can present with psychiatric symptoms are hypo- or hyperparathyroidism and hypo- or hypercortisolism.[20]

Medications

Medications are one of the most common causes of acute psychiatric symptoms in the elderly.[21] Discussion of all the medications that cause behavioral disturbance is beyond the scope of this article; however, polypharmacy, anticholinergic agents, selective serotonin reuptake inhibitors, corticosteroids, benzodiazepines, nonsteroidal anti-inflammatory drugs, and opioids commonly cause altered mental status.[22–24] Furthermore, even medications not prescribed for their anticholinergic effects can have anticholinergic potential, for example, furosemide, digoxin, warfarin, and hydrochlorothiazide.[25] Emergency physicians should suspect medication-related behavioral change in every patient.[26]

Substance Abuse and Withdrawal

Acute intoxication and withdrawal from drugs of abuse can present with confusion, agitation, and psychosis, kicking, bicycling of the legs, or incontinence. Although alcohol is primarily a CNS depressant, alcohol-induced psychopathologic conditions can range from lethargic depression to violent delirium.[27] The most commonly abused stimulants in the United States are cocaine and amphetamines,[16,28] with patients often presenting with a sympathomimetic toxidrome, in addition to agitation, paranoia, and frank psychosis. Patients ingesting sedative hypnotics, such as benzodiazepines and barbiturates, may have a depressed level of consciousness. Hallucinogens, such as phencyclidine, LSD (lysergic acid diethylamide), and other derivatives, are also common drugs of abuse that can present with delirium. Patients may also present with signs and symptoms consistent with drug withdrawal. Those with dependence on sedative hypnotics and alcohol are particularly at risk of progressing to delirium tremens and exhibiting agitation, confusion, and frank psychosis.

CNS Disorders

In young patients, several types of epilepsy can present with psychiatric symptoms. Simple partial seizures may exhibit hallucinations and involuntary crying or laughing. Complex partial seizure presentation can range from automatisms to ambulating aimlessly, disrobing, and dancing.[29] Frontal lobe epilepsy is frequently misdiagnosed as a psychiatric disorder. Symptoms of frontal lobe epilepsy are sudden onset of screaming, kicking, bicycling of the legs, or incontinence.[30] Cerebral tumors, cerebrovascular accidents, and subdural hematomas can also have psychiatric manifestations, based on the location and the structures infiltrated or compressed.[31]

Hydrocephalus, migraine, and other vasculitic phenomena should be considered in the appropriate clinical setting.

CLINICAL EVALUATION

Initial evaluation of the patient should focus on stabilization. The ABCs should be addressed and vital signs should be assessed. Management of acute agitation is not within the scope of this article, but if present, de-escalation techniques should be attempted. If de-escalation techniques fail, the patient should be treated with prompt physical restraint and chemical sedation, followed by release of physical restraints when feasible. A thorough history and physical examination is required to determine the cause of the patient's symptoms. Once a differential diagnosis is generated, ancillary tests must be considered to support the physician's evaluation. Before transferring the patient to a psychiatric facility, treatment plans for each active problem should be generated.

History

The cause of the patient's symptoms is most likely to be elucidated by the history. Obtaining an accurate history from the patient is often difficult; it should be obtained in a calm, nonjudgmental, nonthreatening manner. Some patients may be unable to provide a history secondary to alterations in mental status; other patients may be unwilling to provide an accurate history for fear of legal consequences, shame, or guilt.[32] Collateral history from bystanders, family, health care professionals, police, and emergency medical services is important, especially for patients who are unable to provide sufficient information. All prior documentation, including past medical records and discharge summaries, should be reviewed, providing the physician with additional history.

The history should be directed toward determining the cause of the patient's symptoms. It is essential to have an understanding of the patient's baseline, which is defined as the patient's usual level of alertness, ability to perform activities of daily living, and capacity for social interactions. Once a baseline is established, details of the deviation from baseline must be determined. Differences in the patient's behavior, details on the time of and the events leading to onset of symptoms, and rapidity of progression are necessary to create an accurate assessment.

Because medical conditions can have psychiatric manifestations, the emergency physician must ask pertinent questions to find any evidence of medical illness that may be masquerading as a psychiatric illness. A detailed medication history is a key component of a thorough evaluation, especially in the elderly and those on chronic psychotropic medication. A substance abuse history should be elicited from all patients.

Physical Examination

The physical examination should begin with the vital signs recorded in triage. Studies show triage vital signs are reliable and should not be dismissed.[33] Oxygen saturation and glucose level should be obtained in all patients with altered mental status. Henneman and colleagues[34] reported clinically significant findings in 25% of vital sign measurements in patients presenting with psychiatric symptoms.[2] Psychiatric illnesses should not cause abnormal vital signs; therefore, abnormalities should raise the clinician's suspicion of an organic cause. Vital signs can be a clue to occult infections, withdrawal, cardiovascular disease, substance abuse, and medication overdoses. The emergency physician should be aware of the importance of vital signs and should actively address abnormalities. Observation of general appearance and activity should also be performed. Attention should be paid to the patient's level of grooming, hygiene, and attention, and affect and interactions with other individuals present. Poor grooming and psychomotor retardation or tardive dyskinesia are often clues to chronic psychiatric disorders.

The mental status examination is also highly informative.[34] To evaluate a patient's mental status, a mini-mental status examination (MMSE) can be conducted. However, because MMSEs are not practical in the emergency setting, the physician can apply the Quick Confusion Scale (QCS), which has been validated to assess cognitive function.[35] The QCS is a battery of 6 questions focused on orientation, memory, and concentration.[36] A total score of less than 12 suggests an alteration in cognition (**Table 2**).

A thorough neurologic examination should include an assessment of orientation, memory, motor strength, sensation, cranial nerves, gait, cerebellar functions, and reflexes. Any abnormality or focality should prompt consideration of an organic cause of behavioral disturbance and if appropriate, consideration of subsequent radiological testing. Patients with liver disease, myoclonus, tremor, and automatisms should be assessed for asterixis, which might provide clues to other neurologic processes.

The remainder of the physical examination can provide clues to the cause of the patient's presentation, proceeding in a head-to-toe manner. The head should be inspected for any obvious signs of trauma, including Battle sign and raccoon eyes, and the tympanic membranes visualized for hemotympanum. Prior surgical incisions, indicative of prior craniotomy or shunts, are also important physical findings. Pupillary dilatation or constriction and any abnormality in extraocular movements or nystagmus should be noted. Papilledema or anisocoria should prompt further workup for intracranial processes. The neck should be palpated for masses or thyroid abnormality, auscultated for bruits, and tested for meningeal signs, including nuchal rigidity. Auscultation of the heart, for valvular abnormalities and irregular rhythms, and of the chest, for any obvious sign of pneumothorax, pneumonia, chronic obstructive pulmonary disease, or congestive heart failure, are important. Palpation of the abdomen may

Table 2
Quick confusion scale

Question	Response	Weight	Score
What year is it?	0 or 1	×2	______
What month is it	0 or 1	×2	______
Give memory phrase	John Brown, 42 Market Street, NY		
What time is it?	0 or 1 (if within an hour)	×2	______
Count backward from 20 to 1	0, 1 or 2 (2 if no errors, 1 if 1 error, 0 if 2 or more errors)	×1	______
Say the months in reverse	0, 1 or 2 (2 if no errors, 1 if 1 error, 0 if 2 or more errors)	×1	______
Repeat the phrase	0, 1, 2, 3, 4, or 5 (score for each portion)	×1	______

Data from Stair TO, Morrissey J, Jaradeh I, et al. Validation of the quick confusion scale for mental status screening in the emergency department. Intern Emerg Med 2007;2:130–32; Huff JS, Farace E, Brady WJ, et al. The quick confusion scale in the ED: Comparison with the mini-mental state examination. Am J Emerg Med 2001;19:461–64; and Irons MJ, Farace E, Brady WJ, et al. Mental status screening of emergency department patients: Normative study of the quick confusion scale. Acad Emerg Med 2002;9:989–94.

reveal signs of liver disease, which may be a clue to hepatic encephalopathy. Additional abdominal findings include signs of any obvious surgical pathology and bladder distension or tenderness, which might be present in urinary retention or infection, respectively. Urinary tract infections are commonly found in elderly individuals with behavioral changes. A genitourinary examination should also be performed with special attention to those who report sexual assault. A good skin examination may reveal cellulitis, scabies, frost bite, signs of drug abuse, and signs of trauma.

Overall, the emergency physician should have a preliminary differential diagnosis based on the history and should use the physical examination to strengthen that differential. For example, if a toxicologic cause is suspected, the physical examination should include pupil size, dry or diaphoretic skin, needle marks, urinary retention, and a cardiac examination. On the other hand, if the history suggests an infectious process, the physical examination should evaluate for the source of the potential infection. If the physical examination is not guided by suspicions raised by the history, key findings may be missed.

Laboratory and Ancillary Tests

The need for routine blood tests, electrocardiogram (ECG), and imaging studies in psychiatric patients has been the focus of many studies and much debate. Considerable variation exists between physicians, departments, and institutions in what is generally considered necessary in the medical assessment of patients with acute psychiatric emergencies. The amount of testing performed or required might also be influenced by the type of facility to which the patient is being transferred and the demands of that facility. In general, testing should be guided by pertinent findings in the history and physical examination.

Several studies have reported on clinically significant findings in routine laboratory screening for patients presenting to the ED,[34,37,38] only one of which was prospective.[34] Henneman and colleagues[34] reported clinical significance in 10% of SMA-7 (electrolytes, blood urea nitrogen, creatinine, and glucose) and 5% of complete blood count (CBC) tests, which were ordered in a study group of 100 patients who presented to the ED with new onset psychiatric symptoms; 63% of these patients were found to have an organic cause for their symptoms. This high percentage can be attributed to the study's inclusion criteria for patients in whom a functional cause was considered a possibility.[34] Korn and colleagues[38] reported no clinically significant laboratory tests in their study of 80 ED patients, after excluding those with a significant medical history or significant medical complaints and those with new onset psychiatric complaints. Olshaker and colleagues[37] reported on 345 patients who presented to the ED with a psychiatric complaint and found clinically significant values on SMA-7 and CBC testing in only 8% and 4%, respectively; 19% of these patients were found to have an acute medical condition for which history had a sensitivity of 94%; the sensitivity of laboratory testing was only 20%.[37] The differences between these studies can be attributed to the differences in patient population and in the thoroughness of the initial history and examination.[2]

In awake alert patients with no acute medical complaints, a normal physical examination, and a clear psychiatric cause for presentation, the routine use of laboratory testing is unlikely to result in findings that have clinical significance. In general, there are no data to support routine laboratory testing in psychiatric patients whose history and physical examination exclude significant medical illness. Laboratory testing should be guided by the differential diagnosis formulated after a thorough history and physical examination.[2,37,39] Emergency physicians should consider lowering the threshold to perform additional testing in patients presenting with new onset psychiatric conditions, in patients who are elderly, or when there is clinical uncertainty. In addition, it is reasonable to perform pregnancy testing in all female psychiatric patients of childbearing age.

Some authors have suggested obtaining chest radiographs and ECGs on all patients older than 60 years, based on higher incidence of concurrent medical disease.[2,40] Little data exist to support or oppose the use of routine computed tomographic (CT) head scans in psychiatric patients.[41] Ananth and colleagues[42] studied 34 psychiatric patients to evaluate the utility of routine CT head scans, concluding that routine use of CT was not helpful. In another series of 168 patients with new psychotic illness, only 1.2% of patients had CT scans that had actual implications for patient management.[43] A more recent series, examining 127 young healthy military recruits with new onset psychosis, found no CT scans that were clinically significant.[44] Hufschmidt and Shabarin[45] retrospectively studied 294 elderly patients admitted with a diagnosis of acute confusion, to determine the diagnostic yield of cerebral imaging and to identify clinical markers of patients with a low probability of relevant pathology. They concluded that the likelihood of finding relevant pathology is extremely low when the lack of focal signs is combined with a probable alternate diagnosis. Regardless, it is reasonable for elderly patients with new onset psychiatric complaints, and those with focality on neurologic examination or a history of HIV (human immunodeficiency virus), to undergo CT scanning. This approach seems justified given the potential consequences of missed cerebrovascular accidents, subdural hematoma, or other intracranial processes.

Additional laboratory testing, such as lumbar puncture, should be considered in certain patients. Lumbar puncture is not a routine test; it should be reserved for patients with symptoms suspicious for meningitis or encephalitis. Patients with complaints of headache, photophobia, neck stiffness, vomiting, and fever should be considered for lumbar puncture. A CT head scan should be obtained before a lumbar puncture in patients who are older than 60 years, have an immunocompromised state, have a history of CNS disease, have experienced a seizure within the past week, and have abnormal neurologic findings.[46,47]

The American College of Emergency Physicians (ACEP)'s Clinical Policy recommendation is that there is no role for routine urine toxicologic screening in an alert, awake, and cooperative ED patient.[4] Recommendations are based on a prospective series that found no difference in disposition between mandatory urine toxicologic screening and screening at the physician's discretion.[48] Another study by Eisen and colleagues[49] confirmed that emergency physicians did not change management based on urine toxicology results. ACEP's clinical policy concluded with a recommendation that transfer to a psychiatric facility should not be delayed, if only awaiting urine toxicology results.[4] Blood alcohol levels may also offer little of clinical significance in the ED. Emergency physicians may consider psychiatrists' need for urine toxicologic screens and blood alcohol levels as they can affect later treatment plans. Most emergency physicians would consider it unacceptable to delay transfer to psychiatric care, if these tests are not performed when not clinically indicated.

MANAGEMENT OF PSYCHIATRIC PATIENTS

As mental health care funding continues to decrease, EDs are forced to play an escalating role in managing psychiatric patients. Although some EDs have the resources for "medically cleared" patients to be evaluated by a psychiatrist, studies show that these EDs are the exception. In 2006, Baraff and colleagues[50] surveyed the EDs in California to examine the available resources. Only an estimated 10% of EDs were most patients evaluated by a psychiatrist, and only 34% of the EDs had an on-call psychiatrist.[50,51] Emergency physicians are often expected to care for suicidal and homicidal patients with minimal psychiatric consultation.

Suicidal Patient

Suicide is ranked as the 11th leading cause of death and approximately 39% of suicide victims visit an ED before their death.[52] Emergency physicians have the unique opportunity to intervene early with patients contemplating suicide and to care for patients with injuries from attempted suicide. Recognizing patients who are at high risk of suicide is challenging. It is the emergency physician's responsibility to identify patients who are at a high risk of harming themselves and facilitate appropriate psychiatric treatment.

The management of the suicidal patient begins with placing the patient in a safe setting. Suicidal patients may use shoe laces, belts, keys, and other common objects to inflict self-harm; therefore, their belongings should be searched to remove any possible concealed weapon. Suicidal patients should also be placed in a designated room where they are clearly visible and where there are no scalpels, needles, or any other medical supplies that could be used to inflict harm. Some EDs choose to place suicidal patients on 1:1 observation by designating a staff member to directly watch the patient's activities and prevent any opportunity for self-harm.

The epidemiology of suicide is helpful in assessing these patients. Among adolescents, aged 15 to 24 years, the ratio of suicide completion to attempt ranges from 1:100 to 1:200. However, in the elderly, older than 65 years, the ratio is 1:4.[53] Men commit suicide at a rate 4 times higher than women. The use of firearms is the most common method of suicide among men and poisoning is the most commonly used method among women.[54] Other risk factors for eventual suicide are:[55] male sex, age older than 60 years, widowed or divorced, white or Native American, living alone, unemployed with financial problems, a recent adverse event, clinical depression, schizophrenia, substance abuse, history of suicide attempts or ideation, feelings of hopelessness, panic attacks, severe anxiety, and severe anhedonia.

Taking a good history is the most important part of assessing the suicidal patient. The history should be obtained in a nonjudgmental, compassionate, open-ended manner with careful consideration for the patient's privacy. Intoxication should not hinder the physician from obtaining the history, but it should be repeated when the patient is clinically sober. Identifying intoxicated patients is important, because substance abuse preventive services may be more helpful than admission. Hirschfeld and Russell[55] published an algorithm for assessing suicide risk, which suggests starting with assessment of sociodemographic risk factors (age, gender, race, marital status) and then asking open-ended questions regarding the patient's stressors ("how's life?"). Once the stressors are obvious, the patient should be screened for depression and alcohol abuse. Finally, patients should be asked about suicide directly ("do you have thoughts about killing yourself?," "how do you plan on killing yourself?"). Direct questions about suicide should not be avoided, because they do not cause patients to commit suicide.

If the emergency physician discharges a potentially suicidal patient, as many of the following conditions that can realistically be met should be carefully documented:

- the patient is no longer suicidal
- the patient is medically stable
- the patient will "contract for safety" with the clinician
- the patient is clinically sober

- the suspicion that the patient has access to firearms is low
- the social support, when available, have been contacted
- a follow-up is arranged, when possible.

Unfortunately, there is no single test that identifies patients who are at imminent risk of suicide, and no literature to support the notion that physicians can determine who is at risk and who is not. Overall rates of imminent suicide after ED visits are very low. Furthermore, it is unclear that involuntary admission helps in preventing suicide in any given patient. However, there are some tools to screen for depression and to quantify its severity. Some examples are the Beck Depression Inventory,[56] the Hamilton Depression Scale, the Geriatric Depression Scale, the Suicide Intent Scale, and Beck Hopelessness Scale.[57] These scales are used as an adjunct to good history taking, but they lack strong evidence for accurate identification of patients with an imminent risk.[57]

Despite good history taking and other adjuncts to assessing risk of suicide, emergency physicians cannot accurately predict patient outcomes. The clinician who is in doubt as to whether the patient is at risk of suicide should obtain psychiatric consultation or admit the patient on an involuntary basis. Invariably, some discharged patients will commit suicide, regardless of the physician's efforts to prevent it. Given this risk, it is essential that physicians document their assessment and thought processes. Documentation should include all the low risk features that the physician considered before discharging the patient. "Contracting for safety" is a commonly used approach in which patients enter into a contract with physicians that they will not commit suicide. Although some studies show this act may deter patients from committing suicide, it does not legally exonerate the physician of responsibility for the patient's outcome.

If patients exhibit feelings of hopelessness, and they have a well thought-out suicide plan and persistent suicidal thoughts, the emergency physician should lower the threshold for obtaining psychiatric consultation before discharging the patient, even if it entails committing the patient to obtain psychiatric consultation.

Homicidal Patient

Safety of the staff and other patients is an important consideration before beginning the assessment of the homicidal patient.[58] Similar to suicidal patients, homicidal patients should be separated from their belongings and placed in a room without potentially harmful medical equipment. When interviewing the patient, the physician should always have a quick exit route that cannot be blocked by the patient. Common sense regarding personal safety is essential when interviewing homicidal patients.

Unlike epidemiologic data regarding suicidal patients, data about homicidal patients have focused on long-term prevalence rates. A long-term prevalence rate cannot be applied to the patient in the acute setting, because it does not assess the patient's current risk of homicide.[58] Studies do not provide epidemiologic clues to identify patients that are likely to commit homicide after discharge from the ED. Patients' age, gender, socioeconomic status, and so forth have consistently failed to predict the risk of violence. Furthermore, there are scant data suggesting an association between severity of mental illness and risk of violence. However, lack of previous history of mental illness does not decrease the patient's risk.[59] The most reliable predictor of future violence is a history of violent behavior.[58] Therefore, the physician should dedicate some effort to researching the patient's history of violence. Because acute intoxication may increase the likelihood of violent behavior, acutely intoxicated patients expressing homicidal ideation should not be discharged. These patients should remain in the ED until they are clinically sober and able to undergo a repeat interview to assess for risk.

In 1992, McNiel and colleagues[60] showed that psychiatrists tend to base their decisions to hospitalize violent patients on the potential therapeutic benefit to the patient. Patients whose violent behavior was thought to be secondary to a psychiatric disorder, such as schizophrenia or bipolar disorder, were likely to be hospitalized for treatment. Other violent patients were provided outpatient resources if the psychiatrist did not suspect an underlying cause that needed inpatient treatment.[60] Eventual management of the homicidal patient varies by jurisdiction. In many jurisdictions, imminence of violence requires commitment because of danger to others. Emergency physicians should be aware of the civil commitment laws in their jurisdiction. It is important to know if physicians are legally responsible, in their jurisdiction, for alerting the potential victim or the police. There are no straightforward answers to evaluating homicidal or violent patients. The emergency physician should use all the available resources, such as risk-management officials, hospital security, social work, and psychiatry, to draft a multidisciplinary plan in the management of homicidal patients.

Psychotic Patients

A review of schizophrenia and other conditions responsible for psychosis is beyond the scope of this article. The emergency physician should be able to recognize acutely psychotic patients. It is important to exclude organic causes in patients who present with acute psychosis. Historical clues and collateral information can be invaluable, and the emergency physician should have a higher level of suspicion for organic causes in older psychotic patients without a clear history of psychosis.

Psychotic patients are typically dissociated from reality and report hallucinations (eg, hearing voices) and delusions (eg, the FBI is looking for them). On examination, acutely psychotic patients demonstrate disorganized thinking or behavior, tangential speech, blunted affect, and avolition.[61] Psychotic patients have a high potential for benefit from hospitalization, are often a danger to themselves and others, and have a treatable condition. In most circumstances, psychotic patients are committed for inpatient treatment unless the psychosis is chronic, without acute risk of danger to themselves or others. There should be a low threshold for obtaining psychiatric consultation in psychotic patients.

INVOLUNTARY HOSPITALIZATION

In 1975, the US Supreme Court ruled, in the case of *O'Connor v Donaldson*, that mental illness alone cannot justify confinement against a person's will.[62] To guide the jurisdictions (states), the American Psychiatric Association developed a Model State Law on Civil Commitment of the Mentally Ill.[63] Under the model, a patient's case must meet all six criteria to be eligible for civil commitment: (1) mental illness, (2) danger to self or others, (3) refusal to consent, (4) treatability, (5) lack the capacity to make treatment decisions, and (6) hospitalization is the least restrictive treatment.[62]

Initiation of most involuntary hospitalizations occurs in the ED. To commit a patient, the physician has to complete an initial certificate and hold the patient in a psychiatric facility until further legal proceedings. Then the physician has 72 hours to hold a hearing for involuntary hospitalization or the patient is allowed to leave. This is commonly known as the "72 hour hold".[64] Because involuntary commitment statutes vary from state to state, emergency physicians should be aware of the statutes in their jurisdiction. Although there are no data supporting forced hospitalization to prevent suicide, it may be riskier to discharge a patient than to involuntarily commit the patient.

SUMMARY

Psychiatric emergencies constitute 6% of all ED visits. A focused medical assessment is necessary to identify those patients who cannot be safely treated on a psychiatric ward. The emergency physician should maintain a high index of suspicion for medical conditions that present with psychiatric symptoms. Most of these diagnoses can be made based on a thorough history and physical examination. Laboratory tests and imaging studies are not mandatory for a thorough medical assessment, but they are available to aid the physician in narrowing their differential diagnosis. Once medical illness is identified and treated, emergency physicians should resist using the term "medically clear," and instead document a detailed problem list with specific recommendations for ongoing treatment. In most EDs, emergency physicians evaluate suicidal, homicidal, and psychotic patients to assess the need for hospitalization. Therefore, emergency physicians should be comfortable in evaluating psychiatric patients without a consultant psychiatrist and be aware of the civil commitment laws in their jurisdiction. The importance of thought process documentation on discharged psychiatric patients cannot be overemphasized.

REFERENCES

1. Larkin GL, Claassen CA, Emond JA, et al. Trends in U.S. emergency department visits for mental health conditions, 1992 to 2001. Psychiatr Serv 2005;56:671–7.
2. Gregory RJ, Nihalani ND, Rodriguez E. Medical screening in the emergency department for psychiatric admissions: a procedural analysis. Gen Hosp Psychiatry 2004;26:405–10.
3. Weissberg MP. Emergency room medical clearance: an educational problem. Am J Psychiatry 1979;136:787–90.
4. Lukens TW, Wolf SJ, Edlow JA, et al. Clinical policy: critical issues in the diagnosis and management of the adult psychiatric patient in the emergency department. Ann Emerg Med 2006;47:79–99.
5. Tintinalli JE, Peacock FW IV, Wright MA. Emergency medical evaluation of psychiatric patients. Ann Emerg Med 1994;23:859–62.
6. Larkin GL, Smith RP, Beautrais AL. Trends in US emergency department visits for suicide attempts, 1992–2001. Crisis 2008;29:73–80.
7. Doshi A, Boudreaux ED, Wang N, et al. National study of US emergency department visits for attempted suicide and self-inflicted injury, 1997–2001. Ann Emerg Med 2005;46:369–75.
8. Riba M, Hale M. Medical clearance: fact or fiction in the hospital emergency room. Psychosomatics 1990;31:400–4.
9. Carlson RJ, Nayar N, Suh M. Physical disorders among emergency psychiatric patients. Can J Psychiatry 1981;26:65–7.
10. Hall RC, Gardner ER, Popkin MK, et al. Unrecognized physical illness prompting psychiatric admission: a prospective study. Am J Psychiatry 1981;138:629–35.
11. Hall RC, Gardner ER, Stickney SK, et al. Physical illness manifesting as psychiatric disease. II. Analysis of a state hospital inpatient population. Arch Gen Psychiatry 1980;37:989–95.
12. Anfinson TJ, Kathol RG. Screening laboratory evaluation in psychiatric patients: a review. Gen Hosp Psychiatry 1992;14:248–57.
13. Lipowski ZJ. Delirium in the elderly patient. N Engl J Med 1989;320:578–82.
14. Jacobson S, Schreibman B. Behavioral and pharmacologic treatment of delirium. Am Fam Physician 1997;56:2005–12.

15. Hustey FM, Meldon SW. The prevalence and documentation of impaired mental status in elderly emergency department patients. Ann Emerg Med 2002;39:248–53.
16. Williams ER, Shepherd SM. Medical clearance of psychiatric patients. Emerg Med Clin North Am 2000;18:185–98.
17. O'Brien RF, Kifuji K, Summergrad P. Medical conditions with psychiatric manifestations. Adolesc Med Clin 2006;17:49–77.
18. Skuster DZ, Digre KB, Corbett JJ. Neurologic conditions presenting as psychiatric disorders. Psychiatr Clin North Am 1992;15:311–33.
19. Talbot-Stern JK, Green T, Royle TJ. Psychiatric manifestations of systemic illness. Emerg Med Clin North Am 2000;18:199–209.
20. Geffken GR, Ward HE, Staab JP, et al. Psychiatric morbidity in endocrine disorders. Psychiatr Clin North Am 1998;21:473–89.
21. Blanda MP. Pharmacologic issues in geriatric emergency medicine. Emerg Med Clin North Am 2006;24:449–65.
22. Some drugs that cause psychiatric symptoms. Med Lett Drugs Ther 1998;40:21–4.
23. Drugs that cause psychiatric symptoms. Med Lett Drugs Ther 1993;35:65–70.
24. Gaudreau JD, Gagnon P, Roy MA, et al. Association between psychoactive medications and delirium in hospitalized patients: a critical review. Psychosomatics 2005;46:302–16.
25. Tune L, Carr S, Hoag E, et al. Anticholinergic effects of drugs commonly prescribed for the elderly: potential means for assessing risk of delirium. Am J Psychiatry 1992;149:1393–4.
26. Maldonado JR. Delirium in the acute care setting: characteristics, diagnosis and treatment. Crit Care Clin 2008;24:657–722.
27. Yost DA. Acute care for alcohol intoxication. Be prepared to consider clinical dilemmas. Postgrad Med 2002;112:14–6.
28. Leikin JB. Substance-related disorders in adults. Dis Mon 2007;53:313–35.
29. Moore DP, Jefferson JW. Simple and complex partial seizures. In: Handbook of medical psychiatry. 2nd edition. St Louis (MO): Mosby Inc; 2004. p. 308–11.
30. Sinclair DB, Wheatley M, Snyder T. Frontal lobe epilepsy in childhood. Pediatr Neurol 2004;30:169–76.
31. Bunevicius A, Deltuva VP, Deltuviene D, et al. Brain lesions manifesting as psychiatric disorders: eight cases. CNS Spectr 2008;13:950–8.
32. Kalogerakis MG. Emergency evaluation of adolescents. Hosp Community Psychiatry 1992;43:617–21.
33. Worster A, Elliott L, Bose TJ, et al. Reliability of vital signs measured at triage. Eur J Emerg Med 2003;10:108–10.
34. Henneman PL, Mendoza R, Lewis RJ. Prospective evaluation of emergency department medical clearance. Ann Emerg Med 1994;24:672–7.
35. Stair TO, Morrissey J, Jaradeh I, et al. Validation of the quick confusion scale for mental status screening in the emergency department. Intern Emerg Med 2007;2:130–2.
36. Huff JS, Farace E, Brady WJ, et al. The quick confusion scale in the ED: comparison with the mini-mental state examination. Am J Emerg Med 2001;19:461–4.
37. Olshaker JS, Browne B, Jerrard DA, et al. Medical clearance and screening of psychiatric patients in the emergency department. Acad Emerg Med 1997;4:124–8.
38. Korn CS, Currier GW, Henderson SO. "Medical clearance" of psychiatric patients without medical complaints in the emergency department. J Emerg Med 2000;18:173–6.

39. Dolan JG, Mushlin AI. Routine laboratory testing for medical disorders in psychiatric inpatients. Arch Intern Med 1985;145:2085–8.
40. Kolman PB. The value of laboratory investigations of elderly psychiatric patients. J Clin Psychiatry 1984;45:112–6.
41. Soiza RL, Sharma V, Ferguson K, et al. Neuroimaging studies of delirium: a systematic review. J Psychosom Res 2008;65:239–48.
42. Ananth J, Gamal R, Miller M, et al. Is the routine CT head scan justified for psychiatric patients? A prospective study. J Psychiatry Neurosci 1993;18:69–73.
43. Gewirtz G, Squires-Wheeler E, Sharif Z, et al. Results of computerised tomography during first admission for psychosis. Br J Psychiatry 1994;164:789–95.
44. Bain BK. CT scans of first-break psychotic patients in good general health. Psychiatr Serv 1998;49:234–5.
45. Hufschmidt A, Shabarin V. Diagnostic yield of cerebral imaging in patients with acute confusion. Acta Neurol Scand 2008;118:245–50.
46. Hasbun R, Abrahams J, Jekel J, et al. Computed tomography of the head before lumbar puncture in adults with suspected meningitis. N Engl J Med 2001;345:1727–33.
47. Steigbigel NH. Computed tomography of the head before a lumbar puncture in suspected meningitis – is it helpful? N Engl J Med 2001;345:1768–70.
48. Schiller MJ, Shumway M, Batki SL. Utility of routine drug screening in a psychiatric emergency setting. Psychiatr Serv 2000;51:474–8.
49. Eisen JS, Sivilotti ML, Boyd KU, et al. Screening urine for drugs of abuse in the emergency department: do test results affect physicians' patient care decisions? CJEM 2004;6:104–11.
50. Baraff LJ, Janowicz N, Asarnow JR. Survey of California emergency departments about practices for management of suicidal patients and resources available for their care. Ann Emerg Med 2006;48:452–8, 458.e1-2.
51. Baraff LJ. A mental health crisis in emergency care. Behav Healthc 2006;26:39–40.
52. Gairin I, House A, Owens D. Attendance at the accident and emergency department in the year before suicide: retrospective study. Br J Psychiatry 2003;183:28–33.
53. Goldsmith SK, Pellmar TC, Kleinman AM, et al. Reducing suicide: a national imperative. Washington (DC): National Academy Press; 2002.
54. Centers for Disease Control and Prevention. Web-base injury statistics query and reporting system. National Center for Injury Prevention and Control. 2005. Available at: www.cdc.gov/ncipc/wisqars/default.htm. Accessed February 5, 2009.
55. Hirschfeld RM, Russell JM. Assessment and treatment of suicidal patients. N Engl J Med 1997;337:910–5.
56. Beck AT, Steer RA, Ball R, et al. Comparison of Beck Depression Inventories-IA and -II in psychiatric outpatients. J Pers Assess 1996;67:588–97.
57. Moe J. The suicidal patient. Critical Decisions in Emergency Medicine 2009;23:2–8.
58. Thienhaus OJ, Piasecki M. Assessment of psychiatric patients' risk of violence toward others. Psychiatr Serv 1998;49:1129–30, 1147.
59. Beck J, White K, Gage B. Emergency psychiatric assessment of violence. Am J Psychiatry 1991;148:1562–5.
60. McNiel D, Myers R, Zeiner H, et al. The role of violence in decisions about hospitalization from the psychiatric emergency room. Am J Psychiatry 1992;149:207–12.

61. Edelsohn GA, Gomez JP. Psychiatric emergencies in adolescents. Adolesc Med Clin 2006;17:183–204.
62. Werth JL Jr. U.S. involuntary mental health commitment statutes: requirements for persons perceived to be a potential harm to self. Suicide Life Threat Behav 2001; 31:348–57.
63. Stromberg CD, Stone AA. A model state law on civil commitment of the mentally ill. Harvard J Legis 1983;20:275–396.
64. Reeves RR, Torres RA. Informing ED patients of the initiation of a psychiatric 72-hours hold. Am J Emerg Med 2004;22:495–6.

High-Risk Chief Complaints I: Chest Pain—The Big Three

Kar-mun C. Woo, MD[a], Jeffrey I. Schneider, MD[a,b,*]

KEYWORDS

- Chest pain • Myocardial infarction • Thoracic aortic dissection
- Pulmonary embolism • Tension pneumothorax
- Esophageal rupture • Cardiac tamponade • Risk management

ACUTE CORONARY SYNDROME

A small, but significant percentage of patients discharged from emergency departments (EDs) with "noncardiac chest pain" are ultimately diagnosed with acute coronary syndrome (ACS).[1] This misdiagnosed population accounts for 20% of medical malpractice litigation against ED physicians and, as a result, attempts to obviate this source of significant liability have been at the forefront of risk management strategies for decades.[2] The rate of mistakenly discharged acute myocardial infarctions (MIs) is believed to range between 2% and 8%.[3–5] As the spectrum of ACS has evolved to include unstable angina as well as myocardial infarction, current estimates are that approximately 2% of patients with ACS are inappropriately discharged from the ED.[6] Not surprisingly, discharged patients have nearly twice the morbidity and mortality of those who are appropriately admitted. On the other hand, concern over missing a case of ACS has resulted in increased admission rates for suspected cardiac ischemia, resulting in higher diagnostic sensitivity at the expense of specificity.[7] Rising health care costs and an increasingly litigious environment[8] have spurred a movement in risk management toward attempting to identify a low-risk population who might be safely discharged from the ED.

Clinical Presentation of Acute Coronary Syndrome

The patient with ACS classically is a white man, 60 or more years old, with multiple coronary artery disease (CAD) risk factors, who presents with left-sided chest pressure radiating to the arm with some combination of associated dyspnea, nausea,

[a] Department of Emergency Medicine, Boston Medical Center, Dowling 1 South, 1 Boston Medical Center Place, Boston, MA 02118, USA
[b] Department of Emergency Medicine, Boston University School of Medicine, Boston, MA, USA
* Corresponding author. Department of Emergency Medicine, Boston Medical Center, Dowling 1 South, 1 Boston Medical Center Place, Boston, MA 02118.
E-mail address: jeffrey.schneider@bmc.org (J.I. Schneider).

Emerg Med Clin N Am 27 (2009) 685–712
doi:10.1016/j.emc.2009.07.007
emed.theclinics.com
0733-8627/09/$ – see front matter

lightheadedness, or diaphoresis. The classically *missed* ACS patient is quite different; the patient is more likely to be female, nonwhite, younger (age <55 years), and without a previous history of CAD. The patient is also less likely to identify chest pain as their chief complaint, and may not report other classically associated symptoms of acute cardiac ischemia. (Diabetics and the elderly, surprisingly, are not among the most frequently misdiagnosed patients, perhaps as a result of heightened awareness in this population that has been classically thought to present atypically.) Characteristics of those patients most at risk for missed ACS are presented here.

Atypical presentations

When the Framingham researchers discovered that 25% of the MIs in their cohort of patients had been diagnosed by routine office electrocardiograms (ECGs) *after* the actual event had long been completed, they postulated that these MIs were missed as a result of being "silent" or atypical.[9] Inconsistent methods of defining atypical presentations, however, have resulted in widely varying estimates of its incidence, ranging from 6% to 52%.[10–14] Nevertheless, these studies have identified several populations that are consistently more likely to present in an atypical fashion: females, the elderly, and nonwhite minorities.[15] Painless presentations had the expected association with diabetes but interestingly, heart failure has an even stronger association. Those with a history of hyperlipidemia and tobacco use seem to be *less* likely linked to atypical presentations.

The most commonly reported symptoms in those who had complaints other than chest pain include (from most to least common) dyspnea, diaphoresis, nausea/vomiting, and syncope/presyncope. Patients who do not experience chest pain typically take longer to present to the ED after symptom onset, and are more frequently misdiagnosed at the outset. These patients also are less likely to receive adequate medical therapies and timely interventions when compared with those who present *with* chest pain. Not surprisingly, those with atypical presentations tend to have a higher mortality rate. As the population ages, some have proposed that the incidence of atypical symptoms in those with ACS is likely to increase.

Gender

Women who are ultimately confirmed to have ACS tend to be older, are more likely to have a history of hypertension, and are more likely to delay their presentation to medical providers after symptom onset. At the same time, they are generally less likely to have undergone prior revascularization despite similar rates of prior heart attacks or positive stress tests.[16] Whereas chest pain is still a common chief complaint in women with ACS, it is less common than with men, a disparity that may in part be explained by women's older age and higher prevalence of diabetes on presentation. When present, the chest pain described by women is more likely to be depicted as sharp, stabbing, or transient, and is more likely to radiate to the right arm or shoulder, front neck, or back.[17] Left arm pain and diaphoresis is more common in men whereas women are more prone to gastrointestinal symptoms such as nausea, vomiting,[18] and indigestion. Women are also more likely to report dizziness, fatigue, loss of appetite, and syncope during an acute MI.[17] It is disturbing that women are 3 times as likely to be misdiagnosed with a psychological rather than a cardiac diagnosis.[19]

Race

African Americans who present to the ED with chest pain tend to be younger, are more likely female, and are less likely to have had a history of CAD than their white counterparts,[20] features which may lead clinicians to have a lower index of suspicion for ACS. African Americans also tend to delay their presentations to health care providers.[20]

Their ECGs are more frequently complicated by left ventricular hypertrophy, presumably stemming from a higher rate of hypertension. However, racial inequalities in the clinical presentation may be less pronounced (ie, similar descriptions in the quality, radiation, and duration of chest pain). Unfortunately, there are significant race-related disparities with regards to the management of chest pain patients in the ED, with at least one study reporting lower rates of ordered ECGs, chest radiographs, and cardiac monitoring in African Americans with a chief complaint of chest pain.[21] Pope and colleagues found that nonwhite patients with ACS were more than twice as likely as white patients to be discharged from the ED, and among those with acute MI, 4 times as likely to be sent home. Additional large-population studies are needed to understand the complex socioeconomic, cultural, and biologic factors influencing race-related differences.

Younger patients

Although many population-based studies of missed ACS exclude adults younger than 30 years old, there is literature suggesting that misdiagnosed patients tend to be younger. This finding is especially true for women younger than 55 years. With increasing rates of obesity, insulin resistance, and metabolic syndrome in today's youth, the prevalence of CAD in younger age groups is expected to increase.[22] Although younger patients with ACS are more likely to present with features that are classically associated with ischemic chest pain, their presentations often lack the forewarning of previous anginal symptoms,[23] they are at higher risk of being misclassified as noncardiac chest pain, and they are often recipients of greater damage payments in the event of a bad outcome.[24] With respect to CAD risk factors, family history of premature CAD, smoking, and hyperlipidemia (specifically higher triglycerides or lower high-density lipoprotein levels) are significantly more prevalent in early-onset CAD patients when contrasted with their older-age counterparts, who are more likely hypertensive and diabetic. Younger patients should also be queried regarding recreational drug use and the presence of congenital heart/vascular abnormalities or hypercoagulable syndromes. In a potential approach to risk-stratify younger adults, one group has reported an overall 5% incidence of ACS in adults younger than 40 years old who received an ECG for noncocaine-related chest pain.[25] This risk fell to 1.0% if the patient had no previous cardiac history, a normal ECG, and no conventional CAD risk factors, and further dropped to 0.14% if a first set of cardiac enzymes were negative.[26]

Diagnostic Tests and Their Limitations

History

Numerous studies and meta-analyses have tried to identify which aspects of a patient's history are most critical in determining whether their chest pain is cardiac in origin. ACS-related chest pain classically is described as "pressure," a descriptor that turns out to have minimal utility for predicting true ACS.[27–29] In contrast, pain that is described as sharp, stabbing, pleuritic, or positional is less likely cardiac in nature, with a likelihood ratio (LR) of MI from 0.2 to 0.4.[30] Chest wall tenderness carries a similar LR of 0.3 for ACS. These descriptors of chest pain should be applied cautiously; ischemia is nevertheless diagnosed in 22% of patients who present with sharp or stabbing pain, in 13% of patients with pleuritic pain, and in 7% of patients whose pain is reproducible with palpation.[31,32] Of note, several studies demonstrated a statistically insignificant trend toward *increased* likelihood of ACS when pain was described as burning or indigestion-like. Pain described as similar to or worse than a previous MI should heighten the clinician's concern, as it carries an LR of 1.8 for ACS.[29]

Radiation of chest pain to one, or especially both shoulders/arms (LR 1.4–7.1), or pain produced by exertion (LR 2.5–5.8) is strongly predictive of ACS. The severity of pain and location of chest pain have not been correlated with ACS, although there has been a trend suggesting that a particularly small and localized area of pain (ie, the size of a coin) decreases the likelihood of acute MI.[33] Pain lasting longer than 30 minutes, if ischemic in origin, is more likely to evolve into myocardial infarction. However, pain from esophageal pathology may also persist for prolonged periods, for example in gastroesophageal reflux disease. Brief episodes of pain, lasting a few seconds, are generally considered nonischemic but have not been confirmed in the literature as such. Finally, any clinical suspicion of angina or its equivalents should elicit a brief assessment of the patient's functional status. Doing so may elicit a history that is consistent with unstable angina, and prevent one from inadvertently missing such patients.

Whereas risk factors for the development of CAD have been clearly identified by longitudinal studies such as the Framingham Study,[34] these same risk factors are not necessarily predictive of *acute* ischemia in the emergency department setting, especially when compared with presenting features of chest pain or ECG changes.[35] Except for the presence diabetes or family history of CAD in men only, with a relative risk (RR) of 2.4 and 2.1 for ACS, respectively, none of the other traditional risk factors analyzed (ie, hypertension, hypercholesterolemia, smoking) demonstrated statistically significant associations with acute ischemia. By comparison, the presence of chest pain carried an RR of 12.0 in men and 25.0 in women, whereas ECG changes correlated with an RR of 4.0 to 8.7. Even age greater than 60 and male gender, at respective LRs of 1.5 and 1.3 for acute MIs, pale in comparison to the more robust LRs of 2.2 to 22 for specific ECG changes. Although risk factors *are* correlated with worse prognosis and necessitate more aggressive treatments once ACS is diagnosed, as is used in calculating Thrombolysis in Myocardial Infarction (TIMI) risk scores,[36] one should use caution when relying exclusively on the presence or absence of conventional risk factors in the diagnosis of ACS.

Response to therapy

Medication response has also demonstrated a poor ability to discriminate between cardiac and noncardiac causes of chest pain. For example, nitroglycerin, the hallmark of antianginal therapy, has been shown to provide symptom relief in those with cardiac chest pain as well as in those with esophageal spasm. Multiple studies have demonstrated the lack of utility in assessing response to nitroglycerin[37–39] in determining the cause of chest pain, with, in fact, a trend toward higher response rates from *non*cardiac (41%) versus cardiac (35%) causes of chest pain.

Physician reliance on a patient's response to a "gastrointestinal (GI) cocktail" can similarly be misleading. Numerous case reports have documented patients who responded to a GI cocktail and were subsequently diagnosed with an MI.[40,41] It has been demonstrated physiologically that instillation of hydrochloric acid into the distal esophagus of patients with known CAD significantly reduces coronary blood flow.[42] When patients with known CAD were continuously monitored for both ECG changes and esophageal pH, the frequency and duration of ST depressions correlated with the number of reflux episodes, *all* of which were subsequently improved by omeprazole therapy.[43] Similar reductions in the frequency of anginal episodes and ST depressions were seen in CAD patients subjected to treadmill testing after randomization to omeprazole (versus placebo) therapy.[44] This emerging complex relationship between gastroesophageal reflux and CAD has been termed "linked angina,"[45] and illustrates the danger of relying on a GI cocktail to "rule out" CAD.

Electrocardiogram

Whereas the ECG remains the critical diagnostic tool in the evaluation of potential ACS, it should be interpreted with several caveats in mind. Of importance from a risk management perspective, as many as 53% of missed acute MI and 62% of missed unstable angina (UA) cases have a normal or nondiagnostic ECG on presentation. An ECG provides only a single snapshot of a potentially dynamic process, and comparison with a patient's baseline ECG, whenever available, is crucial for identifying new abnormalities. Continuous ECG monitoring has been shown to identify an additional 16% of acute MIs not seen on initial presenting ECGs,[46] and as a result, some suggest that a repeat ECG be obtained between 15 and 60 minutes later for symptoms consistent with ongoing ischemia.[47] The ECG is also known to underappreciate damage in the right ventricle or posterior basal or lateral walls unless additional leads are requested. The frequent presence of patterns such as left bundle branch blocks or left ventricular hypertrophy can confound interpretation. Finally, the ECG has a highly variable sensitivity and specificity based on how stringently any abnormal findings, many of which may be nondiagnostic for new ischemia, are analyzed. These findings must be taken in the context of a patient's level of risk for acute ischemia.

ED physicians are also susceptible to ECG misclassification; some have reported that as many as 1 in 4 missed MIs might have been prevented by correct ECG interpretation. One retrospective study of admitted patients with acute MI found that 1 in 8 ECGs had demonstrated high-risk abnormalities that were missed in the ED,[48] defined as at least 2 contiguous leads with ST-segment elevation of 0.1 mV or greater, ST-segment depression of 0.05 mV or greater, or T-wave inversions of 0.2 mV or greater. Missed patients tended to be older, are less likely to present with chest pain, and are more likely to have a history of heart failure or other cardiac disease (and thus, more likely to have confounding patterns on ECG). Although ST elevations were less commonly missed than ST depressions or T-wave inversions, they were significantly more likely to be missed when chest pain was not the presenting symptom. Other studies have analyzed disagreements in ST elevations, reporting a 6% to 8% rate of discrepancy between ED attending readings when interpreting whether ST elevations were due to left ventricular hypertrophy, left bundle branch block, benign early repolarization, or acute MI, particularly when the degree of elevation was less than 2 mm or when there was an absence of reciprocal ST changes.[49,50] Of note, inferior lead MIs were found to have a higher rate of misinterpretation.

Cardiac enzymes

The use of a single set of cardiac enzymes in the ED to rule out ACS deserves cautious discussion. Although relatively specific (>85%), biomarkers drawn at presentation are notorious for having a low sensitivity for ACS (<50%).[51] In one prospective study of low-risk (Goldman risk score <4%) chest pain patients with a negative initial troponin, there was a 2.3% rate of acute MI and 1% rate of death at 30 days. The investigators therefore argued that a single troponin, even in low-risk populations, does not enable safe discharge without further testing.[52] However, the timing of biomarker testing is critical; sensitivity of a single troponin for MI within the first hour of symptoms is 10% to 45% (depending on the cutoff criteria used) and increases to more than 90% at 8 or more hours.[53] In contrast, a retrospective study of 588 low-risk patients with nondiagnostic ECGs and negative troponins drawn *6 to 9 hours* after symptom onset reported a 0.3% rate of adverse events and no deaths at 30 days.[54] Low-risk patients were identified by having nondiagnostic ECGs as well as 1 of 2 "low-risk features": (1) patients with CAD risk factors (prior CAD not excluded) who presented with either prolonged/constant atypical symptoms (usually greater than 2 hours) or very atypical symptoms; (2) patients with no CAD risk factors who presented with typical symptoms of myocardial ischemia that were prolonged/continuous. Further prospective and larger studies, as well as standardization and fine-tuning of criteria for low-risk stratification, are needed to validate if this practice is prudent. At this time, the American College of Emergency Physicians (ACEP) endorses with "moderate clinical certainty" that a single negative troponin can effectively rule out acute myocardial infarction if the time of presentation is at least 8 to 12 hours after onset of symptoms.

An accelerated course of serial cardiac biomarkers has been suggested as an alternative strategy to evaluate for an acute MI if the patient presents within 12 hours of symptoms. Investigators have analyzed changes ("deltas") in each of the cardiac biomarkers over shorter intervals of time to assess the safety of more rapid cycling protocols. In particular, a negative myoglobin at zero and 90 minutes, or a negative creatine kinase (CK)-MB at zero and 2 hours, in conjunction with negative troponins, are identified as moderately reliable methods for excluding an acute MI in the ED. Two-hour delta CK-MB levels have demonstrated a 92% to 94% sensitivity and 91% to 95% specificity for acute MI, and seem likely to be more sensitive than delta troponins[55] or delta myoglobins.[56]

Despite the progress being made in this area of ACS research, it is important to remember that in those with UA, single or even serial sets of troponins may be normal despite the presence of unstable atherosclerotic plaque. Thus, the practice of ruling out and discharging ACS from the ED without further provocative testing remains a controversial and continually evolving proposition.

Stress testing

The vast majority of individuals presenting to EDs with chest pain do not have ACS. In one large study of more than 10,000 patients presenting to the ED with symptoms suggestive of ACS, only 8% were ultimately diagnosed with MI and 15% with UA.[57] As hospital and financial resources are not unlimited, and as the cost of health care has become increasingly important, it is incumbent on providers to have an understanding of various stress testing protocols and environments. Provocative testing of ED patients with the goal of early discharge is only appropriate for low- to intermediate-risk patients, because high-risk patients should be admitted for more aggressive diagnostic testing, risk stratification, or therapy. In contrast to previous practice guidelines that recommended stress testing only in patients free of symptoms for at least 48 hours,[58] the American College of Cardiology (ACC) and American Heart Association (AHA) have endorsed stress testing after 6 to 8 hours of observation if repeat ECGs and serial cardiac biomarkers are normal. Numerous studies have confirmed that "early" stress testing in low-risk patients is both safe and effective.[59–61] Some have even proposed protocols that stress low-risk ED chest pain patients directly from the ED *without* serial biomarkers.[62]

The ACC/AHA guidelines alternatively allow for outpatient stress testing within 72 hours if a patient is of sufficiently low-risk. The safety of this recommendation was evaluated in a study of 979 largely insured low-risk patients.[63] Ninety-two percent of patients completed their stress tests as scheduled and 68% were within the 72-hour window. At 6-month follow-up there were no deaths, 0.2% had had MIs, and 2% required coronary intervention. Thus, in a low-risk patient in whom timely follow-up can be assured, outpatient testing may be a feasible option.

Even when diagnostic (a sufficient elevation of heart rate is reached), stress test results must be interpreted carefully and in the context of a patient's pretest probability of CAD.[64] A true negative test at a diagnostic level of stress does have a consistently high negative predictive value (98%–100%) in *appropriately risk-stratified low-risk patients*. (In these studies, patients were variably categorized as low-risk by either predefined criteria, such as the Goldman risk score, or by individual clinician suspicion.) The data from these few studies supports up to a 2% risk of acute MI for the first 6 months following a negative test at a diagnostic level and a mortality rate approaching 0%. Beyond 6 months, the interpretation of prior stress tests is less clear for the patient who returns to the ED. One retrospective study looked at all patients presenting to the ED with chest pain who had a recent negative stress test with imaging; 6% of patients had an MI within 3 years of their testing, a third of which had been sustained in the first year.[65]

Computed tomography coronary angiography

As computed tomography (CT) technology continues to evolve and new applications are found, some have suggested that CT coronary angiography (CTCA) may have an important role in the evaluation of chest pain in ED patients. CTCA allows for the noninvasive evaluation of the extent of calcium deposits and degree of stenosis in the coronary arteries, and has demonstrated a high level of diagnostic accuracy compared with invasive coronary angiography.[66] CTCA boasts a negative predictive value between 97% and 100%[67–69] and an accuracy comparable to stress testing.[70,71] Some have suggested that its high negative predictive value may allow CTCAs to be used to identify patients who may be safely discharged from the ED. In a prospective study of ED patients with TIMI scores 2 or lower, there were no cardiovascular events or nonfatal MIs at 30 days in low-risk patients who were enrolled in an ED protocol using CTCA. The investigators report that relatedly, 75% of patients who would have otherwise been admitted to the hospital were able to be safely discharged after a negative CTCA (defined as <50% degree of stenosis and a calcium score <100).[72]

However, some caution that CTCAs may be harder to interpret in patients with known CAD or older patients who naturally accumulate more coronary calcium over time.[73] Moreover, CTCA cannot identify vulnerable plaques without calcifications, nor can it determine the physiologic significance of "intermediate" lesions. Others warn that the lower specificity of CTCAs (70%–90%) may lead to increased rates of unnecessary invasive cardiac catheterizations, and that the enthusiasm over their potential for quicker disposition in the ED may be at odds with using a new technology whose medical benefit has not yet been fully substantiated in large, prospective, controlled trials.[74] The 2007 ACC/AHA guidelines currently deem CTCA as a "reasonable alternative" to stress testing in low- to intermediate-risk patients following serial ECGs and biomarkers.

Risk Stratification Tools

Clinicians are able to use patient history and physical examination findings in combination with ECG and biomarker results in their evaluation of patients with chest pain. Various prediction models have been proposed, which attempt to quantify the importance of these variables and assist physicians with decisions concerning the management and disposition of these patients, taking into account short- and long-term risks. The validity, use in the ED setting, and impact of several of these commonly discussed models are briefly explored here. Detailed descriptions of these models are beyond the scope of this review and can be found elsewhere.

Agency for Health Care Policy and Research guidelines

The Agency for Health Care Policy and Research (AHCPR) guidelines are aimed at assessing patients' likelihood of ACS due to CAD, and their short-term level of risk for death or nonfatal MI.[75] Created by an expert panel on management of unstable angina in 1994, these widely disseminated recommendations have been repeatedly adopted with each update of the ACC/AHA guidelines for UA and non-ST elevation MIs. Patients with low likelihood of CAD and low level of short-term risk are generally considered safe to discharge to follow-up outpatient stress testing at 72 hours.

Few studies, however, have actually sought to validate this risk prediction model. In addition, critics have noted that its applicability to ED patients may be limited as a cardiac cause of chest pain is assumed in this model, something that cannot always be confirmed in the ED.[76] This model was studied prospectively in the evaluation of 1140 ED patients[77] in whom AHCPR guidelines were used to divide patients into high, intermediate, low, and very low risk categories. ACS was found in 29%, 23%, 12%, and 2%, respectively, in each of these groups. That 2% of ACS events were missed even in the "very low" risk category highlights the model's inadequate sensitivity. Twelve percent of very low- to low-risk patients who were admitted despite AHCPR guidelines were later confirmed to have ACS. Moreover, strict guideline adherence would have resulted in hospitalizing 9% more non-ACS patients. Finally, surveyed physicians expressed—and ultimately demonstrated—their resistance to using these guidelines by admitting and discharging the same percentage of patients in each category regardless of prominent guideline reminders.

Acute Cardiac Ischemic Time-Insensitive Predictive Instrument score

The Acute Cardiac Ischemic Time-Insensitive Predictive Instrument (ACI-TIPI) is a computerized prediction of a patient's probability of acute ischemia.[78] It combines the patient's age, sex, presence/absence of chest or left arm pain, and whether chest discomfort is the primary complaint with specific ECG findings, to compute a percentage probability of ACS that can be automatically printed on top of the patient's ECG. Probability of ACS is divided into low (<10%), intermediate (10%–55%), and high (>55%) risk groups, with the hope that disposition decisions (ie, discharge, admit to monitored bed, admit to intensive care unit setting) could reflect these probabilities.

A controlled prospective clinical trial of 10,689 undifferentiated patients presenting to the ED with symptoms suggestive of acute ischemia (chest/arm/jaw/epigastric discomfort, dyspnea, dizziness, palpitations) evaluated the effect of this prediction tool on patient dispositions.[79] In patients who were ultimately believed not to have ACS, there was a statistically insignificant trend ($P = .09$) toward reduction in coronary care unit (CCU) admissions and increase in hospital discharges, but only in larger hospitals with a higher CCU-to-telemetry bed ratio. At lower levels of physician training, or in cases of stable angina, however, these trends became magnified and statistically significant. A meta-analysis of ACI-TIPI performance has since reported its ability to appropriately triage 97% of patients with ACS and safely reduce unnecessary hospitalizations without increasing the rate of missed ACS patients.[80]

Thrombolysis in Myocardial Infarction risk score

Multiple risk score calculations have been endorsed by the ACC and AHA as reliable predictors of mortality and post-ACS complications. The TIMI risk score, in particular, is worth further discussion, because of the ease of its calculation in the ED compared with other models, and because it has demonstrated utility as a risk stratification tool in ED patients presenting with chest pain even *before* the diagnosis of ACS is confirmed.[81,82] Despite its initial derivation in higher-risk populations already diagnosed with UA or non-ST elevation MI,[83] the TIMI score has shown predictive value for 30-day rates of death, acute MI, and revascularization in ED patients, with a TIMI score of zero demonstrating 2% risk of 30-day events and a score of 6 or 7 predicting 33% to 100% risk. This consistent trend has been mirrored in independent, albeit smaller, ED-based evaluations of the TIMI risk score.[84,85] Investigators caution that because a score of zero still carries a 2% risk of complications, the score's applicability in assessing discharge may be limited. However, the TIMI score's predictive ability may help to further fine-tune the dispositions—intensive care unit or telemetry bed, versus unmonitored wards—of admitted patients from the ED.

Pitfalls and Risk Management Strategies

Critical analyses of malpractice claims for missed MIs yield valuable insights into some factors that might contribute to misdiagnosis or inappropriate discharge. A retrospective examination of 65 closed claim cases of missed MIs revealed that those patients who were misclassified were more likely to be younger and presented with symptoms other than classically described angina. Misdiagnosed patients had fewer ECGs ordered, and these ECGs had higher rates of misinterpretation. Providers for these patients were more likely to have fewer years of ED experience, and were found to have documented less thorough histories and physical examinations.[86] When the Physician Insurers Association of America performed a similar analysis of missed MI cases,[87] they reported that 70% of misdiagnosed MIs had never had a previous history of CAD, that almost half of these patients were younger than 50 years old, and that 1 in 6 patients were younger than 40. These patients were most commonly discharged with a diagnosis of a gastrointestinal disorder (26%) or costochondritis (21%). These disturbing trends seem to be confirmed in the later and wider-based population studies of missed MIs and ACS.

The ED physician should perform a thorough history, but should not be falsely reassured if the patient has no prior history of CAD or any of the other conventionally associated risk factors. A strong index of suspicion for atypical presentations should be maintained, especially in females, nonwhite individuals, elderly patients, and those with a history of diabetes or congestive heart failure. Other high-risk groups include psychiatric patients, "frequent flyers," and intoxicated patients.[88] The ED physician should have a low threshold for obtaining an ECG, even in younger adults with chest-related complaints or patients with chest wall tenderness. Although a normal ECG does not rule out ACS, 1 in 4 cases of misdiagnosed acute MIs may be averted by improved ECG interpretations. As with all strategies aimed at mitigating risk, the ED physician must carefully weigh a patient's clinical presentation in the setting of any diagnostic testing obtained. Although no single test is able to rule out the presence of ACS, the presence of multiple data points that suggest a noncardiac cause of pain, in combination with careful and meticulous charting that clearly explains the thought process of the clinician, will likely be of help in defending cases of missed ACS.

In addition to missed diagnoses, an increasing number of lawsuits are now citing failure to provide treatment in a timely manner as a reason for litigation,[89] with damages not only for death but also reduced viable myocardium as a result of delayed therapy. Failure to comply with the standard of care in the treatment of ACS can result in significant damages. It is incumbent on ED physicians to ensure that guidelines are followed, that consultants see patients within an appropriate timeframe, and that patients are transferred for definitive care when needed. Failure to do so can expose ED practitioners to significant liability.

THORACIC AORTIC DISSECTION

Famously described in 1760 when King George II of England died while straining on the commode, the incidence of thoracic aortic dissection (TAD) is thought to be increasing as the population ages. It has been estimated that more than 2000 new cases of aortic dissection occur per year in the United States. Without treatment, nearly 75% of patients with ascending aortic dissection can be expected to die within 2 weeks,[90] with a mortality of 1% to 3% per hour in the first 48 hours.[91] In contrast, with rapid diagnosis and definitive therapy, 30-day survival rates as high as 90% have been reported.[92,93] Men are affected 3 times as frequently as women,[94] and most of those afflicted are between 50 and 70 years old.[95] African Americans have a higher incidence of aortic dissection than whites, believed to be related to a higher incidence of hypertension.[96] Risk factors for the development of TAD are thought to include hypertension, male gender, cocaine use, advanced age, pregnancy, connective tissue disorders (such as Marfan syndrome or cystic medial necrosis), presence of a bicuspid aortic valve or previous aortic valve replacement, Turner syndrome, weightlifting, and methylenedioxymethamphetamine ("ecstasy") use.[97–99]

Clinical Presentations of Thoracic Aortic Dissection

The diagnosis of TAD is unfortunately often a difficult one to make. Physicians historically are thought to correctly suspect the diagnosis in as few as 15% to 43% of presentations when initially evaluating patients with a dissection.[100] However, as with many clinical entities, a careful history and physical examination can point the clinician toward the correct diagnosis.

As part of the Rational Clinical Examination series in the *Journal of the American Medical Association*, data from 16 studies involving 1553 patients were pooled, and sensitivities for various components of the clinical history and physical examination were reported. The vast majority of patients presented with pain (pooled sensitivity 90%) of severe intensity (90%) that occurred suddenly (84%). Other symptoms, such as abdominal pain, migrating pain, or syncope, were present in a small to moderate percentage of patients. Although the presence of sudden onset of pain was far from diagnostic (positive LR 1.6; 95% confidence interval [CI] 1.0–2.4), the absence of this historical feature did decrease the probability that a patient had a TAD (negative LR 0.2; 95% CI 0.2–0.5). However, the investigators argue that this likely overrepresents the sensitivity due to inclusion bias in this study of patients with TAD.

The pooled sensitivities of many physical examination findings were also poor in this meta-analysis. When present, however, some findings were highly suggestive of TAD. For example, whereas a pulse differential had a sensitivity of only 31%, its presence conferred a positive LR of 5.7 (95% CI 1.4–23.0). Focal neurologic deficits, while similarly only present in 17% of those with TAD, should raise one's suspicion for TAD (positive LR 6.6–33.0). However, it should be noted that the specificity of many of these findings is poor: for example, a 20 mm Hg difference in upper extremity blood pressures may be found in as many as 20% of individuals,[101] and as many as 53% of ED patients may have differences greater than 10 mm Hg.[102]

There are few, if any, historical features and physical examination findings which, when used in isolation, allow the clinician to positively identify those patients with TAD. Whereas there is no *one* historical feature that is pathognomonic for aortic dissection, there is literature that suggests that physicians can improve their diagnostic accuracy by specifically asking about the quality of the patient's pain, the radiation of the pain, *and* the intensity at its onset. In one retrospective study, only 42% of patients who were found to have a TAD were asked all 3 of these questions. When all 3 questions were asked, the clinician's initial diagnostic impression of TAD was correct in 91% of the cases.[103] Unfortunately, the retrospective nature of this study does not rule out the notion that clinicians were simply more likely to inquire about additional findings when they already had a strong clinical suspicion.

Other combinations of findings, such as the presence of sudden-onset pain that is of tearing or ripping quality, blood pressure or pulse differentials, and mediastinal widening on chest radiography, have been found to have a positive LR of 66.0 (95% CI 4.1–1062.0). It is disappointing that the presence of these 3 factors was found in only 27% of patients with TAD.

Diagnostic Tests and Their Limitations

For most ED patients with chest pain, chest radiography and electrocardiography (ECG) are part of the initial diagnostic evaluation. Unfortunately, the sensitivity for TAD of both of these tests is limited. In one study, new Q waves or ST-segment elevation were noted in 7% of admission ECGs in those with TAD, whereas normal ECGs were reported in 8% to 31% of those patients ultimately found to have a TAD. Other nonspecific findings such as left ventricular hypertrophy and atrial fibrillation have also been reported.[104] Perhaps the greatest use of the ECG is to distinguish ST segment elevation myocardial infarction from TAD. Unfortunately however, the conditions are known to coexist, particularly if the dissection extends proximally to include the coronary ostia, most commonly affecting the right coronary artery causing proximal coronary artery occlusion.[105]

Many of those with TAD also do not present with the classically described chest radiograph findings. Again, pooled sensitivities for findings such as an abnormal aortic contour (71%; 95% CI 56%–84%), pleural effusion (16%; 95% CI 12%–21%), displaced intimal calcification (9%; 95% CI 6%–13%), and wide mediastinum (64%; 95% CI 44%–80%) reflect the lack of clinical usefulness of these findings. However, most patients with TAD do have *some* abnormality on chest radiograph (sensitivity 90%), making the disease less likely in those with an entirely normal chest film.[106]

Several imaging modalities, including conventional angiography, ultrasonography (US), CT, and magnetic resonance imaging (MRI), have been used to diagnose aortic dissection. Although an in-depth discussion of each of these imaging techniques is beyond the scope of this review, there are several factors worth noting. The use of conventional aortography, a time-consuming, invasive procedure, which may have limited sensitivity (as low as 88%[107]), has decreased in recent years as the roles of US, CT, and MRI have increased. In one relatively small study in which patients with suspected dissection underwent transesophageal echocardiography (TEE), MRI, *and* CT, the following sensitivities and specificities were reported (**Table 1**):[107]

Table 1
Sensitivity and specificity of imaging modalities for aortic dissection

Testing Modality	Sensitivity (95% CI)	Specificity (95% CI)
CT	100% (89%–100%)	100% (79%–100%)
TEE	100% (89%–100%)	94% (70%–100%)
MRI	100% (89%–100%)	94% (70%–100%)

In many institutions, CT is the diagnostic test of choice due to its easy accessibility, rapid data acquisition, high sensitivity, and ability to simultaneously exclude other morbid causes of chest pain.[108] TEE, although more portable than CT, requires esophageal intubation, may lead to an increase in blood pressure (and a subsequent increase in risk of rupture[109]), and may not provide enough anatomic information to surgeons before operative intervention.[110] The usefulness of MRI is limited by the time needed to complete a study (as long as 30 minutes) and its lack of ready availability in many EDs.

Although laboratory testing has traditionally played only a minor, if any, role in the diagnosis of TAD, some recent literature has suggested that tests such as D-dimer and an immunoassay of smooth muscle myosin heavy chain may be of use. The D-dimer literature is plagued, however, by small sample sizes, inconsistent methodology, and the use of different assays. Whereas most studies report a high sensitivity for D-dimer for the presence of dissection, at least 4 studies report a sensitivity of 94% or less, and 3 of 5 studies with 100% sensitivity have the lower range of their 95% CIs at less than 85%.[111–115] Although a negative D-dimer does make the diagnosis of TAD much less likely, particularly in patients with a low likelihood of disease, there is insufficient evidence to support its use as the *sole* screening test for aortic dissection. Perhaps future study can be directed at using D-dimer in conjunction with other clinical variables or ancillary studies.[116]

There exist a small number of studies advocating the use of smooth-muscle myosin heavy chain protein assays in the diagnosis of aortic dissection. This protein is released from damaged aortic smooth muscle at the onset of dissection, and has a reported sensitivity of 90.9% (95% CI 85%–96.8%) in patients with aortic dissection who presented within the first 3 hours after symptom onset.[117] Limitations of this assay as a diagnostic tool include its limited availability, the small number of patients in which it has been tested, the need for measurement near the onset of symptoms, and its sensitivity for a life-threatening condition of only 90%.

High-Risk Populations

While emergency physicians may suspect TAD in a 70-year-old man with hypertension who presents after the acute onset of chest pain radiating to the back, they must also be wary of the younger patient who presents with concerning symptoms. Analysis of patients younger than 40 years old in the International Registry of Acute Aortic Dissection (IRAD) database reveal that whereas younger individuals with aortic dissection may have presentations and physical examination findings similar to those of their older colleagues, they vary significantly in their risk factor profile. Younger patients were more likely to have a history of Marfan syndrome, bicuspid aortic valve, and prior aortic valve surgery, and were less likely to have hypertension and atherosclerosis.[118] Pregnant women with chest or back pain should also cause clinicians to consider the diagnosis.

Potential Pitfalls

The ED evaluation of chest pain, and in particular the diagnosis of TAD, is fraught with potential pitfalls. There exist no reliable history or physical examination findings that can be trusted to identify those with TAD. Patients with TAD can easily be initially misdiagnosed and thought to have other potentially life-threatening causes of chest pain (most frequently ACS). Inappropriate treatment with antiplatelet, anticoagulant, and fibrinolytic therapies in patients believed to have ACS, but instead found to have TAD can have disastrous consequences. Fibrinolysis in patients eventually found to have TAD has been associated with severe hemorrhagic complications and a fatality rate of 71% (a rate similar to that of untreated TAD and much higher than most studies of current surgical management of the disease). Increasing age and anterior chest pain were highly associated with misdiagnosis, likely reflecting a higher clinician suspicion of ACS.[119]

Risk Management Strategies

The diagnosis of TAD can be a very difficult one to make (in some series the diagnosis is only made at autopsy in as many as 25% of cases).[120] Its presentation can be subtle, and patients may only have complaints that are a consequence of vascular compromise due to the dissection (such as strokelike symptoms, syncope, limb ischemia, gastrointestinal bleeding, and cardiac ischemia), or may even be entirely pain free.[121] Although the "classic" presentation of tearing chest pain that radiates to the back may actually be more uncommon than one would hope,[122] the emergency physician must be vigilant in the rapid evaluation of any patients with any complaint that might suggest TAD. Although there is significant overlap between the presentation of ACS and TAD, it is incumbent on the emergency physician to differentiate between the two as expeditiously as possible. Recognizing that the incidence of MI is nearly 800 times the estimated incidence of acute aortic dissection in the United States, and that ST-elevation MI is an uncommon complication of TAD,[123] some investigators have argued that delaying time-dependent therapy (such as anticoagulation or thrombolysis) to rule out dissection in all patients is short-sighted and impractical.[124] However, further evaluation in those with symptoms of concern for aortic dissection (such as those with a classic presentation, or those presenting with chest pain in association with a neurologic deficit or complaint) is mandatory, as missing the diagnosis is associated with a very high morbidity and mortality. In one series of 33 cases of aortic catastrophes that resulted in litigation, the most common reason for alleged malpractice was failure to diagnose (or delay in diagnosis).[125]

Unfortunately there are no clear, accepted guidelines directing emergency medicine clinicians as to when they should consider the diagnosis of TAD. However, there is evidence suggesting that key aspects of the history and physical examination should lead the physician to at least consider the diagnosis and possibly pursue definitive testing. These critical components include an abrupt onset of pain, pulse or blood pressure differentials, classically described chest radiography findings, or the presence of risk factors such as Marfan syndrome, previous cardiac surgery, or pregnancy. One should also consider the diagnosis of TAD in chest pain patients in whom conventional therapy (nitrates, b-blockers) are ineffective, in those who have chest pain in addition to another complaint (extremity weakness, paresthesias or other neurologic complaints, abdominal pain), or in those who are younger than typical chest pain patients.

PULMONARY EMBOLISM

One of the most common cardiovascular disorders in industrialized countries, venous thromboembolism (including deep vein thrombosis and pulmonary embolism) is thought to affect as many of 5% of people in their lifetime.[126] In the absence of treatment, pulmonary embolism (PE) carries a high morbidity and mortality, is believed to be responsible for 5% to 10% of all in-hospital deaths,[127] is diagnosed after death in 22% of cases,[128] and is thought to account for between 60,000 and 200,000 deaths in the United States annually.[129] Anticoagulant therapy is effective in reducing mortality. Of note, the death rate from acute PE, 15% at 3 months, exceeds that for acute myocardial infarction.

Clinical Presentations of Pulmonary Embolism

As with many other life-threatening disorders, emergency physicians are tasked with distinguishing patients with serious causes of chest pain, such as PE, from the multitude of patients presenting to EDs with less sinister causes of their pain. Unfortunately, the symptoms and signs are highly variable, nonspecific, and are present in many patients with and without PE.[130] In one large, multicenter, prospective study, the most common symptoms were dyspnea at rest or with exertion (73%), pleuritic pain (44%), cough (34%), calf or thigh pain (44%), calf or thigh swelling (41%), and wheezing (21%). Within this same cohort, 54% of patients were tachypneic, 24% were tachycardic, and 17% had decreased breath sounds.[131] The clinical presentation of PE can be as dramatic as cardiovascular collapse and fulminant shock, or as subtle as mild dyspnea or pleuritic chest pain. As history and physical examination findings are unreliable, not sensitive, and not specific, clinicians must rely on ancillary testing to substantiate or confirm the diagnosis of PE.

As with TAD, it is unreasonable, impractical, and unfeasible to obtain confirmatory testing for all patients who present with chest pain. As a result, several criteria or decision rules have been put forth to identify those patients who are in need of further testing. Although many have been proposed and subsequently published, 2 methods seem to be most applicable to ED patients.[132] Both the Wells and colleagues[133] and Wicki and colleagues[134] scoring systems use the presence of certain findings to generate a score that suggests pretest probability for PE. Those who fell into the "low risk" category (40%–49% of patients) had less than a 10% probability of PE, and "high-risk" patients (6%–7%) had a greater than 65% probability of PE. In contrast, "intermediate risk" patients (approximately 50% of patients) had a 20% to 40% probability of PE. In a multicenter study comparing subjective physician judgment of pretest probability of PE to the Wells criteria, the rates of PE in the low-risk groups were 19% for the subjective judgment arm and 28% in the Wells criteria arm. Similar rates of PE were found in the intermediate- and high-risk groups.[135] As with other disease processes, but perhaps more critical in the evaluation of patients with suspected PE, clinicians' suspicion regarding likelihood of a disease is important in determining which, if any, definitive testing is performed.

Diagnostic Tests and Their Limitations

Both the ECG and chest radiograph have limited utility in the diagnosis of PE (other than to perhaps confirm an alternative diagnosis). The classically described ECG finding in PE, S1Q3T3, is rarely seen. More common ECG findings include sinus tachycardia or nonspecific ST- and T-wave changes.[136] Initial chest films are normal in as many as 25% of patients who are ultimately found to have a PE. Again, classic findings such as Hampton hump and Westermark sign are rarely seen.[137]

D-dimer, released during fibrinolysis, has been shown to be a marker of endovascular thrombosis, and as a result has been studied for use in the diagnosis of PE. Several reports indicate that D-dimer may have a role in identifying a population of patients who are at very low risk for PE. D-dimer levels have been found to be elevated in approximately 95% of patients with PE,[138] and patients with a normal D-dimer enzyme-linked immunosorbent assay may have as high as a 95% likelihood of not having PE.[139] More specifically, in patients who are deemed to have a low probability of having a PE, a normal D-dimer confers an LR of 0.27 and a posterior probability of 1.0% (95% CI 0.3%–2.2%).[140] However, the specificity of the D-dimer assay for PE is very poor (particularly in the elderly[141]), and it is not sufficiently sensitive to exclude the diagnosis of PE in *all* patients presenting to the ED with pleuritic chest pain.[142] It is important that D-dimer should *not* be used as a screening tool in anyone other than those who have a low pretest probability of having a PE.[143–145] D-dimer values are known to be higher in pregnancy (after 20 weeks' gestation),[146] in those older than 80 years,[147] and in those with cancer.[148]

In many centers, ventilation/perfusion (V/Q) imaging has largely been replaced by CT pulmonary angiography (CTPA), as V/Q scanning proved to be less than optimal as a diagnostic test (more than half of patients with suspected PE had nondiagnostic scans, and the prevalence of PE in this population was nearly 25%). CT is readily available, interpretation is not complicated by underlying cardiopulmonary disease (as is often a problem with V/Q scanning), and it may identify an alternative diagnosis. Although the literature examining the use of CTPA in the diagnosis of PE suffers slightly from varied methodology, controversy regarding the use of conventional angiography as the "gold standard," and the ever-changing technology of CT imaging, the clinical validity of using CTPA to rule out PE is similar to that reported for conventional pulmonary angiography.[149] A meta-analysis, including 15 studies and 3500 patients, examining the rate of venous thromboembolism after a negative CTPA, reported an overall negative predictive value of 99.1%. The PIOPED II (Prospective Investigation of Pulmonary Embolism Diagnosis II) trial similarly revealed that multidetector contrast-enhanced CT angiography, in combination with a concordant clinical assessment, has a high positive and negative predictive value,[150] and outcome studies have shown that PE can be safely excluded by a negative multislice CTPA.[151,152]

High-Risk Populations

Although presenting symptoms and physical examination findings are unreliable and inconsistent, there are several identifiable risk factors for venous thromboembolism, including recent surgery, trauma, immobility, cancer, neurologic disease with lower extremity paresis, oral contraceptive pills, hormone therapy, and pregnancy.[153,154] It should be noted that older patients with PE are less likely to complain of chest pain, are more likely to be hypoxic, and are more likely to present with syncope.[155]

Potential Pitfalls and Risk Management Strategies

As with several other causes of chest pain, PE presents a diagnostic challenge to ED physicians: its associated symptoms are common and not specific for PE, and both undertreatment (ie, failure to diagnose) and overtreatment (ie, unnecessary anticoagulation) carry significant morbidity. Most patients with symptoms suggestive of the illness do not have PE.[156] This fact must be weighed against the reality that the mortality rate for untreated PE is 18.4%, 7 times greater than that of appropriately treated PE.[157]

As the implementation of specific algorithms and diagnostic tools hinges on the likelihood that a particular patient has a PE, clinicians would be wise to consistently document the absence or presence of risk factors as well as their pretest suspicion that a patient's chest pain is due to PE. Using this pretest probability to determine the diagnostic strategy and rationale for testing is clearly important in cases in which the diagnosis of PE is missed. The related appropriate use of diagnostic tests should be clear. No single test, used in isolation, is sufficiently sensitive to identify all patients with PE in the ED. When there is discordance between clinical probability and the results of objective testing, the posttest probability of PE is neither sufficiently high nor sufficiently low to permit therapeutic decisions.[158] For example, a negative D-dimer in anyone other than a low-risk patient is considered inadequate testing, and in patients with a high probability of having PE, workup should continue even in the presence of a negative CTPA. Finally, as with all other potentially life threatening diseases, maintaining a high index of suspicion for PE is critical (ie, in those with unexplained tachycardia, tachypnea, or hypoxia).[159]

TENSION PNEUMOTHORAX

The *spontaneous* tension pneumothorax is a less discussed and often later-diagnosed entity than its routinely emphasized traumatic counterpart. Primary spontaneous pneumothoraces classically occur in tall, thin males without previous lung disease. Smoking, a history of Marfan syndrome, and family history of spontaneous pneumothorax are also thought to be risk factors for developing the disease. Secondary spontaneous pneumothoraces are defined as being due to underlying lung disease such as chronic obstructive pulmonary disease, infectious or malignant processes, or unusual causes such as catamenial pneumothoraces associated with menses. Although uncommon, all of these types of pneumothoraces have a 1% to 3% potential to convert from a simple to a tension pneumothorax.[160–162]

A tension pneumothorax is most accurately defined as a positive pressure within the intrapleural potential space due to a one-way valve effect between the alveolar/pleural border, but its clinical confirmation varies from the severity of hemodynamic compromise, from a "hiss" of air and clinical improvement on needle decompression or thoracostomy, to mediastinal shift and ipsilateral hyperexpansion on chest radiograph.[163] An awake patient may try to compensate by maximizing inspiratory effort to overcome the positive intrapleural pressure as tension develops, and thus may exhibit normal hemodynamics just before suddenly and rapidly decompensating.

Aside from chest pain and respiratory distress, the classic clinical signs of tension pneumothoraces are not universally present. According to some estimates, only 50% to 75% of awake patients demonstrate tachycardia and decreased air entry on the affected side, whereas hypoxia, tracheal deviation, and hypotension are even less reliable (<25%). Confirmation of ipsilateral hyperresonance, hyperexpansion, and hypomobility, or displacement of cardiac apex, are infrequent (10%) and difficult to fully assess in a critically ill patient. Patients on positive pressure ventilation, however, are more likely to demonstrate many of the classic signs with resultant cardiovascular collapse due to the rapid escalation of intrapleural pressure. In addition, the diagnosis should be strongly considered in those with underlying lung disease, or those on positive pressure ventilation who undergo a rapid or sudden deterioration.

The chest radiograph is traditionally "forbidden" in suspected tension pneumothoraces because of the associated delay in life-saving intervention while awaiting diagnostic confirmation. However, in an awake patient who has not yet developed hypoxia, hypotension, depressed respiratory rate (from fatigue), or altered mental status, a quick confirmatory portable chest radiograph is reasonable to avoid the risk of a potentially unnecessary thoracostomy. Improvement following needle decompression has often been considered a diagnostic test for tension pneumothorax, but is well described in the literature as being an imperfect diagnostic and therapeutic intervention.[164] Thus, lack of a response to needle compression should not prevent tube thoracostomy in the appropriate clinical setting.

ESOPHAGEAL RUPTURE

Full-thickness tears through the esophagus are relatively rare but carry a high morbidity and mortality, presumably due to delayed recognition of the ensuing mediastinitis and septic shock. In one case series of patients with atraumatic esophageal rupture, the median delay from admission to diagnosis was nearly 24 hours.[165] In another case series that included postendoscopic, traumatic, and erosive foreign body origins of esophageal ruptures, a shorter median time to diagnosis was reported, but time to diagnosis still ranged up to 96 hours.[166]

The classic "Mackler's triad" of esophageal rupture—chest pain, vomiting, and subcutaneous emphysema—has been estimated to occur in only 14% of cases. Whereas sudden-onset chest pain or epigastric pain and prior vomiting or retching are considered the 2 key features of esophageal rupture, at least one series reported that less than half of patients complained of vomiting or chest pain.[167] Other less commonly noted symptoms include dyspnea, fever, and dysphagia. Up to two-thirds of patients may demonstrate subcutaneous emphysema on physical examination, whereas Hamman's sign (a crunching sound synchronous with each heart beat) is rare. Other nonspecific signs include tachypnea and tachycardia, with 82% of patients meeting systemic inflammatory response syndrome criteria.

The upright chest radiograph is a useful screening tool for esophageal rupture, as 75% to 90% will be abnormal. Pneumomediastinum, mediastinal widening, hydropneumothoraces (usually left-sided because of the location of the distal esophagus), and pleural effusions are the most common findings. Confirmatory testing usually includes an esophagogram with a water-soluble contrast agent. These agents are less likely to result in irritation and inflammation than barium if there is indeed a leak, but also carry a false negative rate of 10% to 25%. High-density barium adheres better to perforated sites and can diagnose 25% to 50% of esophageal perforations that were not diagnosed by previously performed water-soluble contrast studies.[168] Contrast CT is useful for assessing extraluminal manifestations of perforation,[169] such as air, fluid, or abscesses in the mediastinal, pleural, or pericardial regions. Finally, direct endoscopy most definitively assesses the site of leakage and length of tear.

CARDIAC TAMPONADE

Cardiac tamponade is likely an underrecognized cause of death (particularly in intensive care patients),[170] and should be considered as a cause of unexplained shock in any critically ill patient. Medical conditions at risk for pericardial effusions that can progress to tamponade include acute pericarditis, malignancy, acute myocardial infarction leading to wall rupture, proximal aortic dissection, uremia, congestive heart failure, collagen vascular disease, viral infection (including even the common influenza virus[171]), or bacterial infection (including tuberculosis[172,173]). Iatrogenic causes should also be considered in patients who have recently undergone cardiac surgery, percutaneous coronary intervention,[174] or wire insertion for pacemakers or implantable cardiac defibrillators.[175]

The Rational Clinical Examination series in the *Journal of the American Medical Association* recently explored the utility of specific signs and symptoms for determining whether a patient with a known pericardial effusion has progressed to tamponade.[176] Conscious patients may report shortness of breath (pooled sensitivity 87%–88%) and chest pain (sensitivity 20%), in addition to other nonspecific symptoms, including fever, fullness, nausea, vomiting, or dysphagia. Tachycardia (pooled sensitivity of 77%), tachypnea (80%), and elevated jugular venous pressure (76%) are relatively sensitive signs for tamponade, whereas hypotension (26%) and diminished heart sounds (28%) are less reliable. Hypotension is a late finding and, in fact, some patients may even be *hyper*tensive from increased adrenergic drive and increased peripheral vascular resistance.[177,178] One physical examination finding, an increased pulsus paradoxus, has been shown to be correlated with the progression from effusion to tamponade. A pulsus of 10 mm Hg or greater is associated with a 3.3 LR for tamponade, and a pulsus greater than 12 mm Hg further increases the LR to 5.9. In contrast, a pulsus less than 10 mm Hg lowers the LR to 0.03. This finding, however, may be falsely elevated in lung diseases like chronic obstructive pulmonary disease or massive PE, or minimized by hypotension.[179]

Classically described ECG findings in tamponade are also insensitive. Low voltage is thought to be only 42% sensitive for the presence of cardiac tamponade, whereas electrical alternans is only 16% to 21% sensitive. The chest radiograph finding of cardiomegaly has a pooled sensitivity of 89%. Unfortunately, the often-described "globular" cardiac silhouette, with small yet rapidly accumulating effusions that result in tamponade physiology, may not be present. Finally, whereas echocardiography is crucial for the characterization of a pericardial effusion, echocardiographic signs of tamponade do not always correlate with the clinically significant hemodynamic compromise seen in true tamponade. These signs include the collapse of one or more chambers of the heart (usually starting with the right atrium, then right ventricle or left atrium), inferior vena cava plethora (lack of collapse with inspiration), or changes in venous flow based on respiration or systole versus diastole. In one series of patients with moderate or large pericardial effusions, 90% of patients with tamponade had collapse of one or more cardiac chambers; however, 34% of patients with moderate to large effusions but *no tamponade* also had chamber collapse.[180] The investigators consequently concluded that lack of collapse makes the diagnosis of tamponade unlikely, although this is certainly not definitively diagnostic. A distended inferior vena cava is sensitive (97%) but not specific (40%) for tamponade.[181]

SUMMARY

Patients with chest pain present one of the emergency medicine clinician's greatest challenges. Not only must physicians differentiate between the benign and life-threatening causes of chest pain, they must also quickly identify those patients who would benefit from immediate intervention. Complicating this already difficult task is the fact that therapy for one of these disease processes is contraindicated for another (ie, anticoagulation in a patient presumed to have ACS when in fact they have an aortic dissection). Although it is very important to note that *not* every case of missed ACS, TAD, or PE represents negligence or malpractice, it is critical for clinicians to realize the importance of clear documentation of risk factor assessment and thought processes. When misses do occur, as they will for every emergency physician, it is imperative that the documentation reflects careful, appropriate, and thoughtful management and decision making.

REFERENCES

1. Klompas M. Does this patient have an acute aortic dissection? JAMA 2002; 287(17):2262–72.
2. Mehta RH, Eagle KA. Missed diagnoses of acute coronary syndromes in the emergency room—continuing challenges. N Engl J Med 2000;342(16):1207–10.
3. Schor S, Behar S, Modan B, et al. Disposition of presumed coronary patients from an emergency room: a follow-up study. JAMA 1976;236(8):941–3.
4. Lee TH, Rouan GW, Weisberg MC, et al. Clinical characteristics and natural history of patients with acute myocardial infarction sent home from the emergency room. Am J Cardiol 1987;60:219–24.
5. McCarthy BD, Beshansky JR, D'Agostino RB, et al. Missed diagnoses of acute myocardial infarction in the emergency department: results from a multicenter study. Ann Emerg Med 1993;22:579–82.
6. Pope JH, Aufderheide TP, Ruthazer R, et al. Missed diagnosis of acute cardiac ischemia in the emergency department. N Engl J Med 2000;342:1163–70.

7. Pope JH, Selker HP. Acute coronary syndromes in the emergency department: diagnostic characteristics, tests, and challenges. Cardiol Clin 2005;23:423–51.
8. Beckmann CH. How to avoid being swept away by the rising tide of malpractice litigation. Am J Cardiol 2003;91:585–6.
9. Kannel WB, Abbot RD. Incidence and prognosis of unrecognized myocardial infarction: an update of the Framingham Study. N Engl J Med 1984;311:1144–7.
10. Canto JG, Shlipak MG, Rogers WJ, et al. Prevalence, clinical characteristics, and mortality among patients with myocardial infarction presenting without chest pain. JAMA 2000;283:3223–9.
11. Dorsch MF, Lawrence RA, Sapsford RJ, et al. Poor prognosis of patients presenting with symptomatic myocardial infarction but without chest pain. Heart 2001;86:494–8.
12. Brieger D, Eagle KA, Goodman SG, et al. Acute coronary syndromes without chest pain, an underdiagnosed and undertreated high-risk group: insights from the Global Registry of Acute Coronary Events (GRACE). Chest 2004;126:461–9.
13. Coronado BE, Pope JH, Griffith JL, et al. Clinical features, triage, and outcome of patients presenting to the ED with suspected acute coronary syndromes but without pain: a multicenter study. Am J Emerg Med 2004;22:568–74.
14. Canto JG, Fincher C, Kiefe CI, et al. Atypical presentations among Medicare beneficiaries with unstable angina pectoris. Am J Cardiol 2002;90:248–53.
15. Lee HO. Typical and atypical clinical signs and symptoms of myocardial infarction and delayed seeking of professional care among blacks. Am J Crit Care 1997;6(1):7–13.
16. Arslanian-Engoren C, Patel A, Fang J, et al. Symptoms of men and women presenting with acute coronary syndromes. Am J Cardiol 2006;98:1177–81.
17. Patel H, Rosengreen A, Ekman I. Symptoms in acute coronary syndromes: does sex make a difference? Am Heart J 2004;148:27–33.
18. Milner KA, Funk M, Richards S, et al. Gender differences in symptom presentation associated with coronary heart disease. Am J Cardiol 1999;84:396–9.
19. Kudenchuk PJ, Maynard C, Martin JS, et al. Comparison of presentation, treatment, and outcome of acute myocardial infarction in men versus women (the Myocardial Infarction Triage and Intervention Registry). Am J Cardiol 1996;78: 9–14.
20. Johns PA, Lee TH, Cook F, et al. Effect of race on the presentation and management of patients with acute chest pain. Ann Intern Med 1993;118:593–601.
21. Pezzin LE, Keyl PM, Green GB. Disparities in the emergency department evaluation of chest pain patients. Acad Emerg Med 2007;14:149–56.
22. Egred M, Viswanathan G, Davis GK. Myocardial infarction in young adults. Postgrad Med J 2005;81:741–5.
23. Chen L, Chester M, Kaski JC. Clinical factors and angiographic features associated with premature coronary artery disease. Chest 1995;108(2):364–9.
24. Anonymous. Reduce legal risks of chest pain. ED Manag 1998;10(11):126–8.
25. Walker NJ, Sites FD, Shofer FS, et al. Characteristics and outcomes of young adults who present to the emergency department with chest pain. Acad Emerg Med 2001;8(7):703–8.
26. Marsan RJ, Shaver KJ, Sease KL, et al. Evaluation of a clinical decision rule for young adult patients with chest pain. Acad Emerg Med 2005;12(1):26–32.
27. Goodacre S, Locker T, Campbell S. How useful are clinical features in the diagnosis of acute, undifferentiated chest pain? Acad Emerg Med 2002;9(3):203–8.
28. Chun AA, McGee SR. Bedside diagnosis of coronary artery disease: a systematic review. Am J Med 2004;117:334–43.

29. Swap CJ, Nagurney JT. Value and limitations of chest pain history in the evaluation of patients with suspected acute coronary syndromes. JAMA 2005; 294(20):2623–9.
30. Panju AA, Hemmelgarn BR, Guyatt GH, et al. The rational clinical examination: is this patient having a myocardial infarction? JAMA 1998;280(14):1256–63.
31. Anderson JL, Adams CD, Antman EM, et al. ACC/AHA 2007 guidelines for the management of patients with unstable angina/non-ST-segment elevation myocardial infarction: a report of the American College of Cardiology/American Heart Association Task Force on Practice Guidelines (Writing committee to revise the 2002 guidelines for the management of patients with unstable angina/non-ST-elevation myocardial infarction): developed in collaboration with the American College of Emergency Physicians, American College of Physicians, Society for Academic Emergency Medicine, Society for Cardiovascular Angiography and Interventions, and Society for Thoracic Surgeons. J Am Coll Cardiol 2007;50:652–726.
32. Lee TH, Cook EF, Weisberg M, et al. Acute chest pain in the emergency room: identification and examination of low-risk patients. Arch Intern Med 1985;145: 65–9.
33. Everts B, Karlson BW, Wahrborg P, et al. Localization of pain in suspected acute myocardial infarction in relation to final diagnosis, age and sex, and site and type of infarction. Heart Lung 1996;25:430–7.
34. Gordon T, Sorlie P, Kannel WB. Coronary heart disease, atherothrombotic brain infarction, intermittent claudication—a multivariate analysis of some factors related to their incidence: Framingham Study, 16 year follow-up. Section 27, U.S. Govt. Print. Office; 1971.
35. Jayes RL, Beshansky JR, D'Agostino RB, et al. Do patients' coronary risk factor reports predict acute cardiac ischemia in the emergency department? A multicenter study. J Clin Epidemiol 1992;45(6):621–6.
36. Antman EM, Cohen M, Bernink PJL, et al. The TIMI risk score for unstable angina/non-ST elevation MI: a method for prognostication and therapeutic decision making. JAMA 2000;284(7):835–42.
37. Shry EA, Dacus J, Van De Graaff E, et al. Usefulness of the response to sublingual nitroglycerin as a predictor of ischemic chest pain in the emergency department. Am J Cardiol 2002;90(11):1264–6.
38. Henrikson CA, Howell EE, Bush DE, et al. Chest pain relief by nitroglycerin does not predict active coronary artery disease. Ann Intern Med 2003;139:979–86.
39. Diercks DB, Boghos E, Guzman H, et al. Changes in the numeric descriptive scale for pain after sublingual nitroglycerin do not predict cardiac etiology of chest pain. Ann Emerg Med 2005;45:581–5.
40. Servi RJ, Skiendzielewski JJ. Relief of myocardial ischemia pain with a gastrointestinal cocktail. Am J Emerg Med 1985;3(3):208–9.
41. Dickinson MW. The "GI cocktail" in the evaluation of chest pain in the emergency department. J Emerg Med 1996;14(2):245–6.
42. Chauhan A, Mullins PA, Taylor G, et al. Cardioesophageal reflex: a mechanism for "linked angina" in patients with angiographically proven coronary artery disease. J Am Coll Cardiol 1996;27(7):1621–8.
43. Dobrzycki S, Baniukiewicz A, Korecki J, et al. Does gastro-esophageal reflux provoke the myocardial ischemia in patients with CAD? Int J Cardiol 2005; 104:67–72.
44. Budzynski J, Klopocka M, Pulkowski G, et al. The effect of double dose of omeprazole on the course of angina pectoris and treadmill stress test in patients with

coronary artery disease—a randomised, double-blind, placebo controlled, crossover trial. Int J Cardiol 2007;127:233–9.
45. Smith KS, Papp C. Episodic, postural, and "linked angina". Br Med J 1962; 2(5317):1425–30.
46. Fesmire FM, Percy RF, Bardoner JB, et al. Usefulness of automated serial 12-lead ECG monitoring during the initial emergency department evaluation of patients with chest pain. Ann Emerg Med 1998;31:3–11.
47. Fesmire FM, Decker WW, Diercks DB, et al. Clinical policy: critical issues in the evaluation and management of adult patients with non-ST-segment elevation acute coronary syndromes—from the American College of Physicians clinical polices subcommittee. Ann Emerg Med 2006;48:270–301.
48. Masoudi FA, Magid DJ, Vinson DR, et al. Implications of the failure to identify high-risk electrocardiogram findings for the quality of care of patients with acute myocardial infarction—results of the Emergency Department Quality in Myocardial Infarction (EDQMI) Study. Circulation 2006;114:1565–71.
49. Brady WJ, Perron AD, Ullman E. Errors in emergency physician interpretation of ST-segment elevation in emergency department chest pain patients. Acad Emerg Med 2000;7:1256–60.
50. Erling BF, Perron AD, Brady WJ. Disagreement in the interpretation of electrocardiographic ST segment elevation: a source of error for emergency physicians? Am J Emerg Med 2004;22:65–70.
51. Balk EM, Ioannidis JPA, Salem D, et al. Accuracy of biomarkers to diagnose acute cardiac ischemia in the emergency department: a meta-analysis. Ann Emerg Med 2001;37:478–94.
52. Limkakeng A, Gibler WB, Pollack C, et al. Combination of Goldman risk and initial cardiac troponin I for emergency department chest pain patient risk stratification. Acad Emerg Med 2001;8:696–702.
53. Ebell MH, Flewelling D, Flynn CA. A systematic review of troponin T and I for diagnosing acute myocardial infarction. J Fam Pract 2000;49:550–6.
54. Smith SW, Tibbles CD, Apple FS, et al. Outcome of low-risk patients discharged home after a normal cardiac troponin I. J Emerg Med 2004;26(4):401–6.
55. Fesmire FM. Delta CK-MB outperforms delta troponin I at 2 hours during the ED rule out of acute myocardial infarction. Am J Emerg Med 2000;18:1–8.
56. Fesmire FM, Christenson RH, Fody EP, et al. Delta creatinine kinase-MB outperforms myoglobin at two hours during the emergency department identification and exclusion of troponin positive non-ST-segment elevation acute coronary syndromes. Ann Emerg Med 2004;44:12–9.
57. Pope JH, Ruthazer R, Beshansky JR, et al. Clinical features of emergency department patients presenting with symptoms suggestive of acute cardiac ischemia: a multicenter study. J Thromb Thrombolysis 1998;6:63–74.
58. Braunwald E, Mark DB, Jones RH, et al. Unstable angina: diagnosis and management. Rockville (MD): Agency for Health Care Policy and Research; 1994. Publication No. 94-06062.
59. Zalenski RJ, McCarren M, Roberts R, et al. An evaluation of a chest pain diagnostic protocol to exclude acute cardiac ischemia in the emergency department. Arch Intern Med 157:1085–91.
60. Polanczyk CA, Johnson PA, Hartley LH, et al. Clinical correlates and prognostic significance of early negative exercise tolerance test in patients with acute chest pain seen in the hospital emergency department. Am J Cardiol 1998;81:288–92.
61. Mikhail MG, Smith FA, Gray M, et al. Cost-effectiveness of mandatory stress testing in chest pain center patients. Ann Emerg Med 1997;29(1):88–98.

62. Amsterdam EA, Kirk JD, Diercks DB, et al. Immediate exercise testing to evaluate low-risk patients presenting to the emergency department with chest pain. J Am Coll Cardiol 2002;40:251–6.
63. Meyer MC, Mooney RP, Sekera AK. A critical pathway for patients with acute chest pain and low risk for short-term adverse cardiac events: role of outpatient stress testing. Ann Emerg Med 2006;47:427–35.
64. Duseja R, Feldman JA. Missed acute cardiac ischemic in the ED: limitations of diagnostic testing. Am J Emerg Med 2004;22(3):219–25.
65. Smith SW, Jackson EA, Bart BA, et al. Incidence of myocardial infarction in emergency department chest pain patients with a recent negative stress imaging test [abstract]. Acad Emerg Med 2005;12(5 Suppl 1):51.
66. Raff GL, Gallagher MJ, O'Neill WW, et al. Diagnostic accuracy of noninvasive coronary angiography using 64-slice spiral computed tomography. J Am Coll Cardiol 2005;46:552–7.
67. Hoffman U, Nagurney JT, Moselewski F, et al. Coronary multidetector computed tomography in the assessment of patients with acute chest pain. Circulation 2006;114:2251–60.
68. Rubinshteim R, Halon DA, Gaspar T, et al. Usefulness of 64-slice cardiac computed tomographic angiography for diagnosing acute coronary syndromes and predicting clinical outcome in emergency department patients with chest pain of uncertain origin. Circulation 2007;115:1762–8.
69. Meijboom WB, Mollet NR, Mieghem CAV, et al. 64-slice CT coronary angiography in patients with non-ST elevation acute coronary syndromes. Heart 2007;93: 1386–92.
70. Gallager MJ, Ross MA, Raff GL, et al. The diagnostic accuracy of 64-slice computed tomography coronary angiography compared with stress nuclear imaging in emergency department low-risk chest pain patients. Ann Emerg Med 2007;49:125–36.
71. Goldstein JA, Gallagher MJ, O'Neill WW, et al. A randomized controlled trial of multi-slice coronary computed tomography for evaluation of acute chest pain. J Am Coll Cardiol 2007;49:863–71.
72. Hollander JE, Chang AM, Shofer FS, et al. Coronary computed tomographic angiography for rapid discharge of low-risk patients with potential acute coronary syndromes. Ann Emerg Med 2009;53(3):295–304.
73. Barnett K, Feldman JA. Noninvasive imaging techniques to aid in the triage of patients with suspected acute coronary syndrome: a review. Emerg Med Clin North Am 2005;23:977–98.
74. Newman DH. Computed tomographic angiography for low risk chest pain: seeking passage. Ann Emerg Med 2009;53(3):305–8.
75. Braunwald E, Brown J, Brown L, et al. Unstable angina: diagnosis and management. Clinical practice guideline number 10. Rockville (MD): Agency for Health Care Policy and Research, US Public Health Service, US Department of Health and Human Services; 1994.
76. Hollander JE. Risk stratification of emergency department patients with chest pain: the need for standardized reporting guidelines. Ann Emerg Med 2004; 43(1):68–70.
77. Katz DA, Aufderheid TP, Bogner M, et al. The impact of unstable angina guidelines in the triage of emergency department patients with possible acute coronary syndrome. Med Decis Making 2006;26:606–16.
78. Selker HP, Griffith JL, D'Agostino RB. A tool for judging coronary care unit admission appropriateness, valid for both real-time and retrospective use: a time-insensitive

predictive instrument (TIPI) for acute cardiac ischemia: a multicenter study. Med Care 1991;29(7):610–27.
79. Selker HP, Beshansky JR, Griffith JL, et al. Use of the Acute Cardiac Ischemia Time-Insensitive Predictive Instrument (ACI-TIPI) to assist with triage of patients with chest pain or other symptoms suggestive of acute cardiac ischemia: a multicenter, controlled clinical trial. Ann Intern Med 1998;129(11):845–55.
80. Lau J, Ioannidis J, Balk E, et al. Evaluation of technologies for identifying acute cardiac ischemia in emergency departments. Evidence Report/Technology Assessment Number 26. (Prepared by The New England Medical Center Evidence-based Practice Center under Contract No. 290-97-0019) AHRQ Publication No. 01-E006. Rockville (MD): Agency for Healthcare Research and Quality; May 2001.
81. Pollack CV, Sites FD, Shofer FS, et al. Application of the TIMI risk score for unstable angina and non-ST elevation acute coronary syndrome to an unselected emergency department chest pain population. Acad Emerg Med 2006; 13(1):13–8.
82. Chase M, Robey JL, Zogby KE, et al. Prospective validation of the Thrombolysis in Myocardial Infarction Risk score in the emergency department chest pain population. Ann Emerg Med 2006;48(3):252–9.
83. Antman EM, McCabe CH, Gurfinkel EP, et al. Enoxaparin prevents death and cardiac ischemic events in unstable angina/non-Q-wave myocardial infarction: results of the Thrombolysis in Myocardial Infarction (TIMI) 11B trial. Circulation 1999;100:1593–601.
84. Jaffery Z, Hudson MP, Jacobsen G, et al. Modified thrombolysis in myocardial infarction (TIMI) risk score to risk stratify patients in the emergency department with possible acute coronary syndrome. J Thromb Thrombolysis 2007;24: 137–44.
85. Ramsay G, Podogrodzka M, McClure, et al. Risk prediction in patients presenting with suspected cardiac pain: the GRACE and TIMI risk scores. QJM 2007; 100(1):11–8.
86. Rusnak RA, Stair TO, Hansen K, et al. Litigation against the emergency physician: common features in cases of missed myocardial infarction. Ann Emerg Med 1989;18:1029–34.
87. Acute myocardial infarction study. Rockville (MD): Physician Insurers Association of America; 1996.
88. Croskerry P. Achilles heels of the ED: delayed or missed diagnoses. ED Legal Letter October 2003;109–20.
89. Freas GC. Medicolegal aspects of acute myocardial infarction. Emerg Med Clin North Am 2001;19(2):511–21.
90. Chen K, Varon J, Wenker O, et al. Acute thoracic aortic dissection: the basics. J Emerg Med 1997;15(6):859–67.
91. Meszaros I, Morocz J, Szlavi J, et al. Epidemiology and clinicopathology of aortic dissection. Chest 2000;117(5):1271–8.
92. Kouchokis N, Dougenis D. Surgery of the thoracic aorta. N Engl J Med 1997; 336(26):1876–88.
93. Hagan PG, Nienaber CA, Isselbaher EM, et al. The international registry of acute aortic dissection (IRAD). JAMA 2000;283(7):897–903.
94. Slater E, DeSanctis RW. The clinical recognition of dissecting aortic aneurysm. Am J Med 1976;60:625–33.
95. Massumi A, Mathur VS. Clinical recognition of aortic dissection. Tex Heart Inst J 1990;17:254–6.

96. Levinson D, Edmeades D, Griffith G. Dissecting aneurysm of the aorta: its clinical electrocardiographic and laboratory findings. Circulation 1950;1:360–87.
97. Von Kodolitsch Y, Loose R, Ostermeyer J, et al. Proximal aortic dissection late after aortic valve surgery: 119 cases of a distinct clinical entity. Thorac Cardiovasc Surg 2000;48:342–6.
98. Crawford ES. The diagnosis and management of aortic dissection. JAMA 1990; 264:2537–41.
99. Bordeleau L, Cwinn A, Turek M, et al. Aortic dissection and Turner's syndrome: case report and review of the literature. J Emerg Med 1998;16:593–6.
100. Sullivan PR, Wolfson AB, Leckey RD, et al. Diagnosis of acute thoracic aortic dissection in the emergency department. Am J Emerg Med 2000;18:46–50.
101. Pesola GR, Pesola HR, Lin M, et al. The normal difference in bilateral indirect blood pressure recordings in hypertensive individuals. Acad Emerg Med 2002;9:342–5.
102. Singer AJ, Hollander JE. Blood pressure: assessment of interarm differences. Arch Intern Med 1996;156:2005–8.
103. Rosman HS, Patel S, Bzorak S, et al. Quality of history taking in patients with aortic dissection. Chest 1998;114:793–5.
104. Hirata K, Kyushima M, Asato H. Electrocardiographic abnormalities in patients with acute aortic dissection. Am J Cardiol 1995;76:1207–12.
105. Ohtani H, Kiyokawa K, Asada H, et al. Stanford type A acute dissection developing acute myocardial infarction. Jpn J Thorac Cardiovasc Surg 2000;48:69–72.
106. Gregorio MC, Baumgartner FJ, Omari BO. The presenting chest roentgenogram in acute type A aortic dissection: a multidisciplinary study. Am Surg 2002;68(1): 6–10.
107. Sommer T, Fehske W, Holzknecht N, et al. Aortic dissection: A comparative study of diagnosis with spiral CT, multiplanar transesophageal echocardiography, and MR imaging. Radiology 1996;199:347–52.
108. Moore AG, Eagle KA, Bruckman D, et al. Choice of computed tomography, transesophageal echocardiography, magnetic resonance imaging and aortography in acute aortic dissection: International registry of acute aortic dissection (IRAD). Am J Cardiol 202(89):1235–7.
109. Silvey SV, Stoughton TL, Pearl W, et al. Rupture of the outer partition of aortic dissection during transesophageal echocardiography. Am J Cardiol 1991; 68(2):286–7.
110. Hayter RG, Rhea JT, Small A, et al. Suspected aortic dissection and other aortic disorders: Multi-detector CT in 373 cases in the emergency setting. Radiology 2006;238(3):841–52.
111. Weber T, Högler S, Auer J, et al. D-dimer in acute aortic dissection. Chest 2003; 123:1375–8.
112. Perez A, Abbet P, Drescher MJ. D-dimers in the emergency department evaluation of aortic dissection. Acad Emerg Med 2004;11:397–400.
113. Eggebrecht H, Naber CK, Bruch C, et al. Value of plasma fibrin D-dimers for detection of acute aortic dissection. J Am Coll Cardiol 2004;44:804–9.
114. Wiegand J, Koller M, Bingisser R. Does a negative D-dimer test rule out aortic dissection? Swiss Med Wkly 2007;137:462.
115. Sodeck G, Domanovits H, Schillinger M, et al. D-dimer in ruling out acute aortic dissection: A systematic review and prospective cohort study. Eur Heart J 2007; 28:3067–75.
116. Sutherland A, Escano J, Coon TP. D-dimer as the sole screening test for acute aortic dissection: A review of the literature. Ann Emerg Med 2008;52(4):339–43.

117. Suzuki T, Katoh H, Tsuchio, et al. Diagnostic implications of elevated levels of smooth-muscle myosin heavy-chain protein in acute aortic dissection. Ann Intern Med 2000;133(7):537–41.
118. Januzzi JL, Isselbacher EM, Fatorri R, et al. Characterizing the young patient with aortic dissection: results from the international registry of aortic dissection (IRAD) [abstract 1081–154]. J Am Coll Cardiol 2003;41(6):235A.
119. Hansen MS, Nogareda GJ, Hutchison SJ. Frequency of and inappropriate treatment of misdiagnosis of acute aortic dissection. Am J Cardiol 2007;99:852–6.
120. Spittell PC, Spittell JA, Joyce JW, et al. Clinical features and differential diagnosis of aortic dissection: Experience with 236 cases (1980 through 1990). Mayo Clin Proc 1993;68:642–51.
121. Cohen S, Littman D. Painless dissecting aneurysm of the aorta. N Engl J Med 1964;271:143–5.
122. Alsous F, Silam A, Ezeldin A, et al. Potential pitfalls in the diagnosis of aortic dissection. Conn Med 2003;67(3):131–4.
123. Nallamothu BK, Eagle KA. When zebras run with the horses: The diagnostic dilemma of acute aortic dissection complicated by myocardial infarction. J Interv Cardiol 2002;15:297–300.
124. Piney SP, Wasserman HS. Anterior myocardial infarction, acute aortic dissection and anomalous coronary artery. J Interv Cardiol 2002;15:293–6.
125. Elefteriades JA, Barrett PW, Kopf GS. Litigation in nontraumatic aortic diseases—a tempest in the malpractice maelstrom. Cardiology 2008;109:263–72.
126. Spencer FA, Emery C, Lessard D, et al. The Worcester Thromboembolism Study. A population-based study of the clinical epidemiology of venous thromboembolism. J Gen Intern Med 2006;21:722–7.
127. Goldhaber SZ, Visani L, De Rosa M. Acute pulmonary embolism: clinical outcomes in the International Cooperative Pulmonary Embolism Registry (ICOPER). Lancet 1999;353:1386–9.
128. Heit JA, O'Fallon WM, Petterson TM, et al. Relative impact of risk factors for deep vein thrombosis and pulmonary embolism. Arch Intern Med 2002;162:1245–8.
129. Becattini C, Agnelli G. Acute pulmonary embolism: risk stratification in the emergency department. Intern Emerg Med 2007;2:119–29.
130. Task force on pulmonary embolism. European section of cardiology. Guidelines on diagnosis and management of acute pulmonary embolism. Eur Heart J 2001;21:1301–36.
131. Stein PD, Beemath A, Matta F, et al. Clinical characteristics of patients with acute pulmonary embolism: data from PIOPED II. Am J Med 2007;120:871–9.
132. Clinical Policy. Critical issues in the evaluation and management of adult patients presenting with suspected pulmonary embolism. Ann Emerg Med 2003;41(2):257–70.
133. Wells PS, Ginsberg JS, Anderson DR, et al. Use of a clinical model for safe management of patients with suspected pulmonary embolism. Ann Intern Med 1988;129:997–1005.
134. Wicki J, Pereger T, Junod A, et al. Assessing clinical probability of pulmonary embolism in the emergency ward: a simple score. Arch Intern Med 2001;161:92–7.
135. Sanson B-J, Lijmer JG, Gillavry MRM, et al. Comparison of a clinical probability estimate and 2 clinical models in patients with suspected pulmonary embolism. Thromb Haemost 2000;83:199–203.

136. Stein PD, Henry JW. Clinical characteristics of patients with acute pulmonary embolism stratified according to their presenting syndromes. Chest 1997;112: 974–9.
137. Elliot CG, Goldhaber SZ, Visani L, et al. Chest radiographs in acute pulmonary embolism. Chest 2000;118:33–8.
138. Stein PD, Hull RD, Patel KC, et al. D-dimer for the exclusion of acute venous thrombosis and pulmonary embolism: a systematic review. Ann Intern Med 2004;140(8):589–602.
139. Tapson VF, Carroll BA, Davidson BL, et al. The diagnostic approach to acute venous thromboembolism. Clinical practice guidelines. American Thoracic Society. Am J Respir Crit Care Med 1999;160:1043–66.
140. Kearon C, Ginsberg JS, Jouketis J, et al. An evaluation of D-dimer in the diagnosis of pulmonary embolism: a randomized trial. Ann Intern Med 2006;144(11): 812–21.
141. Brown MD, Vance SJ, Kline JA. An emergency department guideline for the diagnosis of pulmonary embolism: an outcome study. Acad Emerg Med 2005; 12(1):20–5.
142. Hogg K, Dawson D, Mackway-Jones K. The emergency department utility of Simplify D-dimer™ to exclude pulmonary embolism in patients with pleuritic chest pain. Ann Emerg Med 2005;46(4):305–10.
143. Kutinsky I, Blakely S, Roche V, et al. Normal D-dimer levels in patients with pulmonary embolism. Arch Intern Med 1999;159:1569–72.
144. Brown MD, Rowe BH, Reeves MJ, et al. The accuracy of the enzyme-linked immunosorbent assay D-dimer test in the diagnosis of pulmonary embolism: a meta-analysis. Ann Emerg Med 2002;40:133–44.
145. Kabrhel C. Outcomes of high pretest probability patients undergoing D-dimer testing for pulmonary embolism: a pilot study. J Emerg Med 2008;35(4):373–7.
146. Chabloz P, Reber G, Boehlen F, et al. TAFI antigen and D-dimer levels during normal pregnancy and at delivery. Br J Haematol 2001;115:150–2.
147. Righini M, Goehring C, Bounameaux H, et al. Effects of age on the performance of common diagnostic tests for pulmonary embolism. Am J Med 2000;109: 357–61.
148. ten Wolde M, Kraaijenhagen RA, Prins MH, et al. The clinical usefulness of D-dimer testing in cancer patients with suspected deep venous thrombosis. Arch Intern Med 2002;162:1880–4.
149. Quiroz R, Kucher N, Zou KH, et al. Clinical validity of a negative computed tomography scan in patients with suspected pulmonary embolism. JAMA 2005;293:2012–7.
150. Stein PD, Fowler SE, Goodman LR, et al. Multidetector computed tomography for acute pulmonary embolism. N Engl J Med 2006;354:2317–27.
151. Van Belle A, Büller HR, Huisman MV, et al. Effectiveness of managing suspected pulmonary embolism using an algorithm combining clinical probability, D-dimer testing, and computed tomography. JAMA 2006;295:172–9.
152. Perrier A, Roy PM, Sanchez O, et al. Multidetector-row computed tomography in suspected pulmonary embolism. N Engl J Med 2005;28:1760–8.
153. Stone SE, Morris TA. Pulmonary embolism during and after pregnancy. Crit Care Med 2005;33(10):S294–300.
154. Chunilal SD, Wikelboom JW, Attia J, et al. Does this patient have pulmonary embolism? JAMA 2003;290(21):2849–58.
155. Timmons S, Kingston M, Hussain M, et al. Pulmonary embolism: differences in presentation between older and younger patients. Age Ageing 2003;32:601–5.

156. The PIOPED investigators. Value of the ventilation/perfusion scan in acute pulmonary embolism: results of the Prospective Investigation of Pulmonary Embolism Diagnosis (PIOPED). JAMA 1990;263:1753–9.
157. Carson JL, Kelle MA, Duff A, et al. The clinical course of pulmonary embolism. N Engl J Med 1992;326(19):1240–5.
158. Stein PD, Sostman HD, Bounameaux H, et al. Challenges in the diagnosis of acute pulmonary embolism. Am J Med 2008;121(7):565–71.
159. Boie ET. Initial evaluation of chest pain. Emerg Med Clin North Am 2005;23: 937–57.
160. Holloway VJ, Harris JK. Spontaneous pneumothorax: is it under tension? J Accid Emerg Med 2000;17:222–3.
161. Currie GP, Alluri R, Christie GL, et al. Pneumothorax: an update. Postgrad Med J 2007;83:461–5.
162. Weissberg D, Refaely Y. Pneumothorax: experience with 1,199 patients. Chest 2005;117(5):1279–85.
163. Leigh-Smith S, Harris T. Tension pneumothorax—time for a rethink? Emerg Med J 2005;22:8–16.
164. Jones R, Hollingsworth J. Tension pneumothorax not responding to needle thoracocentesis. Emerg Med J 2002;19:176–7.
165. Griffin SM, Lamb PJ, Shenfine J, et al. Spontaneous rupture of the oesophagus. Br J Surg 2008;95:1115–20.
166. Eroglu A, Kurkcuoglu IC, Karaoglanoglu N, et al. Esophageal perforation: the importance of early diagnosis and primary repair. Dis Esophagus 2004;17:91–4.
167. Lemke T, Jagminas L. Spontaneous esophageal rupture: a frequently missed diagnosis. Am Surg 1999;65:449–52.
168. Rubesin SE, Levin MS. Radiologic diagnosis of gastrointestinal perforation. Radiol Clin North Am 2003;41:1095–115.
169. White CS, Templeton PA, Attar S. Esophageal perforation: CT findings. AJR Am J Roentgenol 1993;160:767–70.
170. Nadrous HF, Afess B, Pfeifer EA, et al. The role of autopsy in the intensive care unit. Mayo Clin Proc 2003;78:947–50.
171. Mamas MA, Nair S, Fraser D. Cardiac tamponade and heart failure as a presentation of influenza. Exp Clin Cardiol 2007;12(4):214–6.
172. Gladych E, Goland S, Attali M, et al. Cardiac tamponade as a manifestation of tuberculosis. Southampt Med J 2001;94(5):525–8.
173. Goldberger ZD, Loge AS. Three's company: an unusual clue. Am J Med 2008; 121(9):774–6.
174. Fejka M, Dixon SR, Safian RD, et al. Diagnosis, management, and clinical outcome of cardiac tamponade complicating percutaneous coronary intervention. Am J Cardiol 2002;90:1183–6.
175. Gerson T, Kuruppu J, Olshaker J. Delayed cardiac tamponade after pacemaker insertion. J Emerg Med 2000;18(3):355–9.
176. Roy CL, Minor MA, Brookhart MA, et al. Does this patient with a pericardial effusion have a cardiac tamponade? JAMA 2007;297(16):1810–8.
177. Brown J, MacKinnon D, King A, et al. Elevated arterial blood pressure in cardiac tamponade. N Engl J Med 1992;327(7):463–6.
178. Hoit BD. Pericardial disease and pericardial tamponade. Crit Care Med 2007; 35(8 Suppl):S355–64.
179. Curtiss EI, Reddy PS, Uretsky BF, et al. Pulsus paradoxus: definition and relation to the severity of cardiac tamponade. Am Heart J 1988;115(2):385–90.

180. Merce J, Sagrista-Sauleda J, Permanyer-Miralda G, et al. Correlation between clinical and Doppler echocardiographic findings in patients with moderate and large pericardial effusion: implications for the diagnosis of cardiac tamponade. Am Heart J 1999;138:759–64.
181. Guntheroth WG. Sensitivity and specificity of echocardiographic evidence of tamponade: implications for ventricular interdependence and pulsus paradoxus. Pediatr Cardiol 2007;28:358–62.

High-Risk Chief Complaints II: Disorders of the Head and Neck

Lauren Nentwich, MD[a,*], Andrew S. Ulrich, MD[b]

KEYWORDS

• Headache • Seizure • Acute neurologic deficits • Throat pain
• Neck pain • Ocular emergencies • Difficult airway

Of the many different complaints of patients presenting to the emergency department (ED), some of the most difficult to diagnose and manage involve pathology of the head and neck. Often diagnoses of conditions affecting this part of the body are elusive, and occasionally, even once the diagnosis has been made, the management of these disorders remains challenging. This article addresses some of the high-risk chief complaints of the head and neck regarding diagnosis and management. The high-risk chief complaints that are discussed in this review include headache, seizure, acute focal neurologic deficits, throat and neck pain, ocular emergencies, and the difficult airway.

HEADACHE

Headache is a common complaint of patients presenting to the ED. A query of the National Hospital Ambulatory Medical Care Survey for 1999 to 2001 found that headache accounts for 2.1 million ED visits per year, or 2.2% of total ED visits.[1] Most patients with headache suffer from a benign primary headache, such as migraine, tension-type, cluster, or other primary headaches.[2] However, a smaller but notable percentage of patients (up to 19%) have headaches due to secondary causes including those that are life-threatening and caused by serious intracranial pathology, such as vascular disorders, infections, or tumors.[3] A study of malpractice claims against emergency physicians in Massachusetts found that 3.6% of all claims were in regard to patients with central nervous system (CNS) bleeding, many of whom present with a chief complaint of headache.[4] As such, when treating patients who present with acute headache, it is the primary role of the emergency physician to accurately differentiate between benign headaches and those secondary to intracranial pathology. This section

[a] Department of Neurology, Stroke Research Center, Massachusetts General Hospital, 175 Cambridge Street, Suite 300, Boston, MA 02114, USA
[b] Department of Emergency Medicine, Boston Medical Center, Boston University School of Medicine, 1 Boston Medical Center Place, Boston, MA 02118, USA
* Corresponding author.
E-mail address: lnentwich@partners.org (L. Nentwich).

Emerg Med Clin N Am 27 (2009) 713–746
doi:10.1016/j.emc.2009.08.002
emed.theclinics.com
0733-8627/09/$ – see front matter

discusses the important high-risk features to consider when evaluating patients who present to the ED with headache.

Age

New-onset headache in older patients is worrisome, as age 50 years and older has been shown to be an independent predictor of intracranial pathology.[1,5,6] An analysis of the data from the National Hospital Ambulatory Medical Care Survey from 1999 to 2001 showed that patients with headache who were age 50 years and older had a 6% rate of pathologic findings and an 11% admission rate compared with 1% and 4%, respectively, for younger patients.[1] As such, emergency physicians must be vigilant in the evaluation of older patients presenting with headache, and should maintain a lower threshold for obtaining additional testing. Current recommendations advise that patients older than 50 years presenting with new type of headache but normal neurologic examination should be referred for an urgent neuroimaging study.[7]

History

Onset

Patients who present with a history of acute, sudden-onset severe headache are at increased risk for intracranial pathology. The differential diagnosis for sudden-onset, severe headache is broad and includes many serious causes, such as subarachnoid hemorrhage, intracerebral hemorrhage, cerebral venous sinus thrombosis, arterial dissection, or pituitary apoplexy.[6–8]

The most common serious pathology associated with sudden-onset, severe headache is spontaneous subarachnoid hemorrhage (SAH), and patients classically present with a thunderclap "worst headache of life." In addition to the headache, signs and symptoms of SAH may include nausea or vomiting, photophobia, neck pain or nuchal rigidity, loss of consciousness, or focal neurologic deficits. SAH is a medical emergency that is frequently misdiagnosed, and patients presenting with sudden-onset, severe headache should evoke a high level of suspicion for SAH. Noncontrast cranial computed tomography (CT) is the initial test of choice in making the diagnosis, but the sensitivity of CT in the diagnosis of SAH declines with time from onset of symptoms. In the first 12 hours after SAH, the sensitivity of CT is 98% to 100%, declining to 83% at 24 hours, and to 57% to 85% 6 days after SAH onset. Therefore, lumbar puncture to look for red blood cells (RBCs) or xanthochromia must be performed in all patients with a high suspicion of SAH and a negative cranial CT.[9] Given the high morbidity and mortality of SAH, patients who present with new sudden-onset severe headache should undergo emergent cranial CT and then lumbar puncture for analysis of the cerebrospinal fluid if the cranial CT is normal.[7–9] If both tests are normal then SAH is adequately excluded, and patients may be discharged or undergo further evaluation for other causes of sudden-onset severe headache as clinically indicated.[7]

Response to analgesics

Some clinicians have tried anecdotally to use a favorable response to analgesics as an indication of a benign cause of headache, but this is not a reliable indicator to rule out intracranial pathology. The current understanding of headache suggests a single mechanism for all head pain regardless of the etiology. In addition, the placebo effect in combination with the possible nonspecific sedating effects of the analgesia may produce an altered response. As such, a positive response to therapy cannot be used as a diagnostic indicator of the underlying cause of acute headache, and further evaluation should be pursued as clinically indicated.[7,10]

Physical Examination

Abnormal neurologic examination

A careful neurologic examination is mandatory in all patients who present for evaluation of headache, and an abnormal finding on neurologic examination is the strongest clinical predictor of intracranial pathology.[5,6,11] Ramirez-Lassepas and colleagues[5] reviewed 468 records and found an abnormal finding on neurologic examination to have a highly significant association with intracranial pathology, with a positive predictive value of 39%. Abnormalities can be focal, such as a motor or sensory deficit, or nonfocal, such as altered mental status or papilledema.[5,6,11] Abnormal focal neurologic signs and symptoms usually indicate a stroke or mass lesion. Whereas an abnormal nonfocal neurologic examination can also be seen with these pathologies, it is generally observed in CNS infectious processes, idiopathic intracranial hypertension, or a toxic-metabolic process.[2] Given the strong correlation between abnormal neurologic examination and severe intracranial pathology, a new headache combined with an abnormal neurologic finding is an indication for emergent neuroimaging[7] as well as further testing as clinically indicated.

Associated symptoms

The presence of associated symptoms with headache has been shown in certain studies to be predictive of intracranial pathology. Ramirez-Lassepas and colleagues[5] showed an independent association between the presence of associated symptoms and intracranial pathology but did not describe the associated symptoms. In a prospective observational study of 589 consecutive patients presenting with headache by Locker and colleagues,[6] patients with headache who presented because of associated symptoms were found to have a higher likelihood of intracranial pathology. Of these patients presenting due to associated features, 52% complained of neurologic symptoms other than headache whereas 48% complained of nonneurologic symptoms such as collapse, nausea and vomiting, and nonneurologic symptoms related to otolaryngology, respiratory, or gastrointestinal systems.[6] The American College of Emergency Physicians clinical policy suggests that associated symptoms that should prompt consideration of neuroimaging to evaluate for intracranial pathology include worsening of headache with Valsalva, headache waking patient from sleep, and headache associated with syncope, nausea, or sensory distortion.[7] In patients presenting with headache with other evidence of systemic illness (such as fever, signs of meningeal irritation, or cutaneous rash), a CNS infectious process should be considered.[2]

Medical History

Human immunodeficiency virus infection

Human immunodeficiency virus (HIV) is a neurotrophic virus that easily crosses the blood-brain barrier, accounting for a variety of neurologic complications. CNS complications of HIV infection include HIV encephalopathy, aseptic meningitis, opportunistic infections of the CNS, and neoplasms of the CNS. Many of these entities produce headache, and need to be ruled out when caring for the HIV-infected patients complaining of headache.[12] A prospective descriptive study performed by Rothman and colleagues[13] studied 110 HIV-infected patients to determine predictors of new focal CNS lesions. In their study, 17% of patients were found to have a new focal lesion. The 4 clinical findings that were independently associated with focal findings on cranial CT were new seizure, decreased or altered orientation, headache that was different in quality from prior headaches, and prolonged headache of duration 3 days or longer. In addition, focal motor deficit had a high positive predictive value for a new focal lesion. Current recommendations advise that HIV-infected patients with a new or prolonged headache should be considered for emergent neuroimaging study.[7]

Malignancy

Headache is a common neurologic complaint in patients with cancer. Cancer patients can have multiple serious causes of their headaches, including intracranial metastases and hemorrhage into intracerebral tumor or metastases. Prospective observational studies have found intracranial metastases in 32% to 54% of cancer patients referred for evaluation of new or changed headache.[14,15] When evaluating patients for possible intracranial metastases, magnetic resonance imaging with contrast is the most sensitive and specific test to evaluate for brain metastases. Noncontrast cranial CT may be use as an emergency imaging modality in patients presenting with symptoms suggestive of stroke or CSF flow obstruction. However, noncontrast or contrast CT does not adequately exclude all brain metastases,[16] and contrast-enhanced magnetic resonance imaging (MRI) should be obtained in all cancer patients with new or changed headache.

Pregnancy

The majority of pregnant women with headaches have benign causes.[7] However, women do have an increased risk of both ischemic and hemorrhagic strokes associated with pregnancy, and the 3 days surrounding delivery up to 6 weeks postpartum is the time of highest risk.[17] In addition, pregnancy is considered a risk factor for developing cerebral venous thrombosis,[18] and the initial presentation of eclampsia may be a chief complaint of headache. No firm recommendations for the evaluation of headache in pregnancy exist,[7] but given the increased risk, intracranial pathology as well as preeclampsia should be considered in all pregnant and early postpartum women presenting with headache.

Pediatrics

Headache is a common complaint in children and adolescents. Although most headaches in children are benign due to either primary headache or benign secondary causes, it has been shown that secondary life-threatening headaches occur in 4.1% to 6.9% of children presenting to the ED with a chief complaint of headache. The neurologic etiology of the headaches attributed to dangerous intracranial disease includes subdural hematoma, epidural hematoma, ventriculoperitoneal shunt malformation, brain abscess, brain tumor, pseudotumor cerebri, aseptic meningitis, and brain malformation (such as Chiari type I).[19,20] A retrospective chart review of 277 children presenting to the ED with headache where 6% of the children had a life-threatening headache found several factors associated with life-threatening headache compared with benign headaches. The factors included preschool age, onset of headache attacks less than 2 months before presentation, pain located in the occipital region or patients unable to describe location of pain, patients unable to describe quality of pain, very intense pain, and associated neurologic signs. All children in this study with serious underlying neurologic conditions had objective neurologic signs, such as: papilledema, ataxia, hemiparesis, and abnormal eye movements.[19]

SEIZURE

Seizures are a common presenting complaint to EDs, and by some estimates, seizures account for 1% to 2% of ED visits.[21,22] Epilepsy, a condition resulting in recurrent, unprovoked seizures, effects as many as 4 million people.[23,24] Seizures that occur as a result of insults to the brain or neurologic system, such as anatomic, toxic, or metabolic abnormalities, are referred to as secondary or reactive seizures. One of the primary goals of ED management of seizures is the identification and treatment of reversible causes of secondary seizures. Rapid identification and initiation of treatment is critical to limit or prevent end organ damage or permanent neuronal injury, which can result from prolonged uncontrolled seizure activity. In this section the high-risk features in the evaluation and management of patients who present to the ED with seizures is addressed.

Differentiating Between Primary and Secondary Seizures

Estimated incidence of first-onset seizure accounts for approximately 0.3% of all ED visits. Patients who present with active seizures are often easily identifiable; however, some patients may present after events that are more difficult to categorize as seizures, such as sudden loss of consciousness, myoclonic movements, and incontinence. In these circumstances, patients need to have other conditions ruled out before being diagnosed with first-time seizure.

The most common serious condition that can be misinterpreted as a seizure is syncope.[25] It is essential to appropriately identify syncope, as it carries a high risk for significant morbidity and mortality if unrecognized and misdiagnosed as seizure activity. There can be important clinical signs or preceding events that help differentiate between seizure and syncope. Patients with seizure activity may have prodromal symptoms, including stereotyped smells or taste, lip smacking, or a sensation of "déjà vu." Periseizure activity may include oral trauma such as tongue biting. Postictal confusion or agitation may also be present. To differentiate, syncope is often preceded by lightheadedness, diaphoresis, chest pain, or palpitations. Syncopal episodes may have clear precipitants such as prolonged standing, painful stimuli, sudden neck turning, or micturition. Postsyncopal return to baseline tends to be more rapid than recovery from seizures. In many circumstances patients will be unable to provide critical information, thus it is important to obtain an accurate description from anyone who witnessed the event.

Aside from syncope, several other medical conditions should be included in the differential diagnosis of seizures (**Box 1**).

Evaluation

Laboratory testing

It is recommended that serum electrolytes be checked in patients with new onset seizures, as 2.4% to 8% of patients who present with seizures will have electrolyte abnormalities.

Hypoglycemia is a common cause of seizures. There is no definitive plasma glucose threshold regarding seizures; however, levels approaching 45 mg/dL are considered potential for inducing seizures. Some patients may become ictal at higher levels. Patients with possible seizure activity should have rapid bedside/field finger stick test performed to evaluate for low serum glucose. Rapid infusion of glucose should be initiated and should be repeated if patient remains hypoglycemic. Glucagon, 1 mg intramuscularly or subcutaneously, can be given to hypoglycemic patients without intravenous access as a temporizing measure.

Although rare, various electrolyte disturbances may precipitate seizures. Hypernatremia, usually a result of dehydration, is associated with seizure activity, particularly when serum sodium levels exceed 160 mEq/L. Hyponatremia with levels less than 120 mEq/L is often complicated by seizures. The rate at which sodium rises or falls, and not the actual level, is the best determination of the risk for neurologic sequela. Sodium correction should be performed cautiously.

Box 1
Differential diagnosis of conditions with seizure like symptoms

Breath-holding spells
Episodic dyscontrol syndrome/rage attacks
Fugue states
Hyperventilation
Hypoglycemia
Migraine narcolepsy/cataplexy
Movement disorders
Night terrors
Nonepileptic seizures
Panic attacks
Paroxysmal vertigo
Psychogenic seizures
Syncope
Transient global amnesia
Transient ischemic attack/stroke

From Tarabar AF, Ulrich AS, D'Onofrio G. Seizures. In: Adams JG, editor. Emergency medicine. Philadelphia: Elsevier; 2008. p. 1051–62; with permission.

Hypercalcemia reduces neuronal excitability and is rarely a cause of seizures. However, hypocalcemia, at levels less than 7 mEq/L, is associated with seizure activity. Low calcium levels are found frequently in conjunction with hypomagnesemia, which is also epileptogenic.

Electrocardiogram

An electrocardiogram (ECG) should be obtained in every patient with the first onset of seizures, or with the suspicion of cardiac cause of decreased CNS perfusion. In addition to ischemia, the most important disorders that have to be excluded are related to conduction abnormalities and resultant dysrhythmias, including complete heart block. Widening of QRS complex can occur after an overdose from certain medications, particularly cyclic antidepressants. More specific ECG changes, terminal 40 ms R wave in lead aVR can also assist in identifying cyclic antidepressant toxicity. Prolonged QTc interval can be found in numerous overdoses. Tachyarrhythmias are often seen in the setting of cocaine and methylxanthine toxicity.

Neuroimaging

Although no definitive study demonstrates that it is essential, the standard of care seems to be to obtain a CT scan of the brain in every patient with first onset of seizures. CT scan of the brain should also be obtained in any patient with persistent change of mental status, focal neurologic deficit, or suspicion of organic intracerebral lesion.[26] Early CT scan is essential for identifying surgically correctable causes. If there is a concern for trauma, CT scan should also be used to rule-out cervical spine and intracranial injury.

Electroencephalography

Electroencephalography (EEG) records brain electrical activity and is used for definitive diagnosis of epilepsy and related conditions. The need for EEG in the emergent setting is limited to patients whose seizures are uncontrollable despite aggressive treatment or whose seizure activity is more difficult to diagnose.

Intubated patients, who are paralyzed or have had induction of phenobarbital coma and general anesthesia, should be continuously monitored with EEG to exclude seizure activity, because in these situations they may not able to manifest obvious seizure activity due to neuromuscular paralysis.

Treatment

Airway

One of the primary goals during the evaluation and treatment of seizures is to preserve patent airway and oxygenation, as well as to prevent aspiration in patients who are postictal. This goal can be achieved with simple maneuvers involving administration of supplemental oxygen, and perhaps providing a jaw trust/chin lift, cautiously inserting an oropharyngeal airway, or repositioning the head. Despite the dramatic presentation, including cyanosis, few patients who are actively seizing will require endotracheal intubation.

Pharmacologic treatment

Benzodiazepines should be administered immediately as they have been shown to control the majority of seizures regardless of cause, through increase of γ-aminobutyric acid (GABA) activity. Studies have shown that lorazepam is more effective than diazepam for the initial control of seizures, although both agents are acceptable.[22,24] When intravenous access is difficult, intramuscular or rectal administration of valium or lorazepam are alternative treatment options. Continued seizure activity should be treated with a second dose of benzodiazepines, along with the addition of a second agent. Phenytoin is the second drug of choice, but requires patient monitoring when used intravenously. Early initiation of phenytoin helps achieve a therapeutic level in a timely manner, but delivery is rate limited (no faster than 50 mg/min) to avoid hypotension.

Drug- or Toxin-Induced Seizures

GABA is the chief inhibitory transmitter in the brain. Every drug that can decrease in GABA activity in the CNS can cause seizure. Treatment is generally directed at providing enough GABA stimulus with benzodiazepines. However, certain drugs are associated with particular types of toxicities and they may require specific treatment or antidote (**Table 1**).

Removal of the toxin or drug and secondary decontamination is the hallmark of the treatment of drug- or toxin-induced seizures. Decontamination in the ED typically involves administration of charcoal; however, the clinician should be cautious with those patients who are postictal or who may develop recurrent seizures, as aspiration and need for intubation must be considered.

Cocaine

The most commonly abused substance that causes seizures is cocaine. Benzodiazepines will help to control seizures, agitation, and hyperthermia. It is important to maintain adequate fluid resuscitation to protect against renal damage from potential rhabdomyolysis. If the patient is hyperthermic, cooling measures involving intravenous fluids, ice packs, and even ice baths in the case of refractory hyperthermia should be applied to protect against multi-organ failure and death.

Table 1
Most common drugs associated with seizures

Medication/Drug	Comment
Camphor	Brief, tonic-clonic seizures, usually self limited
Cocaine/amphetamines	Tachycardia, hypertension
Phencyclidine	Rotary nystagmus
Cyclic antidepressants	Can be excluded with ECG Severe toxicity can cause cardiac dysrhythmias Treatment with bicarbonate will control ECG changes, but not the seizures Benzodiazepines are drug of choice
Isoniazid (INH)	Treatment B6
Lindane	Usually ingestion of topical preparation
MDMA (Ecstasy)	Usually associated with hyponatremia Morning after "rave" party Fluid restriction is usually sufficient therapy
Strychnine	Painful muscle spasm.
Theophylline	Wide pulse pressure Tachycardia Hypokalemia Hyperglycemia

From Tarabar AF, Ulrich AS, D'Onofrio G. Seizures. In: Adams JG, editor. Emergency medicine. Philadelphia: Elsevier; 2008. p. 1051–62; with permission.

Alcohol

Alcohol-related seizures (ARS) are defined as adult-onset seizures, generally after the age of 25 years, which occur in the setting of chronic alcohol dependence. ARS are often caused by alcohol withdrawal. However, risk factors such as preexisting epilepsy, structural brain lesions, the use of illicit drugs, or metabolic disorders may also contribute to seizures in patients who drink heavily. ARS are typically brief, have generalized tonic-clonic activity, and occur 6 to 48 hours following the last drink. Sixty percent of patients have multiple seizures without treatment, and the interval between the first and the last seizure is typically less than 6 hours.

The diagnosis of ARS is made only after exclusion of other potential causes. New-onset seizures in an alcohol-dependent patient should prompt a thorough evaluation similar to that described for any person presenting with a new-onset seizure. CT scan of the brain should be performed with a new onset seizure, partial seizure, status epilepticus, and a prolonged postictal state, or if there is evidence of any head trauma. A finger stick for serum glucose determination is important.

In the majority of patients, lorazepam has been shown to prevent subsequent seizures after the first presenting seizure. In a randomized control trial of patients presenting with an ARS, only 3% had a subsequent seizure during a 6-hour observation period, compared with 24% in the placebo group ($P<.001$).[27] Following an observation period of 4 to 6 hours, in the absence of further seizure activity, patients may be safely discharged. These patients ideally should be offered alcohol detoxification programs.

Opioids

Although opioids are not generally associated with the seizures, it is worth mentioning several exceptions including meperidine, propoxyphene, and tramadol. Patients may present with an opioid toxidrome and seizure activity. Of note, administration of naloxone can actually precipitate and worsen meperidine-associated seizures.

3,4-Methylenedioxymethamphetamine

3,4-Methylenedioxymethamphetamine (MDMA; Ecstasy) is an amphetamine-related drug that is associated with seizure activity. Patients who are consuming MDMA typically present with brief tonic-clonic seizure secondary to hyponatremia. MDMA can also lead to transient syndrome of inappropriate antidiuretic hormone secretion (SIADH). Most of these patients can be treated with fluid restriction and observation.

Other medications

Other drugs that can be associated with seizure activity are worthy of mention. Cyclic antidepressants are notorious for their propensity to cause seizures due to GABA inhibition. Seizures are a manifestation of severe toxicity, so it is important to rapidly assess and protect the airway, complete gastrointestinal decontamination, and administer intravenous benzodiazepines, as tricyclic antidepressant overdoses can lead to rapid deterioration. Bicarbonate is the primary treatment of cyclic antidepressant overdose and is effective in treating cardiac conduction abnormalities, but has no role in controlling seizure activity. Isoniazid (INH) overdose should be suspected in the setting of status epilepticus that is not responsive to conventional treatment. Treatment is vitamin B6 (pyridoxine). Methylxanthines (caffeine, theophylline) in overdose are notorious for causing seizures through the antagonism of adenosine. Usually the seizures are short acting and can be controlled with benzodiazepines. However, in severely toxic patients hemodialysis is necessary.

Special Considerations

Status epilepticus

Status epilepticus is defined as seizures that persist more than 20 minutes, as this is the duration seen in animal studies to cause damage to the CNS neurons. However, given the need for earlier intervention to prevent permanent neuronal injury, the operational definition of status epilepticus is continuous seizures lasting at least 5 minutes or 2 or more discrete seizures between which there is incomplete recovery of consciousness.[28]

Status epilepticus has a mortality rate of 20% in adults.[28] Early aggressive administration of intravenous anticonvulsants is the keystone of successful treatment of status epilepticus. **Table 2** summarizes the medications that can be used in the treatment of status epilepticus. Neurology should be consulted early for assistance in management of patients with persistent seizures in possible status epilepticus.

Pregnancy

Pregnancy can precipitate seizure episodes in patients with underlying seizure disorders, and prolonged seizure activity results in increased morbidity and mortality to the fetus. Some women may require a higher dose of antiepileptic medications to maintain therapeutic levels while pregnant.

Eclampsia should be considered in all women of child-bearing age who present with seizures. Eclamptic seizures can occur from the 20th week of gestation up to 6 weeks postpartum, and during this period every new-onset seizure should be initially treated as eclampsia until proven otherwise. The "classic symptoms" of eclampsia are hypertension, proteinuria, and edema, but up to 30% of eclamptic women do not present classically. Pregnant women who have hypertension, proteinuria, headache, visual disturbances, abdominal pain with nausea, or edema should be presumed to have eclampsia until proven otherwise. The treatment of eclampsia is intravenous magnesium, blood pressure control and concomitant delivery of the fetus.

Table 2
Summary of medications used for the treatment of status epilepticus

Medication	Dose (Load)	Dose (Maintenance)	Comments
Diazepam	10 mg over 2 min	Repeat every 5–10 min	Respiratory depression, hypotension
Lorazepam	2–8 mg IV	Repeat once in 10–15 min if seizure persists	Respiratory depression, hypotension
Midazolam	0.1–0.2 mg/kg or 2.25–15 mg IV		Respiratory depression, hypotension
Phenytoin	15–20 mg/kg @ max. rate 50 mg/min	100 mg IV/PO every 6–8 h	Hypotension, ataxia
Fosphenytoin	15–20 mg/kg @ max. rate 150 mg/min		Faster loading time, needs to be metabolized to be effective
Pentobarbital	5–20 mg/kg IV @ 25 mg/min 5 mg/kg is effective for induction anesthesia for most	2.5 mg/kg/h	Severe respiratory depression Faster effect than phenobarbital
Phenobarbital	15–20 mg/kg @ max. 50 mg/min	120–240 mg every 20 min	Severe respiratory depression, hypotension
Propofol	1–2 mg/kg IV	2–4 mg/kg/h	Severe respiratory depression, acidosis (children)
Valproic acid	20 mg/kg at 20 mg/min	Repeat if needed	Only if everything else fails; may be beneficial for the patients who are already on valproic acid but subtherapeutic

IV, intravenous; PO, by mouth

From Tarabar AF, Ulrich AS, D'Onofrio G. Seizures. In: Adams JG, editor. Emergency medicine. Philadelphia: Elsevier; 2008. p. 1051–62; with permission.

Human immunodeficiency virus

People with HIV infection may have a CNS mass or infection as the cause of seizure, which can be the first manifestation of AIDS. HIV-positive patients who present with new-onset seizures, or those that do not have the diagnosis of epilepsy, require CT scan and, if negative, a lumbar puncture. Patients who are HIV positive, as well as those patients who are immunosuppressed, are at risk for numerous infectious entities that may induce seizure activity (**Table 3**).

Central nervous system infection

Patients at high risk of meningitis or encephalitis should be treated with appropriate intravenous antibiotics even before lumbar puncture. Timely administration of

Table 3
Causes of seizures in HIV population

Focal CNS lesions
Cerebral toxoplasmosis
Primary CNS lymphoma
Progressive multifocal leukoencephalopathy
Focal viral encephalitis
Cytomegalovirus
Varicella zoster virus
Herpes simplex virus
Bacterial abscess
Cryptococcoma
Tuberculosis abscess
Mass lesion
Toxoplasmosis
Lymphoma
Meningitis/encephalitis
Cryptococcal
Bacterial/aseptic
Herpes zoster
Cytomegalovirus
HIV encephalopathy/AIDS dementia complex
Progressive multifocal leukoencephalopathy
CNS tuberculosis
Neurosyphilis

From Tarabar AF, Ulrich AS, D'Onofrio G. Seizures. In: Adams JG, editor. Emergency medicine. Philadelphia: Elsevier; 2008. p. 1051–62; with permission.

antibiotics and antiviral medication in patients with CNS infections can improve survival and reduce mortality.

Neurocysticercosis (NCC) is the most common parasitic CNS infection in the world, and has been increasing in the United States since 1980.[29] In endemic areas, namely Latin America, Asia, and Africa, NCC is a frequent cause of late-onset epilepsy. Most of these patients will respond to treatment with phenytoin or carbamazepine. Albendazol is the mainstay antiparasitic treatment for NCC. Patients diagnosed with NCC may require treatment with steroids to control cerebral inflammation and the appropriate medication regimen for meningitis, cysticercal encephalitis, and angiitis.

Intracranial pathology

Patients with intracranial hemorrhage who are anticoagulated or have elevated international normalized ratio may require rapid administration of fresh frozen plasma and vitamin K to prevent further bleeding. It is essential not to delay treatment pending laboratory confirmation of anticoagulated status. Patients with brain tumors, evidence of increased intracranial pressure, or hydrocephalus need immediate attention of neurosurgical service. Administration of steroids may be prudent to reduce the mass effect of intracranial tumors.

Disposition

Every patient with persistent seizures, change of mental status, or significant underlying medical condition should be admitted to the hospital. Patients in status epilepticus should be admitted to the intensive care setting. Patients with chronic seizure disorder can be discharged if they return to their baseline neurologic status. Patients who present with first-onset seizures should have follow-up arranged with a neurologist for further workup and eventual treatment if warranted.

Patients who are discharged should be advised to avoid precipitating factors and informed of the importance of adherence to anticonvulsant regimens. Patients should be given written instructions to avoid driving motor vehicles and not to engage in any activity whereby unexpected seizures with transient loss of consciousness can lead to injury or death. It is important for emergency medicine physicians to be familiar with state and local rules regarding mandatory reporting of seizure patients, as some states require reporting of these patients to motor vehicle departments.

ACUTE FOCAL NEUROLOGIC DEFICITS

An acute neurologic deficit is one that develops in 24 hours or less, with many deficits developing much more rapidly over a period of seconds to minutes. Focal deficits occur when there is an injury or dysfunction in a localized area of the nervous system. Acute focal neurologic deficits may consist of multiple signs and symptoms, including altered level of consciousness or other mental status changes, visual disturbances, cranial nerve abnormalities, weakness or paralysis, sensory abnormalities, speech difficulties, ataxia, neglect, and vertigo.

Patients with acute focal neurologic deficits often present emergently for evaluation, and can pose challenges to the emergency physician in the diagnosis and management of their complaints. The most common cause of acute focal neurologic deficits affecting the head and neck is stroke or transient ischemic attack (TIA). Proper management of patients with stroke requires a rapid and accurate diagnosis by the emergency physician. However, there are many conditions other than acute stroke that cause focal neurologic deficits, some of which are dangerous, and require rapid diagnosis and intervention as well. This section focuses on the high-risk aspects of the diagnosis and management of acute stroke, as well as the differential diagnosis of stroke and other critical conditions to consider in patients presenting with acute focal neurologic deficits.

Stroke

Stroke is defined as the sudden loss of neurologic function caused by an interruption in the blood supply to the brain. Stroke is the third leading cause of death and the leading cause of long-term disability in the United States. Stroke is a common disease affecting approximately 795,000 people in the United States annually.[17] The rapid diagnosis and management of patients who present to the ED with stroke is essential to improving long-term outcomes and lessening the impact of the disease.

The cause of acute stroke is either ischemia or hemorrhage. Diagnosis and management differs, depending on the etiology of the stroke and the stroke type. This section addresses the high-risk features of caring for patients with acute stroke in the ED.

Ischemic stroke

Ischemic stroke is defined as a permanent cerebral injury secondary to prolonged disruption of cerebral flow. Ischemic stroke has 3 different causes: large artery atherosclerosis, embolic events, or small-vessel disease.[30] Approximately 87% of all strokes are ischemic in nature.[17] In patients presenting to the ED with acute-onset neurologic deficits, difficult management decisions occur in both the approach to diagnosis and the treatment of patients with ischemic stroke.

Patients with an anterior circulation strokes often have acute onset of motor and sensory deficits in the contralateral arm, leg, and face, accompanied by aphasia or neglect. As such, the diagnosis in this subset of patients is usually straightforward. However, diagnostic efforts can be complicated by stroke mimics. A variety of conditions mimic ischemic stroke and can be the cause of a patient's acute focal neurologic deficits.[31–37] It is important that the clinician consider and exclude the various stroke mimics in patients presenting with acute focal neurologic deficits. The different causes that can mimic an acute stroke will be discussed in further detail later in this section.

Posterior circulation strokes occur in about 20% of ischemic events, and many remain undiagnosed or incorrectly diagnosed. Dizziness, vertigo, headache, vomiting, double vision, ataxia, numbness, and weakness involving structures on both sides of the body are frequent symptoms in patients with posterior circulation strokes, and should evoke a high degree of suspicion from the physician evaluating the patient. Any patient with suspected posterior circulation stroke should undergo neuroimaging, preferably with MRI, as CT often provides limited visualization of the posterior fossa structures due to artifacts related to the skull.[38] However, it is important to remember that CT is useful in ruling out intracranial hemorrhage in the brainstem and cerebellum, and should be used when clinically indicated.

The treatment of acute ischemic stroke is another potential area of high risk for the emergency physician. The only current Food and Drug Administration approved therapy for the treatment of acute ischemic stroke is intravenous administration of recombinant tissue plasminogen activator (r-tPA) within 3 hours of symptom onset.[39] A recent study has shown that the drug may be safe and effective if given up to 4.5 hours from symptom onset if more stringent patient selection criteria are used.[40] Although the treatment time has been expanded, earlier treatment continues to be associated with more favorable outcomes.[41] However, treatment with intravenous rt-PA can be complicated by symptomatic intracranial hemorrhage, which may be fatal. Given these factors, it is important that all patients presenting with acute ischemic stroke have neuroimaging to exclude intracranial hemorrhage and have an accurately documented time of symptom onset. Urgent neurologic consultation is also recommended for assistance in making the decision on which patients should receive treatment with intravenous r-tPA. Although written consent is not necessary before the administration of intravenous rt-PA for the treatment of ischemic stroke, a full discussion of the potential risks and benefits of treatment with the patient and family members is recommended.[42]

Transient ischemic attack

Although conventional clinical definitions defined TIA as a focal neurologic deficit lasting less than 24 hours, this definition has recently been updated.[43] The new definition for TIA is a "brief episode of neurological dysfunction caused by a focal disturbance of brain or retinal ischemia, with clinical symptoms typically lasting less than 1 hour, and without evidence of infarction."[44] TIAs are an important predictor of stroke, with reports of 90-day risk of stroke in patients who have suffered a TIA as high as 10.5% with 50% of those occurring in the first 2 days.[45] As such, all patients with transient focal neurologic deficits consistent with a TIA should have neurology consultation for further evaluation and ischemic stroke risk reduction. In addition, although there are no established guidelines as to when to admit patients with TIA, it is prudent for the emergency physician to have a low threshold for admitting patients with TIA given the substantial risk of stroke within the first 48 hours.

Hemorrhagic stroke

Hemorrhagic strokes account for approximately 13% of all strokes, with 10% caused by intracerebral hemorrhage (ICH), and the other 3% caused by SAH.[17] The high-risk features of hemorrhagic stroke relate to the diagnosis and early clinical management of patients with hemorrhagic stroke.

ICH is a medical emergency requiring rapid recognition and diagnosis. Frequent early ongoing bleeding often causes progressive clinical deterioration, and patients who suffer a stroke due to ICH have a high mortality rate, approximately 44% to 48% at 1 month.[46] Patients with ICH classically present with sudden neurologic deficits characterized by smooth symptomatic progression over minutes to hours. Patients may have focal neurologic deficits or decreased level of consciousness, depending on the location and size of the hematoma. In addition, patients may only present with nonspecific signs and symptoms, such as headache, vomiting, increased blood pressure, or meningismus, thereby making the diagnosis more elusive. CT and MRI are both first-choice initial imaging options, and either is the essential diagnostic test in the evaluation of patients with potential ICH.[47] Failure to consider ICH and obtain diagnostic neuroimaging in patients with the aforementioned neurologic findings is a high-risk area of emergency medicine. Once diagnosis is reached, urgent consultation with a neurologist or neurosurgeon is essential. Patients with ICH due to iatrogenic anticoagulation must be rapidly reversed.[47] Due to frequent ongoing bleeding, the risk of neurologic and cardiovascular instability in patients with ICH is highest during the first 24 hours, and patients should be admitted to an intensive care unit for frequent monitoring.[48]

The most common cause of SAH is trauma, but spontaneous SAH can by caused by a ruptured aneurysm or arteriovenous malformation. SAH is discussed in detail in the headache section of this article. Patients with SAH classically present with a severe, thunderclap headache with or without focal neurologic deficits. Approximately 20% of patients describe a sentinel headache that occurs within 2 to 8 weeks of overt SAH. SAH is a difficult diagnosis, and is frequently missed by physicians. Patients who present with acute onset of severe headache should evoke a high level of suspicion for SAH. Noncontrast cranial CT is the initial test of choice for making the diagnosis, but its sensitivity declines with the time from onset of symptoms. Lumbar puncture must be performed to look for RBCs and xanthochromia in all patients with a high suspicion of SAH and a negative cranial CT. Patients found to have a SAH should undergo further vascular imaging to look for aneurysms, as well as emergent evaluation by a neurologist or neurosurgeon. Potential for acute neurologic deterioration in patients with SAH is significant. All patients should be emergently evaluated and stabilized, and ultimately monitored in a neurosurgical unit, as failure to detect herniation or worsening neurologic status is another high-risk feature of the management of patients with SAH.[9]

Cerebral venous thrombosis

Cerebral venous thrombosis (CVT) is a rare cerebrovascular disorder and an uncommon cause of stroke. Unlike arterial stroke, CVT most often affects young adults and children. CVT is a challenging diagnosis, as patients' presentations are highly variable and include headache, focal neurologic deficits, seizures, altered mental status, altered level of consciousness, and papilledema.[18] Risk factors for developing a cerebral venous sinus thrombosis include hypercoagulable conditions, pregnancy/puerperium, oral contraceptives, trauma, and infections located near the cerebral sinuses. Routine neuroimaging such as CT or MRI may produce subtle findings that may be missed, but MR venography confirms the diagnosis.[43] It is important to consider the diagnosis in young and middle-aged patients with unusual headache or neurologic deficits in the absence of vascular risk factors, in patients with intracranial hypertension, and in patients with CT evidence of hemorrhagic infarcts, especially if the infarcts are in multiple territories.[22] Once the diagnosis is made, treatment with unfractionated heparin and low molecular weight heparin may be recommended and should be guided by neurology consultation.[43]

Stroke Mimics

A stroke mimic is a nonvascular condition that can simulate the signs and symptoms of a stroke. There are a variety of conditions that can mimic TIA or stroke (**Box 2**). Not only can these conditions complicate diagnostic efforts in the rapid assessment of patients with potential acute stroke, but many stroke mimics are critical diagnoses unto themselves and must be recognized early for proper intervention.

Various studies evaluating the frequency of misdiagnosis of patients presenting with signs and symptoms of acute stroke have found the incidence of stroke mimics to be around 3% to 19%.[32–38] A study by Kothari and colleagues[34] reviewed 446 patients evaluated in the ED with a hospital admission or discharge diagnosis of acute stroke, to determine the ability of emergency physicians to accurately identify patients with stroke. In this study, all of the patients with ICH or SAH were correctly diagnosed by the emergency physician, and 5% (19 of 365) of the patients diagnosed with ischemic stroke or TIA by the emergency physician were discharged with a different final diagnosis. An observational study by Scott and colleagues[36] evaluated 151 consecutive patients with an initial diagnosis of acute ischemic stroke treated with intravenous tPA. Six of 151 (4%) patients had a final diagnosis other that acute ischemic stroke or TIA. These stroke mimics suffered no intracranial hemorrhage, had less disability at discharge, and were younger than patients with acute ischemic stroke or TIA. Another study by Winkler and colleagues[37] evaluated 250 consecutive patients treated with intravenous tPA, and found that 7 (2.8%) had a final diagnosis other than stroke or TIA. All of these patients had a favorable outcome, with none suffering from intracranial hemorrhage.

Given the relative frequency of stroke mimics, it is important that all patients who present with acute focal neurologic deficits should have a thorough evaluation. The first step should be to check blood glucose on arrival. Vital signs should be monitored frequently. Basic laboratory work should include a complete blood cell count, electrolyte levels, coagulation studies, urinalysis, and toxicology screens. Brain imaging should be ordered as indicated. In patients with difficult presentations, neurology consultation is indicated.

OCULAR EMERGENCIES

Ophthalmologic complaints are one of the common presentations to EDs, with estimates as high as 3% of all emergency visits.[49] In the vast majority of these cases, emergency physicians can safely manage these patients. However, prompt and appropriate recognition, and initiation of treatment of entities that are at high risk for vision loss, is essential to mitigate the possibility of serious and permanent visual deficits. The challenge facing emergency physicians is to quickly identify these high-risk injuries and ensure timely ophthalmologic consultation. In most cases, visual or eye complaints should be seen in follow-up by an ophthalmologist, the timing of which can be determined after discussion with the consulting service. This section reviews those injuries that, if missed or have a significant delay in diagnosis, have a high likelihood of resulting in permanent ophthalmologic sequelae.

Box 2
Conditions that can mimic acute ischemic stroke

- Seizure
  - Postictal paralysis
  - Nonconvulsive seizures
- Space-occupying lesions
  - CNS tumor (primary, metastatic)
  - Subdural hematoma
  - Epidural hematoma
  - Cerebral abscess
- Infectious
  - Systemic infection (ie, sepsis)
  - Meningitis
  - Encephalitis
- Toxic-metabolic disturbances
  - Hypoglycemia
  - Hyperglycemia with hyperosmotic coma or DKA
  - Hyponatremia
  - Hepatic encephalopathy
  - Alcohol withdrawal
  - Wernicke encephalopathy
  - Drug toxicity
- Vestibular dysfunction
  - Labyrinthitis
  - Ménière disease
  - Benign positional vertigo
- Demyelinating disease (ie, multiple sclerosis)
- Trauma
- Complicated migraine
- Peripheral nerve neuropathy
- Psychiatric disorders
  - Acute confusional state
  - Somatoform disorders
  - Malingering
  - Dementia
- Hypertensive encephalopathy

Initial Evaluation

A simple but essential part of every ophthalmologic examination is a visual acuity test. In conjunction with vision, pupillary activity, extraocular movements, and fundoscopy should be evaluated. Both the affected and nonaffected eyes should be tested individually, then together to evaluate binocular vision. Pinhole testing corrects most refractive errors, and when vision improves there is likely a problem with the lens. However, when pinhole testing fails to improve vision, the pathology is more likely to be located in the retina or CNS. Fluorescein examination is another critical component of a complete ophthalmologic examination. Fluorescein examination should be performed in all evaluations of ocular trauma, potential foreign bodies, or suspected infections. A variation of the standard fluorescein examination is the Seidel test, screening for globe rupture. Another important component of the ophthalmologic examination is the slit lamp, which allows for a magnified, stereoscopic evaluation of the eye and surrounding structures. The slit lamp is especially useful in the examination of the anterior chamber.[50] Tonometry is essential to diagnose acute angle glaucoma and to establish a baseline intraocular pressure following blunt eye trauma.[51] Lid eversion is useful in the inspection of the tarsal conjunctiva and fornices, as well as being essential for localizing foreign bodies. Ocular ultrasonography is rapidly gaining popularity in the ED evaluation of ophthalmologic complaints. Ocular ultrasonography can be especially useful in the trauma patient, in whom significant periorbital swelling can limit direct visualization of the eye.[52]

High-Risk Diagnoses

When there is suspicion for high-risk ophthalmologic conditions or injuries, emergency ophthalmologic consultation is warranted (**Box 3**). However, there are numerous additional conditions for which ophthalmologic consultation is reasonable and appropriate. In these circumstances, discussion with an ophthalmologist can help determine the subsequent need and urgency of an ophthalmologist's evaluation.

Trauma

Patients with evidence of significant globe trauma, either blunt or penetrating, should be evaluated emergently by ophthalmology. Retrobulbar hemorrhage may be vision threatening, and often requires immediate decompression to ensure adequate blood supply to the optic nerve. In this situation, a lateral canthotomy should be performed as soon as possible. Lacerations involving the nasolacrimal system, the lid margin, or

Box 3
Conditions that warrant emergent ophthalmologic consultation

- Trauma
  - Ruptured globe
  - Lid laceration through margin, nasolacrimal system or canaliculus
- Endophthalmitis
- Angle closure glaucoma
- Acute vision loss
  - Central artery occlusion
  - Optic neuritis
  - Retinal detachment

Data from Magauran B. Conditions requiring emergency ophthalmologic consultation. In: Kahn J, Magauran B, Mattu A, editors. Ophthalmologic emergencies. Emerg Med Clin North Am 2008;(26):233–8.

tarsal plate require specialized repair, and should be performed by plastic surgery or ophthalmology, depending on institutional preference.[53]

Endophthalmitis

Endophthalmitis is the inflammation of the aqueous or vitreous humors. Endophthalmitis can occur as the result of infection, trauma, or postsurgical complications. Suspicion mandates emergent ophthalmologic consultation for treatment options, including surgical intervention.

Acute-angle closure glaucoma

Patients with acute-angle closure glaucoma typically present with general eye pain, often associated with nausea, vomiting, headache, or abdominal pain. Elevated intraocular pressure (IOP) greater than 50 mm Hg may induce optic nerve atrophy if left untreated.[54] Treatment can and should be initiated by emergency physicians, but an ophthalmology consultation is important for monitoring of IOP. Patients refractory to treatment may require urgent surgical intervention.

Acute vision loss

Whether monocular or binocular, acute vision loss should be evaluated by ophthalmology as soon as possible. There are multiple causes, some of which are not directly related to the eye. Pain can help differentiate and direct appropriate treatment. Central artery occlusion results in sudden, painless vision loss. This condition is primarily the result of an embolic event, and immediate ophthalmologic consultation is essential, as irreversible vision loss can occur within 4 hours.[53]

Optic neuritis

In the setting of optic neuritis, patients present with painful eye movements, usually associated with monocular vision loss, visual field deficits, and change in color perception. Vision loss may progress rapidly over hours. Treatment with steroids should be initiated quickly, after consultation with ophthalmology or neurology.

Retinal detachment

Acute retinal detachment typically presents as new onset of floaters, squiggly lines, or "cobwebs" that are associated with visual field deficits. Examination with a standard ophthalmoscope is generally insufficient, as the detachment is likely to be located at the retinal periphery.[54] Eventual visual outcome is associated with the presence of macular involvement and time until repair. Therefore, early ophthalmology consultation is paramount.

Definitive Treatment

Eye irrigation is the immediate and primary treatment for any exposure. In the setting of chemical burns, copious irrigation has shown to have the greatest effect on visual prognosis.[55] Regardless of alkali versus acid exposure, the treatment is the same, and immediately on presentation, irrigation should be initiated. Physical examination should be limited to, at most, a rapid visual acuity and determination of pH. Irrigation should continue for up to 30 minutes after return to normal pH. On discontinuation, the pH should be rechecked 5 to 15 minutes later, to ensure that further chemical has not remained; this is especially important in the setting of alkali burns, where liquefactive necrosis leads to absorption into the anterior chamber.[56]

Removal of ocular foreign bodies is a frequent, but critical task for emergency medicine. It is essential to differentiate those that are superficial, on the surface of the eye, from those that are imbedded within the globe. In the case of the latter, the priority of the emergency physician is to prevent further damage until removal can be performed by an Ophthalmologist. Care should be taken to protect the eye with a shield, elevate the head of the bed, and minimize patient movement. Removal of uncomplicated superficial foreign bodies can be performed on the cooperative patient with the use of local anesthetic and a slit lamp. Removal can often be successful with gentle irrigation. Other techniques include a cotton-tipped applicator or 25-gauge needle held tangentially to the globe.

Paracentesis of the anterior chamber is a technique rarely performed by emergency physicians, but one that can be vision saving in the setting of retinal artery occlusion. In this condition, painless, sudden, monocular vision loss is accompanied by a pale optic disc or cherry-red spot on fundoscopy. Vision loss can be permanent without proper treatment within 48 hours of onset of symptoms.[57] The primary goal of treatment is to increase retinal blood flow or to dislodge the occluding clot. Other therapeutic interventions include digital orbital massage and intravenous acetazolamide, or topical β-blockers to decrease IOP.

Lateral canthotomy is another rarely used but important vision-sparing procedure. Lateral canthotomy is used to emergently relieve retroorbital pressure following blunt trauma, because in the setting of significant retrobulbar hemorrhage the optic nerve can become ischemic in as little as 90 minutes.[58]

In summary, ophthalmologic complaints result in relatively frequent visits to EDs. Familiarity with those entities that are high risk for permanent visual damage is essential for all emergency physicians. Rapid diagnosis, treatment, and ophthalmologic consultation may help increase the chance to avoid serious, permanent vision deficits.

THROAT AND NECK PAIN

The anatomy of the neck is highly complex, with many important structures. Patients' complaints of throat or neck pain can result in diagnoses ranging from benign, self-resolving problems to much more severe, life-threatening conditions with high morbidity and mortality if not diagnosed and treated correctly. This section focuses on some of the high-risk conditions for emergency physicians to consider when evaluating and treating patients presenting with complaints of throat or neck pain.

Throat Pain

Sore throat or throat pain is one of the most common chief complaints of patients treated in an outpatient setting.[59] The differential diagnosis for patients presenting with throat pain is extensive, ranging from benign viral pharyngitis to life-threatening emergent conditions with acute airway obstruction. The majority of patients presenting with sore throat have infectious pharyngitis, and 1.4% of all patients presenting to United States EDs ultimately receive this diagnosis.[49] However, it is the responsibility of the emergency physician to quickly recognize the less common but far more serious causes of throat pain that may cause airway obstruction, as precise and rapid intervention may be life saving. This section discusses the diagnosis and management of high-risk causes of throat pain, including deep neck infections and epiglottitis.

Deep neck infections

Deep neck infections, such as cellulitis or abscesses, are infections that occur in the potential spaces of the facial planes of the neck.[60] These infections are difficult to diagnose due to the complex anatomy of the neck, with the multiple fascial planes forming a framework of at least 11 deep neck spaces. The fascial planes create important barriers and limitations to the spread of infection, but can also serve to direct infectious spread once their natural resistance is overcome.[61] A detailed discussion of the anatomic planes and spaces in the neck is beyond the scope of this review, but a listing of the fascial spaces where deep neck infections can occur is listed in **Box 4**.[62]

This section reviews the signs and symptoms, treatment, and complications of deep neck infections. These infections are high-risk complaints, due to the rapid onset and potential fatal complications if not properly diagnosed and treated.

Signs and symptoms There are numerous signs and symptoms that may be present in patients presenting with deep neck infections. Presenting symptoms may include fever and chills, sore throat, neck pain, odynophagia, dysphagia, neck stiffness, voice changes, tongue base pain, dyspnea, otalgia, and sialorrhea.[62–65] In a retrospective review of 169 cases by Wang and colleagues,[65] the most common presenting symptoms were sore throat (72%) and odynophagia (63%). When peritonsillar abscess was excluded from their analysis, the most common presenting symptoms were neck swelling (70%) and neck pain (63%). Physical signs of patients with deep neck infections include neck swelling, trismus, elevated temperature, tachycardia, drooling, elevation of the floor of the mouth, and bulging of the pharyngeal wall.[62–65] Pain out of proportion to physical findings may suggest the presence of a deep neck infection.

Box 4
Cervical fascial spaces and their synonyms

- Spaces formed by splitting anterior layer
  - Space of parotid gland
  - Space of submaxillary gland
  - Space of body of mandible
  - Masticator space—masseteric, mandibulopterygoid, temporal pouch
- Space deep to the anterior layer of the deep cervical fascia
  - Retropharyngeal space—retrovisceral space, retroesophageal visceral compartment (posterior)
  - Lateral pharyngeal space—parapharyngeal, peripharyngeal, pharyngomaxillary, pterygopharyngeal, pterygomandibular, pharyngomasticatory
    - Anterior—prestyloid
    - Posterior—poststyloid
  - Submandibular space
    - Sublingual—floor of mouth
    - Sumylohyoid—submaxillary, submandibular
- Other spaces
  - Danger space
  - Prevertebral space—paravertebral space
  - Carotid sheath
  - Pretracheal space—visceral compartment (anterior)
  - Peritonsillar space

From Marra S, Hotaling AJ. Deep neck infections. Am J Otolaryngol 1996;17(5):287–98; with permission.

Emergency physicians must be observant for advanced airway signs in patients presenting with possible deep neck infections. Signs such as voice changes, stridor, dyspnea, shortness of breath, and use of accessory muscles signify impending airway obstruction or respiratory arrest, and require immediate intervention.

Treatment The maintenance of a safe and secure airway is the most important therapeutic goal in the management of patients with deep neck infections,[66] as death from loss of an airway can rapidly occur in patients with advanced disease.[67] In many cases of patients with deep neck infection, airway observation in a closely monitored setting may be a reasonable management option, but there is no consensus on the optimal timing of when to observe versus when to intervene.[66] When in doubt, taking control of the airway is the most conservative method, as patients with deep neck infection may progress quickly and airway compromise can occur with little warning.[68]

Indications for immediate aggressive airway management include patients in respiratory distress or impending airway compromise as noted by physical examination or diagnostic imaging.[61] Conventional endotracheal intubation is often difficult in patients with deep neck infections due to distorted airway anatomy, immobility of soft tissues, or trismus. In addition, direct laryngoscopy can be dangerous, as it may precipitate acute airway collapse or can cause rupture of the abscess with subsequent aspiration of pus.[61,66] General anesthesia is also dangerous in advanced cases as it may precipitate complete airway closure, thereby necessitating emergency tracheostomy.[67]

Tracheostomy under local anesthesia has long been considered the gold standard for airway management of patients with deep neck infections, but can be unpractical and risky in certain patients. Blind nasal intubation should never be performed in patients with deep neck infection as it carries risk of damage to the inflamed pharyngeal mucosa, with possible resulting bleeding, abscess perforation, or complete airway obstruction. Awake fiberoptic intubation using topical anesthesia is gaining popularity as the initial choice for airway management, and should be the first approach when it can be performed by an experienced operator. Tracheostomy under local anesthesia should be performed in situations where a fiberoptic bronchoscope is not available, the clinician is not skilled with awake fiberoptic intubation, or attempts at intubation have failed.[61,66,67] Cricothyrotomy or emergency tracheostomy may be performed for emergent airway control when sudden, complete loss of airway necessitates immediate surgical intervention.[61]

Once the airway is determined to be secure, broad systemic antibiotics should be given to patients with presumed or known deep space infection. If treatment is started early when the infection is at the stage of cellulitis, the condition may resolve by fibrosis without abscess formation. However, if the infection is not treated until pus has formed or if antibiotics fail, the abscess must be drained surgically.[69]

Cultures of deep neck abscesses are commonly polymicrobial, reflecting the oropharyngeal and odontogenic nature of these infections. The most frequently isolated aerobic microorganisms are *Streptococcus viridians*, *Klebsiella pneumoniae*, β-hemolytic streptococci, *Staphylococcus aureus*, and *Streptococcus pneumoniae*. The most frequent isolated anaerobic microorganisms include *Prevotella* spp, *Peptostreptococcus* spp, and *Bacteroides* spp.[60,61,63–65,70] *K pneumoniae* is the most common infection in diabetics.[60,61,70]

Early empirical antibiotic coverage should be started immediately. Penicillin with a β-lactamase inhibitor or a β-lactamase-resistant antibiotic combined with an antibiotic that is effective against anaerobes are good initial choices for empirical therapy. If a patient is at risk for methicillin-resistant *S aureus*, adding empirical vancomycin should be considered. The addition of gentamycin for effective gram-negative coverage against *K pneumoniae* is highly recommended for diabetic patients,[61] but special attention should be paid to renal function in these patients.

Evaluation of deep neck infections may be done by ultrasound, plain film radiography, contrast-enhanced CT, or MRI.[61] Contrast-enhanced CT or MRI are useful in characterizing the nature of the deep neck infection and aiding in early recognition of complications. As CT is more available, less expensive, and less time consuming than MRI, contrast-enhanced CT is the standard of care in evaluating deep neck infections.[71]

For many years, open surgical drainage has been the mainstay in the treatment of deep neck infections. However, some centers propose attempting treatment with broad-spectrum intravenous antibiotics alone in certain patients with small abscess who are clinically stable and have no evidence of abscess in "danger spaces" (prevertebral, anterior visceral, and vascular visceral spaces) or in more than 2 places, or have evidence of descending infection.[71] For the emergency physician, it is prudent to consult a surgeon early for assistance in the management of all cases of suspected deep neck infection.

Complications Life-threatening complications of deep neck infection included upper airway obstruction, descending mediastinitis, pleural empyema, pericarditis, pneumonia, jugular vein thrombosis, sepsis, and carotid pseudoaneurysm or rupture.[65] Studies have shown that complicated deep neck infections are associated with patients presenting with neck swelling or respiratory difficulty as well as those found to have an extended space abscess with more than 2 involved spaces. Factors that were found to be less likely associated with a complicated abscess were male gender, presenting complaint of neck pain, and odontogenic causes of infection.[60,65,70]

Epiglottitis

Acute epiglottitis, or supraglottitis, is an inflammatory process of the epiglottis and the adjacent structures that can lead to life-threatening acute respiratory obstruction. In the past, epiglottitis occurred most frequently in children and was associated with *Haemophilus influenzae* type b (Hib) infection.[72] However, since the introduction of the Hib vaccine in the United States in 1985, the incidence of acute epiglottitis in children has decreased while the incidence in adults has remained stable or increased.[73,74]

Acute epiglottitis can be difficult to diagnose, and can lead to rapid and unpredictable airway obstruction. Due to the difficulty of its diagnosis and management, epiglottitis is listed as 1 of 8 high-risk diagnostic categories in a review of malpractice claims filed by emergency physicians in Massachusetts from 1975 to 1993.[4] The emergency physician must maintain a high index of suspicion to make the diagnosis, and then intervene quickly and appropriately. This section reviews the diagnosis and management of acute epiglottitis as well as the high-risk features to be aware of when treating a patient with epiglottitis.

Signs and symptoms Children typically present with fever, irritability, sore throat, and difficulty breathing, with rapidly progressive stridor and respiratory distress.[72,74] Adults generally present with milder disease, and their main complaints are usually sore throat or odynophagia.[74,75] The presence of a severe sore throat in an adult, especially when accompanied by anterior neck tenderness, should prompt the emergency physician to consider epiglottitis in the differential diagnosis.[76] Other signs and symptoms of acute epiglottitis include muffled voice, fever, pharyngitis, tenderness in the anterior neck, drooling, cervical adenopathy, and cough.[74,75] Pain out of proportion to physical findings may suggest epiglottitis.

Diagnosis Diagnosis of epiglottitis is made by history, clinical examination, radiography, and laryngoscopy. Lateral neck soft tissue radiographs may demonstrate obliteration of the vallecula, swelling of the aryepiglottic folds, edema of the prevertebral and retropharyngeal soft tissues, ballooning of the hypopharynx, or an enlarged, thumb-shaped epiglottis in patients with acute epiglottitis.[77] However, these soft tissue neck radiographs are not reliable in the diagnosis of acute epiglottitis due to low sensitivity and specificity. A retrospective chart review by Stankiewicz and colleagues[78] showed that of 30 adults diagnosed with acute epiglottitis, only 1 lateral neck radiograph was read as positive and of 48 children with documented epiglottitis, only 26 lateral neck radiographs were read as abnormal. A retrospective review of hospital records of cases of acute epiglottitis in Rhode Island showed that of 287 soft tissue neck radiographs performed, 247 had findings diagnostic or suggestive of acute epiglottitis, yielding a sensitivity of only 86%.[74]

Diagnosis of acute epiglottitis requires direct visualization of an erythematous and swollen epiglottis and adjacent structures by laryngoscopy. Because of the risk of airway obstruction with direct laryngoscopy, the procedure should be performed in children only when skilled personnel and equipment are available to secure the airway.[72] The procedure should also be performed with extreme caution in adults to avoid sudden airway obstruction.[77] However, in a study of 129 cases of acute epiglottitis in adults by Frantz and colleagues,[75] indirect laryngoscopy did not precipitate airway compromise in any patient. In addition, Mayo-Smith and colleagues[74] reviewed hospital records of 407 cases of epiglottitis in children and adults, and found that direct and indirect laryngoscopic examinations did not precipitate an acute airway obstruction in a single patient.

Management Patients with suspected acute epiglottitis require immediate otolaryngologic consultation, close monitoring of the airway with intubation if necessary, and treatment with intravenous antibiotics.[72,77]

Acute epiglottitis can result in sudden, unpredictable airway obstruction in previously healthy individuals. Younger children (younger than 5 years) are predisposed to sudden airway collapse, and should be immediately intubated in the operating room with an otolaryngologist or surgeon present. In addition, patients with acute airway obstruction or severe respiratory distress at time of presentation should have an airway established immediately, with surgical backup for immediate cricothyrotomy or tracheostomy if intubation fails. Individual with signs and symptoms of impending respiratory distress, including respiratory discomfort, stridor, or drooling, should have an artificial airway established as part of their initial care. In addition, patients who present with symptoms of short durations (<12–24 hours), rapid progression, or with significant enlargement of the epiglottis on radiography or laryngoscopy should strongly be considered for establishment of an urgent artificial airway. Patients with mild symptoms and without respiratory difficulty, stridor, or drooling, and who have only mild swelling on laryngoscopy, may be considered for observation in the intensive care unit without an artificial airway but with high vigilance to the patient's airway patency.[74] The decision to observe the patient without an artificial airway should be made in consultation with an otolaryngologist.

In addition to careful airway management, patients with acute epiglottitis should be started on intravenous antibiotics urgently. Although the Hib vaccination has greatly reduced the Hib infection in children, there is occasional failure of the vaccine, and cases of Hib epiglottitis can still present in both vaccinated and unvaccinated children. Bacteria more commonly associated with epiglottitis include *S pneumoniae*, *S aureus*, and β-hemolytic streptococci. Empirical urgent treatment with cefotaxime, ceftriaxone, or ampicillin/sulbactam is recommended.[72]

Neck Pain

Occult cervical spine injury

The incidence of cervical spine injury following blunt trauma has been estimated to be around 4.3%,[79] and diagnosis of cervical spine injury is a high-risk area, as unrecognized injury can result in catastrophic neurologic disability. The management of potential cervical spine injuries in patients who have sustained major trauma or are comatose involves liberal use of imaging, and maintaining cervical immobilization until consultation with a trauma surgeon. However, in less severe trauma the decision of which stable, alert trauma patients require cervical spine imaging can be a difficult one. Two clinical decision rules have been validated and are sensitive for determining the need for cervical spine imaging in patients with blunt trauma: these are the NEXUS Low-Risk Criteria and the Canadian C-Spine Rule.[80,81]

The NEXUS Low-Risk Criteria requires that cervical spine radiography is indicated for patients with blunt trauma unless they meet the following criteria: no posterior midline cervical spine tenderness, no evidence of intoxication, a normal level of alertness, no focal neurologic deficit, and no painful distracting injuries. This decision instrument was validated in a prospective observational study at 21 centers across the United States, and was found to have a sensitivity of 99% and specificity of 12.9%. The decision instrument identified all 8 of 818 patients who had cervical spine injury, and only 2 of those 8 patients were classified as having a clinically significant injury.[80]

The Canadian C-Spine Rule comprises 3 main questions: (1) is there any high-risk factor present that mandates radiography (ie, age $\geq$65 years, dangerous mechanism, or paresthesias in the extremities)? (2) is there any low-risk factor present that allows safe assessment of range of motion (ie, simple rear-end motor vehicle collision, sitting position in ED, ambulatory at any time since injury, delayed onset of neck pain, or absence of midline C-spine tenderness)? and (3) is the patient able to actively rotate neck 45° to the left and right? In this study, patients had to be alert (GCS = 15) and stable (normal vital signs). Patients were excluded if they did not fulfill the first 2 criteria, were younger than 16 years, were injured more than 48 hours previously, had penetrating trauma, presented with acute paralysis, had known vertebral disease (ankylosing spondylitis, rheumatoid arthritis, spinal stenosis, or previous cervical surgery), had returned for reassessment of the same injury, or were pregnant. In the derivation study, the Canadian C-Spine Rule demonstrated a sensitivity of 100% and specificity of 42.5% for identifying clinically important cervical spine injuries.[81]

These 2 studies were compared in a prospective cohort study conducted in the 9 Canadian EDs where the initial Canadian C-Spine Rule was derived. In this study, the sensitivity of the Canadian C-Spine Rule versus NEXUS was 99.4% versus 90.7%, and the specificity was 45.1% versus 36.8%.[82] Either of these 2 clinical decision rules may be used in evaluating the awake, alert patient who has recently sustained blunt trauma.

Cervicocranial artery dissection

Dissections of the carotid and vertebral arteries usually arise from an intimal tear in the vessel, allowing arterial blood to enter the wall of the artery and form a false lumen, which then results in either stenosis or aneurysmal dilatation of the vessel.[83] Such dissections are relatively common causes of stroke, especially in young patients, via artery-to-artery embolism or stenosis with occlusion of the proximal vessel causing ischemic strokes, or vessel rupture resulting in a hemorrhagic stroke.[43] Although trauma is commonly associated with cervicocranial artery dissections, at least 50% of people with dissections and stroke have no clear history of antecedent neck trauma.[43,84] The high-risk features of cervicocranial artery dissections are related to the subtle clinical presentations of this elusive diagnosis.

Signs and symptoms In carotid artery dissection, the classical clinical presentation is a patient presenting with pain on one side of the head, face, or neck accompanied by a partial Horner syndrome (oculosympathetic palsy, consisting of miosis and ptosis), and followed hours to days later by cerebral or retinal ischemia. This triad is found in less than one-third of patients, but the presence of any 2 elements should strongly suggest the diagnosis. Other local manifestations may include headache (present in approximately 2-thirds of patients), cranial nerve palsies, pulsatile tinnitus, or an objective bruit noted on physical examination.[83]

The initial manifestations of vertebral-artery dissection are less distinct and often present as pain in the back of the neck or head, which is frequently assumed to be musculoskeletal initially, followed by ischemia of the posterior circulation. A headache occurs in about two-thirds of patients and is almost always in the occipital area.[83]

Diagnosis and treatment Diagnosis of cervicocranial dissection can be made via multiple imaging modalities, including angiography, MRI and MR angiography, Doppler sonography, and CT angiography.[85] Once dissection is diagnosed, urgent consultation with a neurologist is required. If intracerebral hemorrhage is excluded, emergent anticoagulation with intravenous heparin may be recommended to prevent thrombotic complications. Most dissections will heal spontaneously, but surgical or endovascular treatment is an option in patients who have failed conservative medical management.[43,83]

DIFFICULT AIRWAY

Airway management is a critical skill for the emergency physician. When intubation is indicated, the most important question the physician can ask is "Is this airway difficult?"[86] A difficult airway is one in which the preintubation examination identifies attributes that may make bag-mask ventilation, laryngoscopy, intubation, the use of an extraglottic device, or surgical airway management more difficult than if those features were not present. A difficult airway can become a failed airway when the initial method chosen for airway management is not successful and an alternative method must be undertaken.[86,87]

Given the high level of acuity and necessity for rapid intervention of many emergency patients requiring airway management, difficult airways are common in the ED, with some estimates as high as 20% of all airways managed in the ED.[86] Despite this fact, the incidence of failed airway is relatively low, around 2% to 3%. An observational study by Sakles and colleagues[88] found that of 610 patients requiring airway control in the ED, only 13 (2.1%) were complicated by a failed airway, with 7 (1%) of those patients requiring rescue by cricothyrotomy. Similar results were seen in a prospective observational study by Bair and colleagues[87] of 7712 intubations in 30 different EDs that were enrolled in the NEAR (National Emergency Airway Registry) project. In this study, a total of 207 (2.7%) of emergency intubations were failed airways requiring rescue technique. Of the 207 failed airways, the majority occurred when rapid sequence intubation (RSI) was not used initially, and consequently RSI was the most common rescue technique accounting for half of all rescued airways. In addition, 44 (0.6%) airways required rescue by surgical intervention (cricothyrotomy or tracheostomy).

Although the failed airway is relatively uncommon in the ED, the morbidity and mortality associated with a failed airway is high. It is essential for emergency physicians to recognize the difficult airway early and thoughtfully plan for its management, so as to minimize the number of failed airways in the ED. This section focuses on the high-risk feature of airway management by discussing predictors of a possible difficult airway as well as alternative airway management techniques that may be used to rescue a failed airway.

Recognizing the Difficult Airway

The failed airway is a dreaded complication of emergency airway management. To minimize failure in airway management, it is important to recognize the difficult airway in advance in order to execute the appropriate plan to maximize airway success.[86] This section discusses how to recognize patients who may be difficult to mask ventilate, perform laryngoscopy on, or intubate, so that the airway management in these patients can be planned to minimize the likelihood of a "can't intubate, can't oxygenate" complication.

Difficult mask ventilation

Mask ventilation is an essential component of airway management,[89] and is of utmost importance in ventilating and oxygenating the patient who is impossible to intubate. The technique for effective mask ventilation is not reviewed here, but should be mastered by all health care providers involved in airway management. This section reviews the predictors of difficult mask ventilation, so that providers can quickly recognize patients who may be difficult to mask ventilate and proceed accordingly.

Difficult mask ventilation may be caused by inadequate mask seal, excessive gas leak, or excessive resistance to the ingress or egress of gas. Signs of inadequate mask ventilation include absent or inadequate chest movement, absent or inadequate breath sounds, auscultatory signs of severe obstruction, cyanosis, gastric air entry or dilatation, decreasing or inadequate oxygen saturation, absent or inadequate exhaled carbon dioxide, absent or inadequate spirometric measures of exhaled gas flow, and hemodynamic changes associated with hypoxemia or hypercarbia.[89]

Several studies have looked at the predictors of difficult or impossible mask ventilation in the anesthesiology setting. A prospective observational study by Langeron and colleagues[90] reported difficult mask ventilation in 75 of 1502 (5%) patients undergoing general anesthesia, with 1 case of impossible ventilation. In this study, the independent factors for difficult mask ventilation were age older than 55 years, body mass index (BMI; calculated as the weight in kilograms divided by height in meters squared) greater than 26 kg/m^2, presence of a beard, lack of teeth, and history of snoring. Similar results were found in a prospective study by Kherterpal and colleagues,[91] which reported 313 of 22,660 (1.4%) patients as difficult to mask ventilate. Independent predictors of difficult mask ventilation were BMI 30 kg/m^2 or greater, presence of a beard, Mallampati score of III or IV, age 57 years or older, severely limited mandibular protrusion, or a history of snoring. Kherterpal and colleagues[92] then evaluated factors associated with impossible mask ventilation in an observational study that reported 77 of 53,041 patients (0.15%) who were impossible to mask ventilate. The 5 independent predictors of impossible mask ventilation were neck radiation changes, male sex, sleep apnea, Mallampati classification of III or IV, and the presence of a beard.

In managing the emergent airway, the validated predictors of difficult mask ventilation are best summarized by Murphy and Walls in the *Manual of Emergency Airway Management* using the mnemonic MOANS (**Box 5**). This mnemonic allows for rapid recall in the ED and can be easily used by any clinician.[86] Although patients who are difficult or impossible to mask ventilate are rare, it is important to recognize

Box 5
Predictors of difficult mask ventilation: MOANS

M—Mask seal

May be complicated by beards, blood on face, or disruption of the lower face

O—Obesity/obstruction

BMI greater than 26 kg/m^2 (including pregnant patients in their third trimester) makes mask ventilation more difficult

Obstruction caused by airway edema, hematomas, tumors, or foreign bodies may complicate mask ventilation

A—Age

Age older than 55 years is associated with a higher risk of difficult mask ventilation due to loss of muscle and tissue tone in the upper airway

N—No teeth

Difficult to obtain an adequate mask seal as the edentulous patient's face tends to cave in

S—Stiff/history of sleep apnea or snoring

Conditions causing stiff lungs resistant to ventilation (ie, reactive airway disease, pulmonary edema, acute respiratory distress syndrome, advanced pneumonia)

History of sleep apnea or snoring

Data from Murphy MF, Walls RM. Identification of the difficult and failed airway. In: Walls RM, Murphy MF. Manual of emergency airway management, 3rd edition. Philadelphia: Lippincott Williams and Wilkins; 2008. p. 81–93.

patients who may be difficult to mask ventilate early, so as to be prepared to use alternative methods to oxygenate and ventilate these patients.

Difficult laryngoscopy and intubation

Unanticipated difficult laryngoscopy and intubation is one of the major challenges of airway management. A landmark article in the *British Medical Journal* by Cass and colleagues[93] in 1956 was the first attempt to identify the anatomic features that may predict difficult intubation. In this article, Cass and colleagues looked at 5 cases of difficult intubation and noted the associated physical features, such as short muscular necks with a full set of teeth, receding lower jaws with obtuse mandibular angles, protruding upper incisors, and poor mobility of the mandible. Since this initial article, numerous investigators have tried to determine with high precision which physical attributes apparent on bedside physical examination could reliably predict successful versus failed laryngoscopy and intubation. Unfortunately, many of these investigations have met with limited or no success,[94–97] and a rapid screening test that is 100% sensitive with a high positive predictive value remains elusive.

In the absence of a proven and validated rule with high sensitivity and specificity in predicting difficult intubation, it is important to have a way to quickly identify those patients who might be difficult to intubate in an emergency setting so that an appropriate plan may be made. The LEMON method (**Box 6**) devised by the US National Emergency Airway Management Course is a simple assessment tool assembled from an analysis of the difficult airway prediction instruments in the anesthesia literature, and is currently undergoing a validation study by the multicenter National Emergency Airway Registry Project (NEAR III).[86] This tool has been favorably assessed in

Box 6
Predictors of difficult laryngoscopy and intubation: LEMON method

L—Look externally

Look at the patient for any external characteristics or a gestalt "feeling" that may indicate difficult laryngoscopy, intubation, or ventilation

E—Evaluate the 3-3-2 Rule

3: Mouth opening—the interincisor distance should be at least 3 finger breadths

3: Length of the mandibular space—the distance between the tip of the mentum and the chin-neck junction (hyoid bone) should be at least 3 finger breadths

2: Position of the glottis in relation to the tongue—the distance between the chin-neck junction (hyoid bone) and the thyroid notch should be at least 2 finger breadths

M—Mallampati score

Reflects the relationships among mouth opening, the size of the tongue, and the size of the oral pharynx

Classes relate to degree of difficulty intubating:

I: Soft palate, uvula, fauces, pillars visible—No difficulty

II: Soft palate, uvula, fauces visible—No difficulty

III: Soft palate, base of uvula visible—Moderate difficulty

IV: Hard palate only visible—Severe difficulty

O—Obstruction/obesity

Upper airway obstruction is always a marker for a difficult airway

Obese patients tend to have poor glottic views by direct laryngoscopy

N—Neck mobility

Cervical spine immobilization makes intubation more difficult. Intrinsic cervical spine immobility (ie, ankylosing spondylitis or rheumatoid arthritis) can make direct laryngoscopy extremely difficult or impossible

Data from Murphy MF, Walls RM. Identification of the difficult and failed airway. In: Walls RM, Murphy MF. Manual of emergency airway management, 3rd edition. Philadelphia: Lippincott Williams and Wilkins; 2008. p. 81–93.

a prospective observational study by Reed and colleagues.[98] In this study, a rapid airway assessment score based on the LEMON method successfully stratified the risk of difficult intubation in the ED, and verified an association between patients with large incisors, a reduced interincisor distance, or a reduced thyroid to floor mouth distance and poor laryngoscopic view (Cormack and Lehane laryngoscopy grades 2, 3, or 4). The LEMON method is a useful tool for the rapid assessment and risk stratification of emergency patients requiring intubation, so that the care of patients who may be at risk of difficult intubation can be managed carefully and a failed airway avoided.

Alternative Techniques for Rescue or Difficult Airways

The most important aspect of emergency airway management is to anticipate and prepare for the difficult airway or the failed airway requiring rescue. There are numerous alternative airway techniques, both invasive and noninvasive, to use in difficult or failed airway situations (**Box 7**).[99] The exact technique by which to perform

Box 7
Alternative techniques for rescue or difficult airways

Endotracheal tube introducers

Blind intubation

–Blind nasotracheal intubation

–Digital tracheal intubation

Fiberoptic intubation

–Flexible

–Rigid and semirigid stylets

Lighted stylet intubation

Video laryngoscopy

Extraglottic devices

–Supraglottic

- Laryngeal mask airway

–Retroglottic

- Esophageal tracheal Combitube
- King LT Airway
- Rush EasyTube

Surgical airway

–Cricothyrotomy

–Needle cricothyrotomy with percutaneous tracheal ventilation

–Tracheostomy

–Translaryngeal guided ("retrograde") intubation

Data from Walls RM, Murphy MF, editors. Manual of emergency airway management, 3rd edition. Philadelphia: Lippincott Williams and Wilkins; 2008.

these alternative techniques is beyond the scope of this review. However, it is the responsibility of every emergency physician to be as well trained as possible in these alternative techniques so as to provide the best possible care to the emergency patient and properly manage the emergency airway.

SUMMARY

Disorders of the head and neck are high-risk areas for the emergency physician. The anatomy is complex and the pathology can be diverse. A high degree of suspicion must be maintained for all potentially life-threatening conditions when patients present with complaints of the head and neck.

REFERENCES

1. Goldstein JN, Camargo CA Jr, Pelletier AJ, et al. Headache in United States emergency departments: demographics, work-up and frequency of pathological diagnoses. Cephalalgia 2006;26(6):684–90.

2. Lipton RB, Bigal ME, Steiner TJ, et al. Classification of primary headaches. Neurology 2004;63(3):427–35.
3. Locker T, Mason S, Rigby A. Headache management—are we doing enough? An observational study of patients presenting with headache to the emergency department. Emerg Med J 2004;21(3):327–32.
4. Karcz A, Korn R, Burke MC, et al. Malpractice claims against emergency physicians in Massachusetts: 1975–1993. Am J Emerg Med 1996;14(4):341–5.
5. Ramirez-Lassepas M, Espinosa CE, Cicero JJ, et al. Predictors of intracranial pathologic findings in patients who seek emergency care because of headache. Arch Neurol 1997;54(12):1506–9.
6. Locker TE, Thompson C, Rylance J, et al. The utility of clinical features in patients presenting with nontraumatic headache: an investigation of adult patients attending an emergency department. Headache 2006;46(6):954–61.
7. Edlow JA, Panagos PD, Godwin SA, et al. Clinical policy: critical issues in the evaluation and management of adult patients presenting to the emergency department with acute headache. Ann Emerg Med 2008;52(4):407–36.
8. Cortelli P, Cevoli S, Nonino F, et al. Evidence-based diagnosis of nontraumatic headache in the emergency department: a consensus statement on four clinical scenarios. Headache 2004;44(6):587–95.
9. Bederson JB, Connolly ES Jr, Batjer HH, et al. Guidelines for the management of aneurysmal subarachnoid hemorrhage: a statement for healthcare professionals from a special writing group of the Stroke Council, American Heart Association. Stroke 2009;40(3):994–1025.
10. Pope JV, Edlow JA. Favorable response to analgesics does not predict a benign etiology of headache. Headache 2008;48(6):944–50.
11. M S, Lamont AC, Alias NA, et al. Red flags in patients presenting with headache: clinical indications for neuroimaging. Br J Radiol 2003;76(908):532–5.
12. Chaisson R, Volberding P. Clinical manifestations of HIV infection. In: Mandell GL, Bennett JE, Dolin R, editors. Mandell, Douglas and Bennett's principles and practice of infectious diseases. 4th edition. New York: Churchill Livingstone; 1995. p. 1217–53.
13. Rothman RE, Keyl PM, McArthur JC, et al. A decision guideline for emergency department utilization of noncontrast head computed tomography in HIV-infected patients. Acad Emerg Med 1999;6(10):1010–9.
14. Christiaans MH, Kelder JC, Arnoldus EP, et al. Prediction of intracranial metastases in cancer patients with headache. Cancer 2002;94(7):2063–8.
15. Argyriou AA, Chroni E, Polychronopoulos P, et al. Headache characteristics and brain metastases prediction in cancer patients. Eur J Cancer Care (Engl) 2006; 15(1):90–5.
16. Baehring J, Quant E, Hochber F. Metastatic neoplasms and paraneoplastic syndromes. In: Goetz CG, editor. Textbook of clinical neurology. 3rd edition. Philadelphia: Saunders Elsevier; 2007. p. 1081–93.
17. Lloyd-Jones D, Adams R, Carnethon M, et al. Heart disease and stroke statistics—2009 update: a report from the American Heart Association Statistics Committee and Stroke Statistics Subcommittee. Circulation 2009;119(3):e21–181.
18. Stam J. Thrombosis of the cerebral veins and sinuses. N Engl J Med 2005; 352(17):1791–8.
19. Conicella E, Raucci U, Vanacore N, et al. The child with headache in a pediatric emergency department. Headache 2008;48(7):1005–11.
20. Kan L, Nagelberg J, Maytal J. Headaches in a pediatric emergency department: etiology, imaging, and treatment. Headache 2000;40(1):25–9.

21. ACE Clinical Policies Committee; Clinical Policies Subcommittee on Seizures. Clinical policy: critical issues in the evaluation and management of adult patients presenting to the emergency department with seizures. Ann Emerg Med 2004; 43(5):605–25.
22. Engel J Jr, Starkman S. Overview of seizures. Emerg Med Clin North Am 1994; 12(4):895–923.
23. Walker MC. The epidemiology and management of status epilepticus. Curr Opin Neurol 1998;11(2):149–54.
24. Dunn MJ, Breen DP, Davenport RJ, et al. Early management of adults with an uncomplicated first generalised seizure. Emerg Med J 2005;22(4):237–42.
25. McKeon A, Vaughan C, Delanty N. Seizure versus syncope. Lancet Neurol 2006; 5(2):171–80.
26. Tarabar A, Ulrich A, D'Onofrio G. Seizures. In: Adams J, Barton E, editors. Emergency medicine. Philadelphia: Saunders/Elsevier; 2008. p. 1051–62.
27. Adams J. Emergency medicine. Philadelphia: Saunders/Elsevier; 2008.
28. Lowenstein DH, Alldredge BK. Status epilepticus. N Engl J Med 1998;338(14): 970–6.
29. Takayanagui OM, Odashima NS. Clinical aspects of neurocysticercosis. Parasitol Int 2006;55(Suppl):S111–5.
30. Jolley S, Allen T. Transient ischemic attack and acute ischemic stroke. In: Adams J, Barton E, editors. Emergency medicine. Philadelphia: Saunders/Elsevier; 2008. p. 1072–82.
31. Goldstein LB, Simel DL. Is this patient having a stroke? JAMA 2005;293(19): 2391–402.
32. Norris JW, Hachinski VC. Misdiagnosis of stroke. Lancet 1982;1(8267):328–31.
33. Allder SJ, Moody AR, Martel AL, et al. Limitations of clinical diagnosis in acute stroke. Lancet 1999;354(9189):1523.
34. Kothari RU, Brott T, Broderick JP, et al. Emergency physicians. Accuracy in the diagnosis of stroke. Stroke 1995;26(12):2238–41.
35. Libman RB, Wirkowski E, Alvir J, et al. Conditions that mimic stroke in the emergency department. Implications for acute stroke trials. Arch Neurol 1995;52(11): 1119–22.
36. Scott PA, Silbergleit R. Misdiagnosis of stroke in tissue plasminogen activator-treated patients: characteristics and outcomes. Ann Emerg Med 2003;42(5): 611–8.
37. Winkler DT, Fluri F, Fuhr P, et al. Thrombolysis in stroke mimics: frequency, clinical characteristics, and outcome. Stroke 2009;40(4):1522–5.
38. Savitz SI, Caplan LR. Vertebrobasilar disease. N Engl J Med 2005;352(25): 2618–26.
39. Tissue plasminogen activator for acute ischemic stroke. The National Institute of Neurological Disorders and Stroke rt-PA Stroke Study Group. N Engl J Med 1995; 333(24):1581–7.
40. Hacke W, Kaste M, Bluhmki E, et al. Thrombolysis with alteplase 3 to 4.5 hours after acute ischemic stroke. N Engl J Med 2008;359(13):1317–29.
41. Marler JR, Tilley BC, Lu M, et al. Early stroke treatment associated with better outcome: the NINDS rt-PA stroke study. Neurology 2000;55(11):1649–55.
42. Adams HP Jr, del Zoppo G, Alberts MJ, et al. Guidelines for the early management of adults with ischemic stroke: a guideline from the American Heart Association/American Stroke Association Stroke Council, Clinical Cardiology Council, Cardiovascular Radiology and Intervention Council, and the Atherosclerotic Peripheral Vascular Disease and Quality of Care Outcomes in Research

Interdisciplinary Working Groups: the American Academy of Neurology affirms the value of this guideline as an educational tool for neurologists. Stroke 2007; 38(5):1655–711.
43. Sacco RL, Adams R, Albers G, et al. Guidelines for prevention of stroke in patients with ischemic stroke or transient ischemic attack: a statement for healthcare professionals from the American Heart Association/American Stroke Association Council on Stroke: co-sponsored by the Council on Cardiovascular Radiology and Intervention: the American Academy of Neurology affirms the value of this guideline. Circulation 2006;113(10):e409–49.
44. Albers GW, Caplan LR, Easton JD, et al. Transient ischemic attack—proposal for a new definition. N Engl J Med 2002;347(21):1713–6.
45. Johnston SC, Gress DR, Browner WS, et al. Short-term prognosis after emergency department diagnosis of TIA. JAMA 2000;284(22):2901–6.
46. Flaherty ML, Haverbusch M, Sekar P, et al. Long-term mortality after intracerebral hemorrhage. Neurology 2006;66(8):1182–6.
47. Broderick J, Connolly S, Feldmann E, et al. Guidelines for the management of spontaneous intracerebral hemorrhage in adults: 2007 update: a guideline from the American Heart Association/American Stroke Association Stroke Council, High Blood Pressure Research Council, and the Quality of Care and Outcomes in Research Interdisciplinary Working Group. Stroke 2007;38(6):2001–23.
48. Qureshi AI, Tuhrim S, Broderick JP, et al. Spontaneous intracerebral hemorrhage. N Engl J Med 2001;344(19):1450–60.
49. Nawar EW, Niska RW, Xu J. National Hospital Ambulatory Medical Care Survey: 2005 emergency department summary. Adv Data 2007;(386):1–32.
50. Broocker G. The ophthalmic examination. In: Wolfson A, Hendey G, Hendry P, et al, editors. Harwood-Nuss' clinical practice of emergency medicine. 4th edition. Philadelphia: Lippincott, Williams & Wilkins; 2005. p. 112–7.
51. Knoop K, Dennis W, Hedges J. Ophthalmologic procedures. In: Roberts J, Hedges J, Chanmugam A, et al, editors. Clinical procedures in emergency medicine. 4th edition. Philadelphia: Saunders/Elsevier; 2004. p.1241–79.
52. Blaivas M, Theodoro D, Sierzenski PR. A study of bedside ocular ultrasonography in the emergency department. Acad Emerg Med 2002;9(8):791–9.
53. Hayreh SS, Zimmerman MB, Kimura A, et al. Central retinal artery occlusion. Retinal survival time. Exp Eye Res 2004;78(3):723–36.
54. Vortmann M, Schneider JI. Acute monocular visual loss. Emerg Med Clin North Am 2008;26(1):73–96, vi.
55. Kuckelkorn R, Kottek A, Schrage N, et al. Poor prognosis of severe chemical and thermal eye burns: the need for adequate emergency care and primary prevention. Int Arch Occup Environ Health 1995;67(4):281–4.
56. Magauran B. Conditions requiring emergency ophthalmologic consultation. Emerg Med Clin North Am 2008;26(1):233–8, viii.
57. Babineau MR, Sanchez LD. Ophthalmologic procedures in the emergency department. Emerg Med Clin North Am 2008;26(1):17–34, v-vi.
58. Colby K. Approach to the ophthalmologic patient. In: Beers M, Porter R, Jones T, et al, editors. The Merck manual of diagnosis and therapy. 18th edition. Whitehouse Station (NJ): Merck Research Laboratories, Division of Merck & Co., Inc.; 2006. p. 867–928.
59. Cooper RJ, Hoffman JR, Bartlett JG, et al. Principles of appropriate antibiotic use for acute pharyngitis in adults: background. Ann Intern Med 2001;134(6):509–17.
60. Lee JK, Kim HD, Lim SC. Predisposing factors of complicated deep neck infection: an analysis of 158 cases. Yonsei Med J 2007;48(1):55–62.

61. Vieira F, Allen SM, Stocks RM, et al. Deep neck infection. Otolaryngol Clin North Am 2008;41(3):459–83, vii.
62. Marra S, Hotaling AJ. Deep neck infections. Am J Otolaryngol 1996;17(5): 287–98.
63. Bottin R, Marioni G, Rinaldi R, et al. Deep neck infection: a present-day complication. A retrospective review of 83 cases (1998–2001). Eur Arch Otorhinolaryngol 2003;260(10):576–9.
64. Eftekharian A, Roozbahany NA, Vaezeafshar R, et al. Deep neck infections: a retrospective review of 112 cases. Eur Arch Otorhinolaryngol 2009;266(2):273–7.
65. Wang LF, Kuo WR, Tsai SM, et al. Characterizations of life-threatening deep cervical space infections: a review of one hundred ninety-six cases. Am J Otolaryngol 2003;24(2):111–7.
66. Karkos PD, Leong SC, Beer H, et al. Challenging airways in deep neck space infections. Am J Otolaryngol 2007;28(6):415–8.
67. Ovassapian A, Tuncbilek M, Weitzel EK, et al. Airway management in adult patients with deep neck infections: a case series and review of the literature. Anesth Analg 2005;100(2):585–9.
68. Shockley WW. Ludwig angina: a review of current airway management. Arch Otolaryngol Head Neck Surg 1999;125(5):600.
69. Brook I. Microbiology and management of peritonsillar, retropharyngeal, and parapharyngeal abscesses. J Oral Maxillofac Surg 2004;62(12):1545–50.
70. Huang TT, Liu TC, Chen PR, et al. Deep neck infection: analysis of 185 cases. Head Neck 2004;26(10):854–60.
71. Boscolo-Rizzo P, Marchiori C, Zanetti F, et al. Conservative management of deep neck abscesses in adults: the importance of CECT findings. Otolaryngol Head Neck Surg 2006;135(6):894–9.
72. Alcaide ML, Bisno AL. Pharyngitis and epiglottitis. Infect Dis Clin North Am 2007; 21(2):449–69, vii.
73. Frantz TD, Rasgon BM. Acute epiglottitis: changing epidemiologic patterns. Otolaryngol Head Neck Surg 1993;109(3 Pt 1):457–60.
74. Mayo-Smith MF, Spinale JW, Donskey CJ, et al. Acute epiglottitis. An 18-year experience in Rhode Island. Chest 1995;108(6):1640–7.
75. Frantz TD, Rasgon BM, Quesenberry CP Jr. Acute epiglottitis in adults. Analysis of 129 cases. JAMA 1994;272(17):1358–60.
76. Carey MJ. Epiglottitis in adults. Am J Emerg Med 1996;14(4):421–4.
77. Shores C. Infections and disorders of the neck and upper airway. In: Tintinalli JE, Kelen GD, Stapczynski JS, editors. Emergency medicine: a comprehensive study guide. 6th edition. New York: McGraw-Hill; 2004. p. 1494–501.
78. Stankiewicz JA, Bowes AK. Croup and epiglottitis: a radiologic study. Laryngoscope 1985;95(10):1159–60.
79. Grossman MD, Reilly PM, Gillett T, et al. National survey of the incidence of cervical spine injury and approach to cervical spine clearance in U.S. trauma centers. J Trauma 1999;47(4):684–90.
80. Hoffman JR, Mower WR, Wolfson AB, et al. Validity of a set of clinical criteria to rule out injury to the cervical spine in patients with blunt trauma. National Emergency X-Radiography Utilization Study Group. N Engl J Med 2000; 343(2):94–9.
81. Stiell IG, Wells GA, Vandemheen KL, et al. The Canadian C-spine rule for radiography in alert and stable trauma patients. JAMA 2001;286(15):1841–8.
82. Stiell IG, Clement CM, McKnight RD, et al. The Canadian C-spine rule versus the NEXUS low-risk criteria in patients with trauma. N Engl J Med 2003;349(26):2510–8.

83. Schievink WI. Spontaneous dissection of the carotid and vertebral arteries. N Engl J Med 2001;344(12):898–906.
84. Bassi P, Lattuada P, Gomitoni A. Cervical cerebral artery dissection: a multicenter prospective study (preliminary report). Neurol Sci 2003;24(Suppl 1):S4–7.
85. Provenzale JM. MRI and MRA for evaluation of dissection of craniocerebral arteries: lessons from the medical literature. Emerg Radiol 2009;16(3):185–93.
86. Murphy M, Walls R. Identification of the difficult and failed airway. In: Walls R, Murphy M, editors. Manual of emergency airway management. 3rd edition. Philadelphia: Lippincott Williams & Wilkins; 2008. p. 81–93.
87. Bair AE, Filbin MR, Kulkarni RG, et al. The failed intubation attempt in the emergency department: analysis of prevalence, rescue techniques, and personnel. J Emerg Med 2002;23(2):131–40.
88. Sakles JC, Laurin EG, Rantapaa AA, et al. Airway management in the emergency department: a one-year study of 610 tracheal intubations. Ann Emerg Med 1998; 31(3):325–32.
89. American Society of Anesthesiologists Task Force on Management of the Difficult Airway. Practice guidelines for management of the difficult airway: an updated report by the American Society of Anesthesiologists Task Force on Management of the Difficult Airway. Anesthesiology 2003;98(5):1269–77.
90. Langeron O, Masso E, Huraux C, et al. Prediction of difficult mask ventilation. Anesthesiology 2000;92(5):1229–36.
91. Kheterpal S, Han R, Tremper KK, et al. Incidence and predictors of difficult and impossible mask ventilation. Anesthesiology 2006;105(5):885–91.
92. Kheterpal S, Martin L, Shanks AM, et al. Prediction and outcomes of impossible mask ventilation: a review of 50,000 anesthetics. Anesthesiology 2009;110(4): 891–7.
93. Cass NM, James NR, Lines V. Difficult direct laryngoscopy complicating intubation for anaesthesia. Br Med J 1956;1(4965):488–9.
94. Savva D. Prediction of difficult tracheal intubation. Br J Anaesth 1994;73(2): 149–53.
95. Tse JC, Rimm EB, Hussain A. Predicting difficult endotracheal intubation in surgical patients scheduled for general anesthesia: a prospective blind study. Anesth Analg 1995;81(2):254–8.
96. Iohom G, Ronayne M, Cunningham AJ. Prediction of difficult tracheal intubation. Eur J Anaesthesiol 2003;20(1):31–6.
97. Shiga T, Wajima Z, Inoue T, et al. Predicting difficult intubation in apparently normal patients: a meta-analysis of bedside screening test performance. Anesthesiology 2005;103(2):429–37.
98. Reed MJ, Dunn MJ, McKeown DW. Can an airway assessment score predict difficulty at intubation in the emergency department? Emerg Med J 2005;22(2): 99–102.
99. Walls RM, Murphy MF. Manual of emergency airway management. 3rd edition. Philadelphia: Lippincott Williams & Wilkins; 2008.

High-Risk Chief Complaints III: Abdomen and Extremities

Karis Tekwani, MD, Rishi Sikka, MD*

KEYWORDS

- Abdominal complaints • Extremity complaints
- Risk management • Orthopedic injuries • Soft tissue injuries

Abdominal and extremity complaints are a frequent reason for presentation to the emergency department (ED). Although these are common complaints, several abdominal and extremity disease entities may be missed or subject to delayed diagnosis. The failure to diagnose and treat in a timely and appropriate fashion can result in significant patient morbidity, mortality, and expose the ED physician to litigation.

This article provides an overview of the diagnosis and management of several high-risk abdominal and extremity complaints in pediatric and adult patients. These disease entities include appendicitis, abdominal aortic aneurysm (AAA), mesenteric ischemia, bowel obstruction, retained foreign body, hand and finger lacerations, fractures, and compartment syndrome. Each section focuses primarily on the pitfalls in diagnosis by highlighting the limitations of history, physical examination findings, and diagnostic testing. At the end of each section, there is a summary of specifics to facilitate timely diagnosis and to mitigate any potential risk exposure to the ED physician.

ACUTE APPENDICITIS

Acute appendicitis is a common disease entity encountered in the ED, with more than 250,000 new cases annually in the United States.[1] Failure to make a timely diagnosis can result in appendiceal perforation and an increase in patient morbidity and mortality.[1] Certain populations are especially at risk for these complications from a delayed diagnosis or misdiagnosis. In women, the most common misdiagnoses are pelvic inflammatory disease, gastroenteritis, urinary tract infection, ruptured ovarian follicle, and ectopic pregnancy.[1] In children and the elderly, delays in the

No outside funding or support was received for this article.
Department of Emergency Medicine, Advocate Christ Medical Center, 4440 West 95th Street, Oak Lawn, IL 60453, USA
* Corresponding author.
E-mail address: sikka@att.net (R. Sikka).

Emerg Med Clin N Am 27 (2009) 747–765
doi:10.1016/j.emc.2009.07.006
emed.theclinics.com

diagnosis of appendicitis are common because of atypical presentations and difficulty in obtaining an accurate history and physical examination.[1] In these populations, the delayed diagnosis results in a substantially higher rate of appendiceal perforation, perhaps as high as 50% when compared with 26% in the general population.[2] To avoid these adverse outcomes, the ED physician must maintain a heightened clinical suspicion while understanding the limitations and confounders associated with the history, physical examination, and diagnostic results.

History and Physical Examination

Management of acute abdominal pain begins with an accurate history and physical examination. Although no one feature generally clinches the diagnosis of acute appendicitis, a combination of signs and symptoms can increase clinical suspicion. The three most predictive signs and symptoms of acute appendicitis are right lower quadrant (RLQ) pain, abdominal rigidity, and periumbilical pain migrating to the RLQ.[1,3] The duration of illness can also be useful, as patients with acute appendicitis often (but not always) have a shorter duration of pain than those with other causes of acute abdominal pain. To better quantify these clinical findings, several scoring systems have been developed to predict the likelihood of acute appendicitis. One of these methodologies is the MANTRELS scoring system. This score is derived from a constellation of patient findings and results, including migration of pain to the RLQ, anorexia, nausea and/or vomiting, tenderness in the RLQ, rebound on palpation, elevated temperature, leukocytosis, shift of white blood cell (WBC) count to the left.[4] However, neither the MANTRELS score nor other clinical algorithms have been shown prospectively to have enough sensitivity to reliably exclude the diagnosis of appendicitis. The elderly particularly provide a diagnostic challenge to clinical assessment and scoring because they are more likely to present with generalized and longer duration of pain, distention, rigidity, decreased bowel sounds, and often lack fever, leukocytosis, or localized tenderness.[5–7]

Laboratory Evaluation

Several laboratory tests including complete blood count, urinalysis, and urine pregnancy test are often used in the initial evaluation of acute abdominal pain. Studies have shown that a single WBC count of more than 10,000 cells/μL in adults is neither sensitive nor specific in the diagnosis of appendicitis; sensitivities range from 68% to 88%, and specificities range from 50% to 76%.[8–12] The same holds true for children; a single WBC count of more than 15,000 cells/μL has sensitivities that range from 19% to 60% and specificities that range from 84% to 100%.[8,9,13,14] However, the sensitivity of the WBC count increases the longer the symptoms have been present, with a sensitivity of nearly 90% when symptoms have been present for 48 hours.[15] However, a WBC count in isolation is rarely helpful for the detection of acute appendicitis.

Urinalysis is another test that rarely changes management in acute appendicitis. Patients presenting to the ED with undifferentiated lower abdominal pain often have a urinalysis performed to exclude alternate causes of the pain. However, irritation of the ureter from an inflamed appendix can lead to vague urinary complaints, and pyuria, hematuria, or bacteriuria can be seen in up to 40% of patients with acute appendicitis.[16] Therefore, in spite of an abnormal urinalysis, if a clinical suspicion of appendicitis still exists, then additional workup should be pursued.

C-reactive protein (CRP) is another laboratory test that has been proposed for use in the diagnosis of appendicitis. CRP has been found to increase markedly only after appendiceal perforation or abscess formation, and therefore, a normal value in isolation has minimal utility in excluding uncomplicated appendicitis.[17] However, when used in combination with the leukocyte count, multiple studies have found acute appendicitis to be unlikely with a normal leukocyte count and a normal CRP.[17–19]

Radiologic Evaluation

Various imaging techniques are available to clinicians when the diagnosis of acute appendicitis is being entertained, including ultrasound (US), computed tomography (CT), and magnetic resonance imaging (MRI). The choice of imaging modality depends on several patient-specific factors, operator and/or reader proficiency, and inherent technology limitations.

CT is the most commonly used imaging modality for the diagnosis of acute appendicitis; there are various protocols available that involve scanning the abdomen and pelvis or just the pelvis with different routes of contrast administration (intravenous, oral, and rectal). Historically, the most common scan involves the use of intravenous and oral contrast, and the entire abdomen and pelvis are imaged; this approach allows for the detection of alternate causes and the location of the appendix when it is in a nonstandard location.[2] This technique is shown to have 94% sensitivity and 89% specificity, and alternate diagnoses were obtained in 66% of patients.[1,2] An alternative CT technique involves administration of intravenous and rectal contrast and focused scanning of the pelvis. This focused technique has a sensitivity and specificity of 98%. However, an alternative diagnosis was detected in only 39% of cases that were negative for appendicitis.[2] Similarly, another well-studied technique is noncontrast CT of the abdomen and pelvis, which yields a sensitivity of 96% and specificity of 99%. This technique yields an alternate diagnosis in only 35% of cases.[2] An increasingly used technique involves CT scan of the abdomen and pelvis with intravenous contrast only, eliminating the time required to administer oral contrast. This technique is nearly 100% sensitive and 97% specific for the diagnosis of acute appendicitis.[20] However, CT technique is largely institution dependent, and varies based on the radiologist's comfort level with and preferences for different techniques.

CT is not without risks, particularly in children and pregnant women. It has been estimated that a single abdominal CT done within the first year of life contributes 0.35% to the background lifetime risk for cancer mortality, and it is a potentially avoidable risk in children.[2] In pregnant women, a single abdominal CT performed during the first trimester has been shown to double the likelihood of childhood cancer (from 1 to 2 in 600) as a result of fetal exposure to radiation in utero.[2]

As a result of these risks, US has become an alternative to CT, particularly in the pediatric and pregnant female population. US, in the hands of a skilled operator, has been shown to have a pooled sensitivity of 88% and specificity of 94% in children and a pooled sensitivity of 83% and specificity of 93% in adults.[21] Although helpful when positive, a normal appendix is visualized in less than 5% of patients, and clinicians are reluctant to end the workup based on a nonvisualized appendix.[1] In addition, US has shown pelvic pathology in 33% of female patients undergoing evaluation for acute appendicitis.[1]

MRI can be used in the diagnosis of acute appendicitis. However, it is rarely useful in the emergency setting because of the high cost, long duration of study, and limited availability. Its use is limited to pregnant females with a nondiagnostic US, with the recommendation to avoid gadolinium during pregnancy and especially during the first trimester.[2]

Overall, CT with intravenous and oral contrast is recommended in most adult patients when the diagnosis of acute appendicitis is not straightforward and when alternate diagnoses, such as colitis, diverticulitis, small bowel obstruction (SBO), inflammatory bowel disease, adnexal cysts, acute cholecystitis, acute pancreatitis, or ureteral obstruction, are being considered. In pregnant women and pediatric patients, US can be a safe and effective first-line imaging option. Regardless of the diagnostic strategy used, patients with ongoing pain and abdominal tenderness on physical examination, in whom imaging is nondiagnostic or unable to visualize the appendix, surgical consultation and admission for serial examinations is appropriate.

Special Circumstances: Children

Children pose a diagnostic challenge for several reasons, including inability to communicate clearly, fear response to health care professionals, and atypical presentations. Initial misdiagnosis rates range from 28% to 57% for children younger than 12 years and nearly 100% for children 2 years of age or younger.[15] The most common misdiagnoses of childhood appendicitis are gastroenteritis, upper respiratory tract infection, and unknown abdominal pain.[15] Because of the delay in diagnosis, appendiceal perforation is nearly universal in children 3 years of age and younger.[15]

Signs and symptoms are not as useful in the pediatric population as in the adult population, but a meta-analysis showed the presence of fever (likelihood ratio 3.4), rebound tenderness (likelihood ratio 3.0), and involuntary guarding (likelihood ratio 1.6–2.6) to be useful predictors of acute appendicitis.[22] In children younger than 2 years, the most common signs and symptoms are abdominal pain (89%–100%), vomiting (66%–100%), fever (80%–87%), and anorexia (53%–60%).[15] As children approach school age, they are able to verbalize symptoms, and the presentation becomes more typical.

Risk Management Strategy

A high index of suspicion should be maintained for appendicitis in children or the elderly, given the more atypical and delayed presentations. Laboratory evaluation should not be relied on solely to rule out appendicitis. Despite increasing reliance on CT, clinicians should not hesitate to admit for observation patients with a normal CT but a strong clinical suspicion or ongoing pain, or those patients in whom the appendix was not visualized on CT. It is also important to clearly document serial abdominal examinations and any discussions with consultants or primary care physicians. If discharging a patient with acute abdominal pain and an unrevealing workup, it is necessary to ensure that their pain is improving, they can tolerate oral intake, they have appropriate and timely follow-up (call the primary care physician if possible), they are given explicit discharge instructions to return if worse, and they have a support system (family or friends) available to observe the patient.

ABDOMINAL AORTIC ANEURYSM

AAA is an important cause of abdominal pain in older adults, and has a high mortality rate if not diagnosed and treated. Rupture or impending rupture of an AAA is a true abdominal emergency, with nearly 15,000 deaths resulting from AAA rupture annually.[23] Among these deaths, 25% occur before reaching the hospital, 51% after reaching the hospital but before surgery, and the remainder during or after emergent surgical repair of a ruptured AAA.[24] However, most AAAs are asymptomatic, and the physical examination lacks sensitivity. Therefore, it is important for ED physicians to facilitate appropriate treatment and disposition once AAA has been diagnosed.[23] Aneurysms greater than 5.5 cm in diameter are at a high risk of rupture and are considered for elective repair; when incidental AAAs are detected by ED physicians, patients with aneurysms less than 5.5 cm should be referred to a primary care physician for monitoring, and to a vascular surgeon when the aneurysm is 5.5 cm or greater in diameter.[25] Much of the research on this topic has been done on men, and it is suggested that women undergo elective repair when the aneurysm is 4.5 to 5 cm.[24]

History and Physical Examination

There has been a trend toward increased screening for AAA. Therefore, some patients will present to the ED with a known diagnosis of AAA. However, a significant number of patients will not have known disease, and an assessment of a patient's risk factors may be useful. Major risk factors for AAA include age greater than 65 years, male gender, smoking, hypertension, peripheral vascular disease, and a family history of AAA.[5,23] Smoking is the strongest independent risk factor for AAA, with 90% of patients with AAA having a history of tobacco use.[5]

Most nonruptured AAAs are asymptomatic. When symptoms do occur, pain is usually the chief complaint, typically described as a steady and gnawing pain in the hypogastrium or lower back[24] or a vague chronic abdominal or back pain.[25] The classic triad of hypotension, abdominal or back pain, and pulsatile abdominal mass presents in only 25% to 50% of patients with ruptured AAA.[5] AAA should be considered in any older adult with abdominal, back, testicle, groin, leg, or buttock pain.[23] AAA can also present with flank pain, especially on the left side and thus is at risk of being misdiagnosed as renal colic. Other clinical findings seen less frequently include signs of retroperitoneal hematoma, scrotal or groin abnormalities, bruits, neuropathy, or lower extremity edema.

In older patients presenting to the ED with abdominal pain, a detailed abdominal examination should always include assessment of the size of the aorta. The sensitivity for palpation of AAA increases with the diameter of the aneurysm; sensitivity is 69% for lesions 4.0 to 4.9 cm and 76% to 82% for lesions more than 5 cm.[23,25] However, a normal physical examination should not be solely relied on to exclude AAA.

Radiologic Evaluation

US is the simplest and the least expensive method of diagnosing AAA and can be used at the bedside in a hemodynamically unstable patient. In addition to obtaining an estimated diameter of the aorta, US allows for rapid determination of free fluid in the abdomen and pelvis. US is the method of choice for diagnosing and screening, and has a sensitivity of nearly 100% in diagnosing AAA.[26,27]

Compared with US, CT has the benefit of establishing a diagnosis of AAA rupture and assisting surgeons in determining which method of repair is best (endovascular vs open) by better defining the shape, extent, and anatomic relationships of the aneurysm.[24,25] CT measurements tend to be larger than US measurements by a mean of 3 to 9 mm.[24] CT is also useful in the outpatient setting for serially monitoring the size of the aneurysm. Overall, in the ED setting, CT with intravenous contrast is most useful for the hemodynamically stable patient with suspected AAA rupture. CT without intravenous contrast is capable of diagnosing the presence or absence of AAA and large amounts of free fluid in the abdomen; however, CT is not able to diagnose a leaking AAA or active extravasation. CT should never delay definitive care in patients who are clinically unstable with a increased likelihood of rupture.

MRI combined with magnetic resonance angiography (MRA) offers an alternative to CT when the patient has contraindications dye (such as renal insufficiency or allergy). MRI and/or MRA has similar sensitivity for the detection of AAA but is more time consuming and less readily available in the emergency setting.

Risk Management Strategy

ED clinicians should seriously consider the diagnosis of AAA in any patient older than 50 years who presents with abdominal pain, back pain, or syncope. AAA should also be in the differential when evaluating patients with atypical symptoms, such as hip, groin, flank, or isolated quadrant pain. Although rare in people younger than 50 years, it should be considered in younger patients who have a family history of aneurysm. Be wary of diagnosing flank pain as renal colic, especially in the elderly or first-time diagnosis of renal colic, without appropriately ruling out AAA. The physical examination is not sufficiently sensitive to allow for the exclusion of an AAA as a cause of a patient's symptoms. Surgical consultation should not be delayed for CT in hemodynamically unstable patients with increased suspicion for AAA rupture.

MESENTERIC ISCHEMIA

Acute mesenteric ischemia is an uncommon but often fatal cause of acute abdominal pain in older adults with an overall mortality of 60% to 80%. Mesenteric ischemia occurs when the mesenteric blood supply fails to meet the demand of the bowel, leading to ischemia and necrosis. There are FOUR major causes of acute mesenteric ischemia: arterial embolism (50%), arterial thrombosis (25%), nonocclusive ischemia (20%), and venous thrombosis (5%).[5] The high mortality associated with mesenteric ischemia may be attributed to the nonspecific clinical presentation and difficulty recognizing the condition before bowel infarction occurs.[28]

History and Physical Examination

Mesenteric ischemia tends to be a disease of older adults. Some historical features that might prompt consideration of mesenteric ischemia include history of heart failure, cardiac arrhythmias, recent myocardial infarction, hypercoagulable state, valvular disorders, vasopressor use, or hypotension.[29] The classic presentation of acute mesenteric ischemia is severe, diffuse abdominal pain out of proportion to physical examination findings.[5] However, pain is often atypical and vague, and other associated symptoms such as nausea, vomiting, diarrhea, and/or bloating often confound the presentation.[5,30] Patients with arterial embolus may experience sudden, severe abdominal pain with a rapid, forceful bowel evacuation, whereas patients with venous thrombosis may have a more indolent course of colicky abdominal pain.[29] Only 25% of patients will have occult blood positive stools.[5] Patients showing signs of shock, distention, and peritoneal irritation have already reached the late stages of the disease process.[5]

Chronic mesenteric ischemia occurs most commonly in elderly women, often with a history of smoking or atherosclerotic disease, and presents as colicky postprandial epigastric pain radiating to the back, that begins 15 to 30 minutes after eating and lasts 1 to 3 hours.[26,29,31] Patients develop a fear of eating and thus develop anorexia and weight loss. The physical examination is normally unremarkable.

Laboratory Evaluation

There are no laboratory tests that are sensitive or specific for the diagnosis of acute mesenteric ischemia.[29] Leukocytosis, metabolic acidosis, elevated serum lactate, and amylase may be present. However, all of these findings may be absent in the early stages of ischemia.[5,29]

Radiologic Evaluation

Plain abdominal radiographs have limited use in the evaluation of acute mesenteric ischemia because the findings are nonspecific; up to 25% of plain films are normal in early disease.[28] The main use of plain films is to exclude other diagnoses, such as obstruction or perforation. The characteristic thumb printing or thickening of bowel loops occurs in less than 40% of patients. Air in the portal system is another very late finding that is associated with poor outcomes.[28]

Abdominal CT alone without angiography has poor sensitivity and specificity in the diagnosis of most types of acute mesenteric ischemia.[28] Some CT findings that would prompt further evaluation include thickened bowel walls, engorgement of mesenteric vessels, intramural hematoma, dilated bowel loops, pneumatosis, mucosal enhancement, or portal venous gas.[28,30,31]

As a result, multidetector CT angiography has evolved as the imaging modality of choice to diagnose acute mesenteric ischemia and has come to replace mesenteric angiography as the gold standard. Multidetector CT angiography should be performed with intravenous and intraluminal contrast.[29] Studies have suggested that the use of low-attenuation contrast agents, such as water or methylcellulose, may be superior to the conventional use of barium because the intestinal wall enhancement can be assessed more easily.[29,31] CT angiography allows for direct visualization of vascular occlusion and when combined with detection of other abnormalities of the bowel wall, provides the best sensitivity for diagnosing acute mesenteric ischemia.[30]

Doppler US has been used primarily in the diagnosis of chronic mesenteric ischemia and can detect stenosis of more than 50% in the mesenteric vessels. An optimal study requires restriction of oral intake for 8 hours, and thus it is rarely useful in the emergency setting for the detection of acute mesenteric ischemia.[28] Likewise, MRI has not been studied sufficiently in the acute setting to determine its usefulness in the detection of acute mesenteric ischemia and is not recommended at this time.[30]

Treatment

ED management begins with early and aggressive resuscitation, including intravenous fluid hydration (with central venous pressure monitoring if necessary), administration of broad spectrum antibiotics, and prevention of propagation of disease by reduction of vasospasm.[28] If no contraindications exist, intravenous heparin should be started. If vasopressors are indicated, dopamine or epinephrine should be the first-line choices, and pure α-adrenergic agents should be avoided because of the potential to cause increased vasospasm and worsening ischemia.[28] Peritoneal signs generally mandate emergency laparotomy. Despite advances in imaging, conventional angiography still remains the lone diagnostic modality that offers potential therapeutic options.[30]

Risk Management Strategy

Acute mesenteric ischemia is a difficult diagnosis to make; therefore, it is necessary to maintain a high index of suspicion when evaluating abdominal pain in the elderly population in the setting of a compatible history and/or presence of risk factors. Mortality is 50% when the diagnosis occurs within 24 hours after the onset of symptoms but rises to greater than 80% when the diagnosis is delayed. If acute mesenteric ischemia is high on the differential, surgical consultation should be obtained early in the process. CT alone is not sufficient to rule out acute mesenteric ischemia, as the CT manifestations can be nonspecific. If sufficient suspicion is present, as in a clinically high-risk patient with a compatible history of acute diffuse abdominal pain out of proportion to the physical examination or ongoing pain despite analgesia, imaging with multidetector CT angiography should undertaken. Again, given the difficulty in diagnosing this disease process, documentation of repeat abdominal examinations, patient reassessment, any discussions with consultants, and clinical decision making is essential.

BOWEL OBSTRUCTION

SBO is a common cause of abdominal pain and is responsible for 15% of emergency admissions for acute abdominal pain.[32] When the bowel is occluded, it allows the build up of bacteria, which produces gas that causes pressure and necrosis to the bowel wall.[32] In a simple obstruction, the bowel is occluded at one point, and in a closed-loop obstruction the bowel segment is occluded at two points, such as with an incarcerated hernia or volvulus.[32] Most SBOs result from postoperative adhesions, followed by hernias, neoplasms, and strictures caused by Crohn disease or medications.[32]

Morbidity and mortality associated with SBO result if surgical therapy is delayed when a complete mechanical obstruction is misdiagnosed as either a partial mechanical obstruction or pseudoobstruction.[32] The goals when evaluating a patient with possible obstruction should focus on differentiating mechanical obstruction from ileus, determining the cause of obstruction, discriminating partial from complete obstruction, and differentiating simple from strangulating obstruction.[33]

History and Physical Examination

The clinical presentation of bowel obstruction varies depending on the severity, duration, and type of obstruction. The classic presentation is colicky abdominal pain, nausea and emesis, abdominal distention, and progressive obstipation.[32] Pain is usually sudden, sharp, and periumbilical, and may progressively diminish as a result of bowel fatigue or may be partially relieved by emesis.[32] The pain becomes more intense and unremitting as the disease progresses to ischemia or perforation.[32] Depending on the location of the obstruction, patients may present with more frequent (every 3–4 minutes) pain intervals with bilious emesis for proximal obstructions versus less frequent (every 15–20 minutes) pain intervals with feculent emesis for distal obstructions.[32] However, occasionally, patients with SBO will present with no history of pain.

Historical features that increase the risk of bowel obstruction include prior SBO, prior abdominal surgeries, cancer, radiation, hernias, or inflammatory bowel disease.[32] Inability to pass flatus may be an indication of transition from partial to complete SBO. Once the patient develops high fever, rigors, or systemic toxicity, it is likely that the bowel is becoming necrotic.[32]

Several physical examination findings may increase the suspicion for SBO. The abdomen should be inspected for abdominal scars and hernias, with particular attention to the groin. A rectal examination should also be performed to exclude obstruction from mass or fecal impaction.

The classic physical examination findings are a distended abdomen with abdominal tympany and high-pitched (tinkling) hyperactive bowel sounds with borborygmi corresponding to paroxysms of abdominal pain. The abdomen is generally diffusely and mildly tender, and peritoneal signs are absent unless bowel necrosis or perforation has occurred.[32] A nontender abdomen is not uncommon in patients with SBO. The longer the duration of pain, the more progressively hypoactive the bowel sounds become because of bowel fatigue.[32] Overall, patients often appear ill and volume depleted.

Laboratory Evaluation

There are no laboratory tests that are either sensitive or specific in the diagnosis of bowel obstruction. The most common laboratory abnormalities are electrolyte imbalances or azotemia due to the third spacing of fluids.[32] Patients may also have leukocytosis, neutrophilia, acidosis, and elevated amylase and/or lactate levels. However, none of these are diagnostic for bowel obstruction.[32]

Radiologic Evaluation

Plain abdominal radiographs are often the initial imaging method for the detection of bowel obstruction and are diagnostic in 50% to 70% of cases. The diagnosis requires a dilated, gas-filled, proximal bowel and a collapsed, gasless, distal bowel.[32,34] Plain films are as sensitive (86%) as CT to differentiate high-grade obstruction versus non-obstruction.[33] However, they do not reveal the cause of obstruction, and a negative abdominal plain radiograph does not rule out bowel obstruction.

Patients with inconclusive plain films should have a CT with oral and intravenous contrast. CT is 82% sensitive in ruling out high-grade obstruction. However, one of the limitations of CT is its low sensitivity (<50%) in detecting low-grade or partial SBO.[33,35] With new multidetector row CT, sensitivity is improved to 92% for complete SBO.[36] CT can detect the site, level, and cause of obstruction in addition to closed-loop obstructions and strangulation.[34,35] In patients with suspicion for low-grade or partial SBO, CT should be supplemented with a contrast study, ideally enteroclysis or CT enteroclysis, which has a much higher sensitivity (89%) for the detection of partial SBO.[34,35]

Abdominal US is as sensitive and more specific than plain abdominal radiographs, but it is rarely used because other tests are more accurate.[32] MRI is an alternative to CT, with similar sensitivity and ability to identify the cause, but has the limitations of increased time to diagnosis and variable availability in the emergency setting.[33]

Treatment

Patients with findings of SBO and fever, leukocytosis, acidosis, ongoing pain, or peritonitis warrant surgical consultation and possible exploration.[33] Patients lacking the aforementioned signs, with either partial or complete SBO, may undergo conservative therapy with intravenous fluids, antiemetics, bowel rest, and nasogastric tube decompression.[33] However, 30% of patients with complete SBO treated conservatively will eventually require surgical intervention.[33] Patients treated conservatively, who fail to improve within 48 hours, should also undergo surgical intervention.[33] Controversy exists over the use of broad-spectrum antibiotics and the use of long tube decompression, and there are no controlled data to support or refute either.[33]

Risk Management Strategy

Mortality dramatically increases from 3% to 8% with simple SBO to 20% to 37% once strangulation has occurred.[36] Therefore, the goal is to detect bowel obstruction as early as possible and institute appropriate therapy. CT has a low sensitivity for the detection of low-grade and partial SBO; therefore, low-grade SBO should be considered in any case of undiagnosed acute abdominal pain.[37] CT will also miss a number of closed-loop obstructions. If an increased clinical suspicion of SBO exists, urgent surgical consultation is advisable. As in the case with the high-risk abdominal complaints, if the patient is discharged, serial examinations, thought processes, and discussions with consultants should be clearly documented, and the patient should be given timely and specific instructions.

RETAINED FOREIGN BODY

Lacerations account for more than 4 million ED visits annually.[38] These lacerations may often be caused and complicated by the presence of a foreign body.[39] Foreign bodies are often difficult to identify on the first presentation. In one review, 38% of foreign bodies in the hand were missed by the initial evaluating clinician.[40] These retained foreign bodies may result in delayed wound healing, infection, allergic reaction, tissue damage, and disability.[41–43] There may also be malpractice implications. Wounds have been identified as a frequent cause of malpractice litigation in emergency medicine.[44] The cornerstone of identifying and mitigating the risk associated with retained foreign bodies rests on an appropriate history, focused wound exploration, and the liberal use of diagnostic imaging.

History and Physical Examination

The evaluation begins with a thorough history, with an emphasis on the mechanism of injury. Certain mechanisms and anatomic locations are more highly associated with the presence of a retained foreign body. These high-risk mechanisms include motor vehicle collisions and puncture wounds.[45] With respect to patient anatomy, wounds to the head and hands have been most commonly associated with retained glass.[45,46]

An additional factor to consider in the history is the patient's perception of a retained foreign body. In a prospective study of patients with wounds caused by glass, the patient's perception of a retained foreign body had a positive predictive value of 31%. However, in this particular study, relying on patient perception alone would have missed 57% of all foreign bodies.[45] A patient's lack of perception of a foreign body is not sufficient to rule out its presence.

It is apparent that the patient history needs to be augmented with a focused wound exploration. This exploration should be conducted under optimal lighting conditions with minimal wound bleeding to enhance the recognition of retained foreign bodies.[47] This exploration should also ideally include probing and visualization of the bottom of the wound. Probing and visualization of the bottom of the wound have been associated with a negative predictive value of a foreign body of between 93% and 98%.[45,48] An incomplete wound examination, without probing or visualization of the bottom of the wound, may miss up to 31% of retained foreign bodies.[45]

Radiologic Evaluation

Plain film radiography is the primary modality in the diagnosis of radiopaque, retained foreign bodies. Approximately 0.6% to 4.3% of superficial wounds have a retained foreign body detected by radiography after adequate exploration or visualization.[49] In a review of retained glass, standard two-view radiography detected 99% of glass pieces bigger than 2 mm.[50] Smaller pieces were less frequently visualized. Glass pieces of 1 mm and 0.5 mm were visualized with plain radiographs 83% and 61% of the time, respectively.[50] In contrast, plain radiographs are inadequate for the detection of radiolucent foreign bodies such as plastic, wood, and vegetative material.[40]

US is probably the preferred imaging modality in cases with a suspected radiolucent foreign body. Literature on animal models and clinical settings has established the utility of US in identifying both radiopaque and radiolucent foreign bodies.[43] The sensitivity of US ranges from 43% to 98%, and specificity ranges from 59% to 98%.[43]

Compared with plain film radiography, CT can detect radiopaque and radiolucent foreign bodies. Although CT is better at the detection of radiolucent foreign bodies, it still has only a modest sensitivity.[51,52] CT also has disadvantages with respect to its cost and radiation exposure of the patient. As a result, CT is not routinely recommended in the workup and should probably be confined to cases with a high clinical suspicion and negative radiograph and US results.[43,53]

Risk Management Strategy

The history and physical examination are not sufficiently sensitive to rule out the presence of a retained foreign body. A suspicion of a retained foreign body due to the mechanism of injury, patient perception or findings on wound exploration, should be followed up with liberal use of imaging. Plain film radiographs are the mainstay for the diagnosis of retained radiopaque foreign bodies, including glass. US is an evolving modality that has particular applications in the diagnosis of radiolucent foreign bodies. If a foreign body is not identified, the patient should be instructed about the possibility of a missed foreign body and to return for signs of pain or localized infection. In addition, all patients should be instructed about the importance of timely follow-up, regardless of the results of imaging and wound exploration.

HAND AND FINGER LACERATIONS

Lacerations to the hand and fingers may often present dramatically with attendant patient anxiety. In this setting, it is important for the clinician to adhere to a focused and methodologic approach for workup to avoid missing a tendon or nerve injury.

History and Physical Examination

The most important component of the examination is the performance and documentation of a thorough neurovascular examination. This should include testing of the motor and sensory branches of the median, radial, and ulnar nerves, two-point discrimination of the fingertips, and capillary refill. Digital nerve injuries should be suspected when two-point discrimination is greater on one side of the volar pad than the other or when it is greater than 10 mm.[54] In addition, flexor and extensor tendon testing, passively and against resistance, should be performed at the distal interphalangeal, proximal interphalangeal, and metacarpalphalangeal joints. Partial tendon tears may only be revealed through testing strength against resistance across the joint.

The components of a good wound examination include adequate lighting and a bloodless field. Suboptimal lighting and bleeding within the wound can hinder the identification of injury. If necessary, to improve the field of the wound, a tourniquet can be applied to the finger, or a blood pressure cuff may be inflated over the forearm. During the exploration, careful attention should be paid to the continuity of the extensor and flexor tendons and the integrity of all joints.

Treatment

Extensor tendon injuries can be repaired by an experienced ED physician, in consultation with a hand surgeon.[54] If the tendon is not repaired, the wound should be closed, and the finger splinted in a position of function with a follow-up by a hand surgeon. In contrast, flexor tendon injuries always require operative repair. However, similar to delayed repair of extensor tendon injuries, in flexor tendon injuries the wound should be closed and the finger splinted in flexion. Follow-up by a specialist should occur within 2 to 3 days, with repair ideally within 7 days.[54] Digital nerve lacerations can also undergo delayed repair using microsurgical techniques, although long-term deficits may persist.[54]

In the case of tendon and nerve lacerations, it is recommended that a discussion occur with the referring specialist before the patient is discharged, to establish additional preferences on antibiotics, wound care, and timing of follow-up. In addition, the patient should be explicitly advised on the nature of their potential injury and the possibility of functional and neurologic deficits even with a timely follow-up.

Risk Management Strategy

A complete neurovascular examination and a thorough wound exploration are important to avoid missing a nerve or tendon injury. The patient should also be instructed that despite best efforts, a nerve or tendon injury might be missed. The patient should be instructed to look for localized neurologic deficits or pain. In addition, the importance of early follow-up should be particularly emphasized.

FRACTURES

Fractures and suspected fractures are a common reason for an ED visit. In 2004, approximately 3.9 million ED visits were because of fractures.[55] Certain types of fractures may be missed and are prone to significant complications from delayed diagnosis. Fractures at particular risk of an initial missed diagnosis include pediatric growth plate injury, pediatric supracondylar fracture, and occult hip fracture in the elderly.

Pediatric Growth Plate Injuries

Pediatric physis injuries typically occur between the ages of 10 and 16 years, most often in the distal radius.[56] Although physis injuries are common, they are prone to be missed initially. Missed physis injuries can result in premature closure with complete arrest of continued bone growth. A strategy to avoid missing a physis injury rests on an appreciation of growth plate anatomy, the mechanism of injury, and subtle physical examination findings.

History and physical examination

The Salter-Harris classification system is most frequently used to describe physis injury.[57] This scheme categorizes pediatric fractures into five distinct categories:

1. Type I fractures involve a separation through the physis, causing a separation of the epiphysis from the metaphysis. They are most often seen in infants and toddlers.[56]
2. Type II fractures involve a fracture through the physis and the metaphysis. They account for most physeal injuries.[56]
3. Type III fractures are intraarticular fractures through the epiphysis and physis.
4. Type IV fractures extend through the epiphysis, physis, and metaphysis.
5. Type V fractures involve a crush injury to the physis and are often diagnosed after the initial presentation.[56]

The higher the Salter-Harris classification number, the more likely the vascular supply to the physis is injured and the greater the possibility of a physeal arrest.[57,58]

Salter-Harris injuries may often be the result of mechanisms that would typically cause ligament sprain or joint dislocations in adults.[56] Even minor trauma or repetitive stress can result in a physeal injury.[56] Further confounding the diagnosis, the physical examination findings may only include tenderness over the physis.

Radiologic evaluation

Plain films are the preferred imaging modality for physis injury. Unfortunately, the physis is radiolucent and a fracture may be missed. This is particularly true of the Salter-Harris type I and type V injuries. If initial radiographs are negative but a fracture is suspected, then advanced imaging with MRI, US, or bone scintigraphy may be used. However, these additional imaging modalities are unlikely to change the initial treatment, and they are generally not warranted within the ED.[56]

Treatment

Salter-Harris type I fractures and type II fractures without significant displacement or angulation can be treated with splint immobilization and elevation. Patients with Salter-Harris type III and type IV fractures require orthopedic consultation in the ED to ensure adequate anatomic alignment to prevent future bone growth arrest.[56] Patients with Salter-Harris type V fractures are rarely diagnosed in the ED. Because these fractures are usually accompanied by growth arrest, they require orthopedic consultation.[56]

Risk management strategy

If the diagnosis of a sprain is being considered in a pediatric patient, the physician should also consider the possibility of a physeal injury.[56] In particular, a patient with negative radiographs and tenderness over the physis should be assumed to have a Salter-Harris type I injury and requires splinting and timely follow-up.

Supracondylar Fracture

Supracondylar fracture is the most common pediatric elbow fracture.[59] The presentation spans the spectrum of obvious clinical deformity to subtle radiologic findings. Regardless of the initial appearance, this injury can be associated with significant complications, including vascular injury, compartment syndrome, Volkmann ischemic contracture, and neurologic injury. The incidence of these sequelae can be reduced through prompt identification of the subtle presentation and early aggressive treatment in the ED.[59]

History and physical examination

The classic mechanism of injury associated with a supracondylar fracture is a fall on the outstretched hand. There may be pain on supination or an inability to supinate. In some patients, the symptoms may present initially similar to a nursemaid's elbow, with the arm in pronation and refusal to use or flex the elbow.[60] However, these two entities can be distinguished by their different mechanisms of injury.[59]

The physical examination should focus on the neurovascular status of the extremity and hand. Nerve injuries are common. The incidence varies in the literature: median nerve 28% to 60%, radial nerve 26% to 61%, and ulnar nerve 11% to 15%.[59,61–63] In general, the median nerve is considered the most common nerve to be injured, particularly the anterior interosseus branch.[61] This branch provides only motor innervation and may be overlooked during the examination. It can be tested by having the patient make an OK sign and testing for strength.[59]

Radiologic evaluation

Significantly displaced fractures (type III) are easy to identify on plain radiographs. However, nondisplaced or minimally displaced fractures (types I and II) are more difficult to see and often have subtle or indirect radiographic findings. Several of these subtle findings involve the anterior and posterior fat pads around the elbow. In a supracondylar fracture, the anterior fat pad may become more elevated and appear like the sail of a sailboat (sail sign). A posterior fat pad is normally not present on the lateral projection of the elbow. Its presence should be considered evidence of the presence of a fracture.

Treatment

Type I fractures with no displacement are stable and can be placed in a long-arm posterior splint with the elbow flexed to 90°. Although complications are rare, orthopedics consultation and a brief period of ED observation are advised.[59] In contrast, type II and type III fractures are more unstable and may have or lead to neurovascular compromise. Orthopedic consultation and admission are recommended to observe for neurovascular deficits and the development of compartment syndrome.[59] If neurovascular compromise is noted on the initial ED evaluation and orthopedics consultation is not immediately available, the ED physician should consider prompt reduction.[59]

Risk management strategy

Supracondylar fractures are always high on the differential diagnosis when a child presents with an appropriate mechanism of injury and elbow pain. A careful neurovascular examination, including that of the anterior interosseous branch of the median nerve, should be documented. A nondisplaced fracture may have only subtle radiologic signs, including the sail sign and posterior fat pad sign. Fractures with displacement or neurovascular compromise require orthopedics consultation and admission. In those patients with negative radiographs but a fracture is suspected, the elbow should be splinted, with rapid orthopedics follow-up for repeat evaluation and radiographs.

Hip Fracture

Hip fracture is a public health problem that affects more than 300,000 persons annually in the United States and contributes billions to health care costs.[64] Although most cases are clinically obvious, subtle presentations can occur. These occult presentations may lead to delayed diagnosis, with accompanying increases in patient morbidity and mortality.[64]

History and physical examination

The classic presentation for a hip fracture is an elderly person with an inability to ambulate after a fall. Often, their hip is abducted and externally rotated, and a leg length discrepancy may be present. However, this is in sharp contrast to the patient with an occult hip fracture. An occult hip fracture should be suspected in an elderly patient who can ambulate but has a vague sense of pain in their buttocks, knees, or thighs. Passive range of motion on physical examination may also be normal.[64]

Radiologic evaluation

Plain film radiography is the cornerstone of diagnosis. However, in some cases the radiographs may be normal or indeterminate. If a clinical suspicion persists, additional imaging, including CT, bone scanning, and MRI, should be pursued. Although there is debate on the merits of each, some authors advocate MRI as a more accurate and a potentially less expensive alternative to CT and bone scanning.[64,65] However, its availability at all times through the ED might be limited.

Risk management strategy

Patients with hip fracture may have occult and subtle clinical presentations. It is important to consider hip fracture in the differential of lower extremity pain in elderly individuals even with the ability to ambulate. In all cases of suspected hip fracture, if plain films are unremarkable then additional imaging and workup is warranted.

COMPARTMENT SYNDROME

Compartment syndrome is a potentially limb- and life-threatening condition. The failure to diagnose this condition is a common cause of medical litigation and is associated with significant malpractice liability.[66] The cornerstone of this diagnosis rests on early recognition and an appreciation of the subtle physical examination findings.

History and Physical Examination

Pain, particularly out of proportion to the mechanism of injury, is commonly considered to be the most fundamental clinical finding. However, many experts consider this to be unreliable and caution against overreliance on the lack of pain.[67,68] Pain may not be present because of concomitant nerve injury or because the patient is severely injured and impaired and may not be able to articulate the presence of pain.[69,70] Pain that is out of proportion to the physical findings is not sensitive, but when it is present, is suggestive of compartment syndrome.

The traditional pentad of findings in compartment syndrome is pain, paresthesias, paresis, pallor, and pulselessness. Overall, the positive predictive value of clinical findings is low, between 11% and 15%.[66] The absence of findings appears to be more useful in excluding the diagnosis, with a negative predictive value of 97% to 98%.[66] The most reliable and earliest physical finding is sensory deficits, in particular diminished sensation.[69,70] Pallor and pulselessness are late physical findings and should not be relied upon solely to exclude the diagnosis.[70]

Diagnosis and Treatment

The diagnosis of compartment syndrome is based on the measurement of intracompartmental pressure. Intracompartmental pressure may be measured with pressure monitors, the needle technique, the wick catheter, or the slit catheter. Pressure monitors, such as the Stryker (Kalamazoo, MI), are easiest and used most frequently.[69] To use one of these self-contained pressure monitors, the skin is initially cleansed and prepared using an aseptic solution. An 18-gauge needle is attached to the monitor and inserted into the suspected compartment. A small amount of saline is injected, and the pressure is measured.[69]

Normal tissue pressure is between 0 and 10 mm Hg. At 20 mm Hg, capillary blood flow may be compromised, and at 30 to 40 mm Hg muscle and nerve tissue become necrotic. There is debate regarding the compartment level pressure that requires fasciotomy. Some advocate an absolute pressure standard, whereas others feel the compartment pressure needs to be interpreted in light of the blood pressure.[69] However, several absolute indications for fasciotomy have been identified: clinical signs of compartment syndrome, compartment pressure greater than 30 mm Hg in a patient with a clinical picture of compartment syndrome, and interrupted arterial flow to an extremity for more than 4 hours.[71]

Risk Management Strategy

Pain should not be considered the only or principle finding of compartment syndrome. Neurologic findings are more common and appear early in the course of the illness. An appropriate clinical scenario with neurologic findings should prompt measurement of compartment pressures to establish the diagnosis. Compartment pressure readings should be interpreted with specialist consultation to determine the need for fasciotomy.

SUMMARY

Abdominal and extremity complaints in the ED may present from a spectrum of benign to life-threatening diagnoses. Establishing the presence of a high-risk, potentially compromising abdominal or extremity diagnosis first requires an understanding of the limitations of historical and physical examination findings. This knowledge can be augmented with a strategy using liberal imaging criteria. However, the limitations of diagnostic testing, including laboratory and imaging results, need to be considered in the ultimate disposition. Throughout the workup process, it is also important to document repeat examinations, the diagnostic thought process, and communication with consulting and admitting services. A high clinical suspicion in spite of an inconclusive workup, grounded in the evidence of disease pathology and presentation, mandates judicious use of consultant services and consideration of admission. If a decision is made to discharge the patient, it is important to provide carefully worded discharge instructions and a clear plan for follow-up. Adherence to these strategies should mitigate the risks associated with the workup and diagnosis of high-risk abdominal and extremity complaints.

REFERENCES

1. Paulson EK, Kalady MF, Pappas TN. Clinical practice. Suspected appendicitis. N Engl J Med 2003;348(3):236–42.
2. Rybkin AV, Thoeni RF. Current concepts in imaging of appendicitis. Radiol Clin North Am 2007;45(3):411–22, vii.
3. Old JL, Dusing RW, Yap W, et al. Imaging for suspected appendicitis. Am Fam Physician 2005;71(1):71–8.
4. Alvarado A. A practical score for the early diagnosis of acute appendicitis. Ann Emerg Med 1986;15(5):557–64.
5. Lyon C, Clark DC. Diagnosis of acute abdominal pain in older patients. Am Fam Physician 2006;74(9):1537–44.
6. McKay R, Shepherd J. The use of the clinical scoring system by Alvarado in the decision to perform computed tomography for acute appendicitis in the ED. Am J Emerg Med 2007;25(5):489–93.
7. Schneider C, Kharbanda A, Bachur R. Evaluating appendicitis scoring systems using a prospective pediatric cohort. Ann Emerg Med 2007;49(6):778–84, 84 e1.
8. Miskowiak J, Burcharth F. The white cell count in acute appendicitis. A prospective blind study. Dan Med Bull 1982;29(4):210–1.
9. Lau WY, Ho YC, Chu KW, et al. Leucocyte count and neutrophil percentage in appendicectomy for suspected appendicitis. Aust N Z J Surg 1989;59(5):395–8.
10. Dueholm S, Bagi P, Bud M. Laboratory aid in the diagnosis of acute appendicitis. A blinded, prospective trial concerning diagnostic value of leukocyte count, neutrophil differential count, and C-reactive protein. Dis Colon Rectum 1989; 32(10):855–9.
11. Amland PF, Skaane P, Ronningen H, et al. Ultrasonography and parameters of inflammation in acute appendicitis. A comparison with clinical findings. Acta Chir Scand 1989;155(3):185–9.
12. Andersson RE, Hugander AP, Ghazi SH, et al. Diagnostic value of disease history, clinical presentation, and inflammatory parameters of appendicitis. World J Surg 1999;23(2):133–40.
13. Doraiswamy NV. Leucocyte counts in the diagnosis and prognosis of acute appendicitis in children. Br J Surg 1979;66(11):782–4.

14. Peltola H, Ahlqvist J, Rapola J, et al. C-reactive protein compared with white blood cell count and erythrocyte sedimentation rate in the diagnosis of acute appendicitis in children. Acta Chir Scand 1986;152:55–8.
15. Rothrock SG, Pagane J. Acute appendicitis in children: emergency department diagnosis and management. Ann Emerg Med 2000;36(1):39–51.
16. Puskar D, Bedalov G, Fridrih S, et al. Urinalysis, ultrasound analysis, and renal dynamic scintigraphy in acute appendicitis. Urology 1995;45(1):108–12.
17. Gronroos JM, Gronroos P. Leucocyte count and C-reactive protein in the diagnosis of acute appendicitis. Br J Surg 1999;86(4):501–4.
18. Sengupta A, Bax G, Paterson-Brown S. White cell count and C-reactive protein measurement in patients with possible appendicitis. Ann R Coll Surg Engl 2009;91(2):113–5.
19. Khan MN, Davie E, Irshad K. The role of white cell count and C-reactive protein in the diagnosis of acute appendicitis. J Ayub Med Coll Abbottabad 2004;16(3):17–9.
20. Mun S, Ernst RD, Chen K, et al. Rapid CT diagnosis of acute appendicitis with IV contrast material. Emerg Radiol 2006;12(3):99–102.
21. Doria AS, Moineddin R, Kellenberger CJ, et al. US or CT for diagnosis of appendicitis in children and adults? A meta-analysis. Radiology 2006;241(1):83–94.
22. Bundy DG, Byerley JS, Liles EA, et al. Does this child have appendicitis? JAMA 2007;298(4):438–51.
23. Upchurch GR Jr, Schaub TA. Abdominal aortic aneurysm. Am Fam Physician 2006;73(7):1198–204.
24. Isselbacher EM. Thoracic and abdominal aortic aneurysms. Circulation 2005;111(6):816–28.
25. Sakalihasan N, Limet R, Defawe OD. Abdominal aortic aneurysm. Lancet 2005;365(9470):1577–89.
26. Hermsen K, Chong WK. Ultrasound evaluation of abdominal aortic and iliac aneurysms and mesenteric ischemia. Radiol Clin North Am 2004;42(2):365–81.
27. Sparks AR, Johnson PL, Meyer MC. Imaging of abdominal aortic aneurysms. Am Fam Physician 2002;65(8):1565–70.
28. Oldenburg WA, Lau LL, Rodenberg TJ, et al. Acute mesenteric ischemia: a clinical review. Arch Intern Med 2004;164(10):1054–62.
29. Levy AD. Mesenteric ischemia. Radiol Clin North Am 2007;45(3):593–9, x.
30. Herbert GS, Steele SR. Acute and chronic mesenteric ischemia. Surg Clin North Am 2007;87(5):1115–34, ix.
31. Horton KM, Fishman EK. Multidetector CT angiography in the diagnosis of mesenteric ischemia. Radiol Clin North Am 2007;45(2):275–88.
32. Cappell MS, Batke M. Mechanical obstruction of the small bowel and colon. Med Clin North Am 2008;92(3):575–97, viii.
33. Diaz JJ Jr, Bokhari F, Mowery NT, et al. Guidelines for management of small bowel obstruction. J Trauma 2008;64(6):1651–64.
34. Nicolaou S, Kai B, Ho S, et al. Imaging of acute small-bowel obstruction. AJR Am J Roentgenol 2005;185(4):1036–44.
35. Maglinte DD, Heitkamp DE, Howard TJ, et al. Current concepts in imaging of small bowel obstruction. Radiol Clin North Am 2003;41(2):263–83, vi.
36. Qalbani A, Paushter D, Dachman AH. Multidetector row CT of small bowel obstruction. Radiol Clin North Am 2007;45(3):499–512, viii.
37. Maglinte DD, Kelvin FM, Rowe MG, et al. Small-bowel obstruction: optimizing radiologic investigation and nonsurgical management. Radiology 2001;218(1):39–46.

38. McCaig LF, Burt CW. National hospital ambulatory medical care survey: 2002 emergency department summary. Adv Data 2004;340:1–34.
39. Hollander JE, Singer AJ, Valentine S, et al. Wound registry: development and validation. Ann Emerg Med 1995;25(5):675–85.
40. Anderson MA, Newmeyer WL 3rd, Kilgore ES Jr. Diagnosis and treatment of retained foreign bodies in the hand. Am J Surg 1982;144(1):63–7.
41. Browett JP, Fiddian NJ. Delayed median nerve injury due to retained glass fragments. A report of two cases. J Bone Joint Surg Br 1985;67(3):382–4.
42. Lammers RL. Soft tissue foreign bodies. Ann Emerg Med 1988;17(12):1336–47.
43. Blankenship RB, Baker T. Imaging modalities in wounds and superficial skin infections. Emerg Med Clin North Am 2007;25(1):223–34.
44. Karcz A, Korn R, Burke MC, et al. Malpractice claims against emergency physicians in Massachusetts: 1975–1993. Am J Emerg Med 1996;14(4):341–5.
45. Steele MT, Tran LV, Watson WA, et al. Retained glass foreign bodies in wounds: predictive value of wound characteristics, patient perception, and wound exploration. Am J Emerg Med 1998;16(7):627–30.
46. Gron P, Andersen K, Vraa A. Detection of glass foreign bodies by radiography. Injury 1986;17(6):404–6.
47. Capellan O, Hollander JE. Management of lacerations in the emergency department. Emerg Med Clin North Am 2003;21(1):205–31.
48. Avner JR, Baker MD. Lacerations involving glass. The role of routine roentgenograms. Am J Dis Child 1992;146(5):600–2.
49. Weinberger LN, Chen EH, Mills AM. Is screening radiography necessary to detect retained foreign bodies in adequately explored superficial glass-caused wounds? Ann Emerg Med 2008;51(5):666–7.
50. Courter BJ. Radiographic screening for glass foreign bodies–what does a "negative" foreign body series really mean? Ann Emerg Med 1990;19(9):997–1000.
51. Ginsburg MJ, Ellis GL, Flom LL. Detection of soft-tissue foreign bodies by plain radiography, xerography, computed tomography, and ultrasonography. Ann Emerg Med 1990;19(6):701–3.
52. Russell RC, Williamson DA, Sullivan JW, et al. Detection of foreign bodies in the hand. J Hand Surg Am 1991;16(1):2–11.
53. Flom LL, Ellis GL. Radiologic evaluation of foreign bodies. Emerg Med Clin North Am 1992;10(1):163–77.
54. Tintinalli J. Emergency medicine: a comprehensive study guide. 6th edition. New York: McGraw-Hill; 2004. p. 305–12.
55. McCaig LF, Nawar EW. National hospital ambulatory medical care survey: 2004 emergency department summary. Adv Data 2006;372:1–29.
56. Perron AD, Miller MD, Brady WJ. Orthopedic pitfalls in the ED: pediatric growth plate injuries. Am J Emerg Med 2002;20(1):50–4.
57. Salter RB, Harris WR. Injuries involving the epiphyseal plate. J Bone Joint Surg Am 1963;45:587–622.
58. Robertson WW Jr. Newest knowledge of the growth plate. Clin Orthop Relat Res 1990;253:270–8.
59. Wu J, Perron AD, Miller MD, et al. Orthopedic pitfalls in the ED: pediatric supracondylar humerus fractures. Am J Emerg Med 2002;20(6):544–50.
60. Della-Giustina K, Della-Giustina DA. Emergency department evaluation and treatment of pediatric orthopedic injuries. Emerg Med Clin North Am 1999;17(4):895–922, vii.
61. Lyons ST, Quinn M, Stanitski CL. Neurovascular injuries in type III humeral supracondylar fractures in children. Clin Orthop Relat Res 2000;376:62–7.

62. Campbell CC, Waters PM, Emans JB, et al. Neurovascular injury and displacement in type III supracondylar humerus fractures. J Pediatr Orthop 1995;15(1):47–52.
63. Brown IC, Zinar DM. Traumatic and iatrogenic neurological complications after supracondylar humerus fractures in children. J Pediatr Orthop 1995;15(4):440–3.
64. Brunner LC, Eshilian-Oates L, Kuo TY. Hip fractures in adults. Am Fam Physician 2003;67(3):537–42.
65. Cannon J, Silvestri S, Munro M. Imaging choices in occult hip fracture. J Emerg Med 2009;37:144–52.
66. Ulmer T. The clinical diagnosis of compartment syndrome of the lower leg: are clinical findings predictive of the disorder? J Orthop Trauma 2002;16(8):572–7.
67. Johnson GW Jr. The 'occult' compartment syndrome [editorial]. J Trauma 1989;29(1):135.
68. Wright JG, Bogoch ER, Hastings DE. The 'occult' compartment syndrome. J Trauma 1989;29(1):133–4.
69. Perron AD, Brady WJ, Keats TE. Orthopedic pitfalls in the ED: acute compartment syndrome. Am J Emerg Med 2001;19(5):413–6.
70. Hoover TJ, Siefert JA. Soft tissue complications of orthopedic emergencies. Emerg Med Clin North Am 2000;18(1):115–39, vi.
71. Mabee JR. Compartment syndrome: a complication of acute extremity trauma. J Emerg Med 1994;12(5):651–6.

Afterword: High Success Approach

Emergency physicians care for a high volume of critically ill and injured patients, generally with no prior knowledge of patients' histories and, usually, with little or no warning of patients' arrival. Despite the careful, knowledgeable, compassionate practice of most emergency physicians, bad outcomes will occur. There is no way to completely avoid being named in a malpractice suit because a patient, patient's family, or patient's estate may sue despite the emergency physician's best efforts. However, there are some principles that may help minimize adverse outcomes and avoid litigation.

PRIORITIES

When evaluating a patient, the clinician should try to consider all threats to life, organ, and limb, and systematically rule them out. Many entities can be ruled out by history and physical; some will require ancillary testing or even admission. Mentally considering life, organ, and limb threats is probably the best way to avoid missing them.

High-risk Areas

Keeping in mind certain high-risk areas in the practice of emergency medicine can help the emergency physician avoid adverse outcomes that may lead to litigation.

Change of shift

One of these high-risk areas is change of shift, when a patient is already given a diagnosis and the patient is not re-evaluated by the new clinician. Sometimes the patient is discharged without a careful review of the chart or the labs and radiographs, so important findings may be missed.

Repeat visits

A patient who returns to the emergency department (ED) for re-evaluation within 72 hours of an ED evaluation represents a high-risk area. These patients are often written off as problem patients who did not follow instructions properly. Many of repeat patients need a re-evaluation because their discharge instructions were inadequate, their disease worsened, or the initial diagnosis was not correct. A repeat visit should be viewed by the clinician as an opportunity.

Private patients

Private patients fall into a high-risk area because sometimes the emergency physician does not realize that he is responsible for them. Under the Emergency Medical Treatment and Active Labor Act, a medical screening examination for medical emergency must be performed while waiting for the patient's private physician to arrive. The responsibility for the patient is shared between the emergency physician and private physician, and communication between the two may help avoid adverse

Emerg Med Clin N Am 27 (2009) 767–770
doi:10.1016/j.emc.2009.08.004

outcomes. Private physician's patients coming to the ED for a specific treatment must still be evaluated.

Admitted patients

Patients who are admitted to the hospital may have to wait in the ED for an inpatient bed for prolonged periods. The ED often does not have the physician and nursing resources to re-evaluate and care for admitted patients. The patients and families are often ignored, and if the patient's condition changes it may go undetected, leading to possible adverse outcomes and angry patients and families.

Against medical advice or refusal of care

It is important to ascertain and document that the patient understands his or her medical condition, the recommended treatment, the risks and benefits of the treatment, the risks of refusing treatment, and alternate treatment plans. It is the clinician's responsibility to determine that the patient has the capacity to refuse care or leave against medical advice.

Red Flags

It is important to recognize red flags when they appear.

Myocardial ischemia

In considering myocardial ischemia, recognize that classic symptoms, ischemic EKG changes, diaphoresis, history of coronary artery disease, and radiation of pain place patients at high risk.

Thoracic aortic dissection

When evaluating a chest pain patient, certain findings place patients at high risk for thoracic aortic dissection (TAD): pain of sudden onset at maximum severity, associated neurologic signs and symptoms, chest pain associated with syncope, presumed acute coronary syndrome not responding to treatment or with normal ECG and normal 6-hour troponin, family history of TAD, pregnancy, and new aortic insufficiency murmur.

Subarachnoid hemorrhage

In evaluating a patient with headache, recognize that sudden onset of a severe headache may represent a subarachnoid hemorrhage (SAH), and that family history of SAH dramatically increases the risk.

Abdominal aortic aneurysm

Recognize that abdominal pain, back pain, or flank pain with hypotension is a red flag for abdominal aortic aneurysm.

Pulmonary embolism

Remember to consider pulmonary embolism when there is unexplained tachycardia, tachypnea, hypoxemia, wheezing, or hypotension.

If the clinician is unable to exclude a life threatening diagnosis by history or physical, and there is still a doubt about whether it is safe to discharge the patient, it is safer to work up or admit the patient.

Communication

Communicating your thoughts with the patient, patient's family, and patient's primary care provider (PCP) is also a priority. Introducing yourself to the patient and family in a professional manner, and making it clear that you are the doctor taking care of the patient is helpful in establishing effective communication. Some patients may prefer to accept a small amount of risk rather than undergoing a test or an admission. It is preferable to discuss openly your thought process with the patient and to involve the patient, family, and even the PCP in the decision. This open discussion may help prevent litigation in the event of an unexpected bad outcome.

Documentation

Careful documentation on the chart of your thought process, of why you do or do not think a patient has certain diagnoses, is also helpful from a medical legal point of view. It is also important to document your conversations regarding testing, therapy, and admission with the patient, the patient's family, and patient's PCP. This communication and documentation may help you demonstrate that there was no negligence in working up complaints that subsequently turned out to be more serious. A chart thoroughly demonstrating your reasoning is especially essential when potentially life-threatening chief complaints such as chest pain, shortness or breath, or headache are felt to be of benign causes.

It is helpful to address inconsistencies in the chart, rather than ignoring them. For example, when the triage note states one chief complaint and you work up a different chief complaint.

Documenting serial examinations in some detail is extremely helpful, and is far superior to simply checking a box that states "patient improved." It is also important to document the patient's condition on discharge from the ED, even for admitted patients.

Discharge Instructions

For patients being discharged, careful documentation of the treatment, including new prescriptions, reconciliation with existing medications, and the follow-up plan is essential. It is also essential that the patient and family understand the treatment (including medication reconciliation) and the follow-up plan, and are able to implement it. Document on the chart that the patient and family understand the treatment and follow-up plan and are comfortable with it. It should be stated and documented for all patients discharged from the ED that they should return to the ED immediately if they worsen.

SUMMARY

Unfortunately, bad outcomes will continue to occur in emergency medicine, despite the best efforts of the competent emergency physician. It is to be hoped that this issue provides some information that will help patients avoid bad outcomes and help emergency physicians avoid litigation.

Jonathan S. Olshaker, MD, FACEP, FAAEM
Department of Emergency Medicine
Boston Medical Center
Boston University School of Medicine
1 Boston Medical Center Place
Boston, MA 02118, USA

Brendan G. Magauran Jr, MD, MBA
Department of Emergency Medicine
Boston Medical Center
Boston University School of Medicine
1 Boston Medical Center Place
Boston, MA 02118, USA

Joseph H. Kahn, MD, FACEP
Department of Emergency Medicine
Boston Medical Center
Boston University School of Medicine
1 Boston Medical Center Place
Boston, MA 02118, USA

E-mail addresses:
jonathan.olshaker@bmc.org (J.S. Olshaker)
brendan.magauran@bmc.org (B.G. Magauran Jr)
joseph.kahn@bmc.org (J.H. Kahn)

Index

Note: Page numbers of article titles are in **boldface** type.

Emerg Med Clin N Am 27 (2009) 771–779
doi:10.1016/S0733-8627(09)00133-3 emed.theclinics.com

B

C

D

E

I

J

L

P

Q

R

United States Postal Service

Statement of Ownership, Management, and Circulation
(All Periodicals Publications Except Requestor Publications)

1. Publication Title: Emergency Medicine Clinics of North America
2. Publication Number: 0 0 0 - 7 1 4
3. Filing Date: 9/15/09
4. Issue Frequency: Feb, May, Aug, Nov
5. Number of Issues Published Annually: 4
6. Annual Subscription Price: $229.00
7. Complete Mailing Address of Known Office of Publication (*Not printer*) (*Street, city, county, state, and ZIP+4®*)
   Elsevier Inc.
   360 Park Avenue South
   New York, NY 10010-1710
   Contact Person: Stephen Bushing
   Telephone (Include area code): 215-239-3688
8. Complete Mailing Address of Headquarters or General Business Office of Publisher (*Not printer*)
   Elsevier Inc., 360 Park Avenue South, New York, NY 10010-1710
9. Full Names and Complete Mailing Addresses of Publisher, Editor, and Managing Editor (*Do not leave blank*)
   Publisher (*Name and complete mailing address*)
   John Schrefer , Elsevier, Inc., 1600 John F. Kennedy Blvd. Suite 1800, Philadelphia, PA 19103-2899
   Editor (*Name and complete mailing address*)
   Patrick Manley, Elsevier, Inc., 1600 John F. Kennedy Blvd. Suite 1800, Philadelphia, PA 19103-2899
   Managing Editor (*Name and complete mailing address*)
   Catherine Bewick, Elsevier, Inc., 1600 John F. Kennedy Blvd. Suite 1800, Philadelphia, PA 19103-2899
10. Owner (*Do not leave blank. If the publication is owned by a corporation, give the name and address of the corporation immediately followed by the names and addresses of all stockholders owning or holding 1 percent or more of the total amount of stock. If not owned by a corporation, give the names and addresses of the individual owners. If owned by a partnership or other unincorporated firm, give its name and address as well as those of each individual owner. If the publication is published by a nonprofit organization, give its name and address.*)

Full Name	Complete Mailing Address
Wholly owned subsidiary of	4520 East-West Highway
Reed/Elsevier, US holdings	Bethesda, MD 20814

11. Known Bondholders, Mortgagees, and Other Security Holders Owning or Holding 1 Percent or More of Total Amount of Bonds, Mortgages, or Other Securities. If none, check box ☐ None

Full Name	Complete Mailing Address
N/A	

12. Tax Status (*For completion by nonprofit organizations authorized to mail at nonprofit rates*) (*Check one*)
    The purpose, function, and nonprofit status of this organization and the exempt status for federal income tax purposes:
    ☐ Has Not Changed During Preceding 12 Months
    ☐ Has Changed During Preceding 12 Months (*Publisher must submit explanation of change with this statement*)

13. Publication Title: Emergency Medicine Clinics of North America
14. Issue Date for Circulation Data Below: August 2009

15. Extent and Nature of Circulation			Average No. Copies Each Issue During Preceding 12 Months	No. Copies of Single Issue Published Nearest to Filing Date
a. Total Number of Copies (*Net press run*)			2120	1939
b. Paid Circulation (By Mail and Outside the Mail)	(1)	Mailed Outside-County Paid Subscriptions Stated on PS Form 3541. (*Include paid distribution above nominal rate, advertiser's proof copies, and exchange copies*)	1162	1079
	(2)	Mailed In-County Paid Subscriptions Stated on PS Form 3541 (*Include paid distribution above nominal rate, advertiser's proof copies, and exchange copies*)		
	(3)	Paid Distribution Outside the Mails Including Sales Through Dealers and Carriers, Street Vendors, Counter Sales, and Other Paid Distribution Outside USPS®	337	324
	(4)	Paid Distribution by Other Classes Mailed Through the USPS (e.g. First-Class Mail®)		
c. Total Paid Distribution (*Sum of 15b (1), (2), (3), and (4)*) ►			1499	1403
d. Free or Nominal Rate Distribution (By Mail and Outside the Mail)	(1)	Free or Nominal Rate Outside-County Copies Included on PS Form 3541	103	107
	(2)	Free or Nominal Rate In-County Copies Included on PS Form 3541		
	(3)	Free or Nominal Rate Copies Mailed at Other Classes Through the USPS (e.g. First-Class Mail)		
	(4)	Free or Nominal Rate Distribution Outside the Mail (Carriers or other means)		
e. Total Free or Nominal Rate Distribution (Sum of 15d (1), (2), (3) and (4)			103	107
f. Total Distribution (Sum of 15c and 15e) ►			1602	1510
g. Copies not Distributed (See instructions to publishers #4 (page #3)) ►			518	429
h. Total (Sum of 15f and g)			2120	1939
i. Percent Paid (15c divided by 15f times 100) ►			93.57%	92.91%

16. Publication of Statement of Ownership
    ☐ If the publication is a general publication, publication of this statement is required. Will be printed in the **November 2009** issue of this publication. ☐ Publication not required
17. Signature and Title of Editor, Publisher, Business Manager, or Owner
    Stephen R. Bushing – Subscription Services Coordinator
    Date: September 15, 2009
    I certify that all information furnished on this form is true and complete. I understand that anyone who furnishes false or misleading information on this form or who omits material or information requested on the form may be subject to criminal sanctions (including fines and imprisonment) and/or civil sanctions (including civil penalties).

Printed and bound by CPI Group (UK) Ltd, Croydon, CR0 4YY
03/10/2024
01040462-0004